T0177274

# Introductory Statistics for Data Analysis

Warren J. Ewens • Katherine Brumberg

# Introductory Statistics for Data Analysis

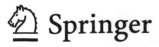 Springer

Warren J. Ewens
Department of Statistics and Data Science
University of Pennsylvania
Philadelphia, PA, USA

Katherine Brumberg
Department of Statistics and Data Science
University of Pennsylvania
Philadelphia, PA, USA

ISBN 978-3-031-28191-4      ISBN 978-3-031-28189-1   (eBook)
https://doi.org/10.1007/978-3-031-28189-1

Mathematics Subject Classification: 62-01

© The Editor(s) (if applicable) and The Author(s), under exclusive license to Springer Nature Switzerland AG 2023
This work is subject to copyright. All rights are solely and exclusively licensed by the Publisher, whether the whole or part of the material is concerned, specifically the rights of translation, reprinting, reuse of illustrations, recitation, broadcasting, reproduction on microfilms or in any other physical way, and transmission or information storage and retrieval, electronic adaptation, computer software, or by similar or dissimilar methodology now known or hereafter developed.
The use of general descriptive names, registered names, trademarks, service marks, etc. in this publication does not imply, even in the absence of a specific statement, that such names are exempt from the relevant protective laws and regulations and therefore free for general use.
The publisher, the authors, and the editors are safe to assume that the advice and information in this book are believed to be true and accurate at the date of publication. Neither the publisher nor the authors or the editors give a warranty, expressed or implied, with respect to the material contained herein or for any errors or omissions that may have been made. The publisher remains neutral with regard to jurisdictional claims in published maps and institutional affiliations.

This Springer imprint is published by the registered company Springer Nature Switzerland AG
The registered company address is: Gewerbestrasse 11, 6330 Cham, Switzerland

# Preface

We take "data analysis" to be the analysis of data to obtain information of scientific and social value. Much of the data currently considered derive from a sample, and the randomness in the selection of that sample means that Statistics is a key component in data analysis, since Statistics is the science of analyzing data derived from some random process such as sampling.

Our aim in this book is to give a precise account of introductory Statistics theory suitable for those wishing to analyze data from a variety of fields, including medicine, biology, economics, social sciences, the physical sciences, and engineering. However, the examples given in the book are often simple ones involving flipping a coin, rolling a die, and so on. This is because we do not want the complexities that arise in any given scientific field to obscure the basic principles that we describe. We have emphasized concepts and the basics of the statistical theory, first because they are central to any data analysis, and second because in our teaching experience, this is what students find most difficult to understand.

This implies that we have occasionally been pedantic in presenting some theoretical concepts. For example, we have been careful to distinguish between the concepts of a mean and an average. The conflation of these two words, sometimes in the same paragraph in published papers, has led in our experience to much confusion for students. Similarly, we distinguish carefully between the concepts of a random variable, of data, and of a parameter, using notation that helps in making this distinction. On the other hand, we have not been pedantic in stating the requirements, for example, needed for the Central Limit Theorem to hold.

We have followed a two-track approach in this book. A student not interested in the computing aspects of the material can follow one track and ignore all references to R. For a student interested in a computing approach to some parts of the material discussed, an additional approach using R has been provided. The non-computing part of the book is self-contained and can be read without any reference to R. All examples and problems in this book contain small data sets so that they can be analyzed with just a simple calculator.

We have often given detailed answers to the problems since this allows them to be considered as instructive examples rather than as problems. We have also provided flowcharts that help put the material discussed into perspective.

We are well aware of the practical aspects of data analysis, for example of ensuring that the data analyzed form an unbiased representative sample of the population of interest and that the assumptions made in the theory are justified, and have referred to these and similar matters several times throughout the book. However, our focus is on the basic theory, since in our experience this is sometimes little understood, so that incorrect procedures and inappropriate assumptions are sometimes used in data analysis.

Any errors or obscurities observed in this book will be reported at the webpage https://kbrumberg.com/publication/textbook/ewens/. Possible errors can be reported according to the instructions on the same webpage.

Philadelphia, PA, USA                                    Warren J. Ewens
January, 2023                                        Katherine Brumberg

# Contents

# Part I
# Introduction

# Chapter 1
# Statistics and Probability Theory

## 1.1 What is Statistics?

The word "Statistics" means different things to different people. For a baseball fan, it might relate to batting averages. For an actuary, it might relate to life tables. In this book, we mean the scientific definition of "Statistics", which is *Statistics is the science of analyzing data in whose generation chance has played some part.* This sentence is the most important one in the entire book, and it permeates the entire book. Statistics as we understand it via this definition has become a central area of modern science and data analysis, as discussed below.

Why is Statistics now central to modern science and data analysis? This question is best answered by considering the historical context. In the past, Mathematics developed largely in association with areas of science in which chance mechanisms were either non-existent or not important. Thus in the past a great deal of progress was made in such areas as Physics, Engineering, Astronomy and Chemistry using mathematical methods which did not allow any chance, or random, features in the analysis. For example, no randomness is involved in Newton's laws or in the theory of relativity, both of which are entirely deterministic. It is true that quantum theory is the prevailing paradigm in the physical sciences and that this theory intrinsically involves randomness. However, that intrinsic level of randomness is not discussed in this book.

Our focus is on more recently developed areas of science such as Medicine, Biology and Psychology, in which there are various chance mechanisms at work, and deterministic theory is no longer appropriate in these areas. In a medical clinical trial of a proposed new medicine, the number of people cured by the new medicine will depend on the choice of individuals in the trial: with a different group of individuals, a different number of people cured will probably be seen. (Clinical trials are discussed later in this book.) In areas such as Biology, there are many random factors deriving from, for example, the random transmission of genes from parent to offspring, implying that precise statements concerning the evolution of a

© The Author(s), under exclusive license to Springer Nature Switzerland AG 2023
W. J. Ewens, K. Brumberg, *Introductory Statistics for Data Analysis*,
https://doi.org/10.1007/978-3-031-28189-1_1

population cannot be made. Similar comments arise for many other areas of modern science and indeed in all areas where inferences are to be drawn from data in whose generation randomness played some part.

The data in "data analysis" are almost always a sample of some kind. A different sample would almost certainly yield different data, so that the sampling process introduces a second chance element over and above the inherent randomness in areas of science described above. This means that in order to make progress in these areas, one has to know how to analyze data in whose generation chance mechanisms were at work.

This is where Statistics becomes relevant. The role played by Mathematics in Physics, Engineering, Astronomy and Chemistry is played by Statistics in Medicine, Economics, Biology and many other associated areas. Statistics is fundamental to making progress in those areas. The following examples illustrate this.

*Example 1.1.1* In a study to examine the effects of sunlight exposure on the growth of a new type of grass, grass seeds were sown in 22 identical specifically designed containers. Grass in 11 of these containers were exposed to full sunlight during the growing period and grass in the remaining 11 containers were exposed to 50% shade during the growing period. At the end of the growing period, the biomass in each container was measured and the following data (in coded units) were obtained:

Full sun: 1903, 1935, 1910, 2096, 2008, 1961, 2060, 1644, 1612, 1811, 1714

50% Shade: 1759, 1718, 1820, 1933, 1990, 1920, 1796, 1696, 1578, 1682, 1526

$$(1.1)$$

There are clearly several chance mechanisms determining the data values that we observed. A different experiment would almost certainly give different data. The data do not immediately indicate an obvious difference between the two groups, and in order to make our assessment about a possible difference, we will have to use statistical methods, which allow for the randomness in the data. The statistical analysis of data of this form is discussed in Sects. 8.5 and 13.2.

*Example 1.1.2* The data from the 2020 clinical trial of the proposed Moderna COVID vaccine, in which 30,420 volunteers were divided into two groups, 15,210 being given the proposed vaccine and 15,210 being given a harmless placebo, are given below. The data are taken from L. R. Baden et al. *Efficacy and Safety of the mRNA-1273 SARS-CoV-2 Vaccine*, New England Journal of Medicine 384:403-416, February 2021.

|  | Did not develop COVID | Did develop COVID | Total |
|---|---|---|---|
| Given proposed vaccine | 15,199 | 11 | 15,210 |
| Given placebo | 15,025 | 185 | 15,210 |
| Total | 30,224 | 196 | 30,420 |

The way in which data such as those in this table are analyzed statistically will be described in Chap. 10. For now, we note that if this clinical trial had been carried out on a different sample of 30,420 people, almost certainly different data would have arisen. Again, Statistics provides a process for handling data where randomness such as this arises.

These two examples are enough to make two important points. The first is that because of the randomness inherent in the sampling process, no exact statements such as those made, for example, in Physics are possible. We will have to make statements indicating some level of uncertainty in our conclusions. It is not possible, in analyzing data derived from a sampling process, to be 100% certain that our conclusion is correct. This indicates a real limitation to what can be asserted in modern science. More specific information about this lack of certainty is introduced in Sect. 9.2.2 and then methods for handling this uncertainty are developed in later sections.

The second point is that, because of the unpredictable random aspect in the generation of the data arising in many areas of science, it is necessary to first consider various aspects of probability theory in order to know what probability calculations are needed for the statistical problem at hand. This book therefore starts with an introduction to probability theory, with no immediate reference to the associated statistical procedures. This implies that before discussing the details of probability theory, we first discuss the relation between probability theory and Statistics.

## 1.2   The Relation Between Probability Theory and Statistics

We start with a simple example concerning the flipping of a coin. Suppose that we have a coin that we suspect is biased towards heads. To check on this suspicion, we flip the coin 2000 times and observe the number of heads that we get. Even if the coin is fair, we would not expect, beforehand, to get exactly 1000 heads from the 2000 flips. This is because of the randomness inherent in the coin-flipping operation. However, we would expect to see approximately 1000 heads. If once we flipped the coin we got 1373 heads, we would obviously (and reasonably) claim that we have very good evidence that the coin is biased towards heads. The reasoning that one goes through in coming to this conclusion is probably something like this: "if the coin is fair, it is extremely unlikely that we would get 1373 or more heads from 2000 flips. But since we did in fact get 1373 heads, we have strong evidence that the coin is unfair."

Conversely, if we got 1005 heads, we would not reasonably conclude that we have good evidence that the coin is biased towards heads. The reason for coming to this conclusion is that, because of the randomness involved in the flipping of a coin, a fair coin can easily give 1005 or more heads from 2000 flips, so that observing 1005 heads gives no significant evidence that the coin is unfair.

These two examples are extreme cases, and in reality we often have to deal with more gray-area situations. If we saw 1072 heads, intuition and common sense might not help. What we have to do is to calculate the probability of getting 1072 or more heads *if the coin is fair.* Probability theory calculations (which we will do later) show that the probability of getting 1072 or more heads from 2000 flips of a fair coin is very low (about 0.0006). This probability calculation is a *deduction, or implication.* It is very unlikely that a fair coin would turn up heads 1072 times or more from 2000 flips. From this fact and the fact that we did see 1072 heads on the 2000 flips of the coin, we make the statistical *induction*, or *inference*, that we can reasonably conclude that we have significant evidence that the coin is biased.

The logic is as follows. Either the coin is fair and something very unlikely has happened (probability about 0.0006) or the coin is not fair. We prefer to believe the second possibility. We do not like to entertain a hypothesis that does not reasonably explain what we saw in practice. This argument follows the procedures of modern science.

In coming to the opinion that the coin is unfair we could be incorrect: the coin might have been fair and something very unlikely might have happened (1072 heads). We have to accept this possibility when using Statistics: we cannot be certain that any conclusion, that is, any statistical induction or inference, that we reach is correct. This problem is discussed in detail later in this book.

To summarize: probability theory makes *deductions*, or *implications*. Statistics makes *inductions*, or *inferences*. Each induction, or inference, is always based both on data and the corresponding probability theory calculation relating to those data. This induction might be incorrect because it is based on data in whose generation randomness was involved.

In the coin example above, the statistical induction, or inference, that we made (that we believe we have good evidence that the coin is unfair, given that there were 1072 heads in the 2000 flips) was based entirely on the probability calculation leading to the value 0.0006. In general, no statistical inference can be made without first making the relevant probability theory calculation. This is one reason why people often find Statistics difficult. In doing Statistics, we have to consider aspects of probability theory, and unfortunately our intuition concerning probability calculations is often incorrect.

Here is a more important example. Suppose that we are using some medicine (the "current" medicine) to cure some illness. From experience we know that, for any person having this illness, the probability that this current medicine cures any patient is 0.8. A new medicine is proposed as being better than the current one. To test whether this claim is justified, we plan to conduct a clinical trial in which the new medicine will be given to 2000 people suffering from the disease in question. If the new medicine is equally effective as the current one, we would, beforehand, expect it to cure about 1600 of these people. Suppose that after the clinical trial is conducted, the proposed new medicine cured 1643 people. Is this significantly more than 1600? Calculations that we will do later show that the probability that we would get 1643 or more people cured with the new medicine *if it is equally effective as the current medicine* is about 0.009, or a bit less than 0.01. Thus if the new medicine did indeed cure 1643 or more people, we might claim that we have good evidence that it is better than the current one. Intuition probably does not help here and a probability calculation followed by a statistical inference based on that calculation is necessary.

The relation between probability theory and Statistics will be discussed in more detail in Chap. 9 in connection with the statistical theory of hypothesis testing. Despite the fact that the reason why we discuss probability theory is that it is basic to the statistical calculations considered later, for the next few chapters we discuss probability theory on its own, without considering its relation to Statistics.

## 1.3 Problems

**1.1** This problem is intended to illustrate the relation between probability (involving a deductive calculation) and Statistics (involving an inductive statement). This relation will be discussed at length in the Statistics part of the book.

It has been claimed, on the basis of the physical and geometrical properties of a thumbtack, that if it is thrown in the air it has a probability 3/4 of landing "point up" (as opposed to "point down"). We want to test this claim.

If this claim is true and the thumbtack is to be thrown in the air 4000 times, the probability that the number of times that it will land "point up" is between 2929 and 3071 is about 0.99. This statement is a *deduction*, or *implication*, that is, a statement deriving from probability theory. For now we take it on trust: later we will see how this probability calculation is made. The thumbtack is now thrown 4000 times and it is observed that it lands "point up" 3082 times. What reasonable *induction*, or *inference*, that is, statistical statement, do you think you can make about the claim that the thumbtack will land "point up" with probability 3/4? (Whatever your answer is, *it must depend on the probability theory calculation given above.*)

**1.2** This problem is also intended to illustrate the relation between a probability calculation and a statistical induction (or inference). We are interested in whether a newborn is equally likely to be a boy as a girl. If a newborn is indeed equally likely to be a boy as a girl, then in a well-conducted representative unbiased sample of 10,000 newborns, the probability that the number of boys will be between 4825 and 5175 is about 0.9996 (we will learn how to calculate this later). In a well-conducted representative unbiased sample of 10,000 newborns we observed 5202 boys. What reasonable statistical induction can make about the view that a newborn is equally likely to be a boy as a girl?

**1.3** These non-statistical examples are intended to illustrate the relation between a deductive statement starting with "if", which is taken as being true, and the corresponding inductive statement, based on the deductive statement together with an observation (or data). In each case, indicate the words that should appear in "...".

(a) Susan always looks at the weather forecast before going to work. If the forecast predicts rain, she will take her umbrella to work. I observe that she did not take her umbrella to work. Therefore...

(b) If he has the ace of spades, he will play it. I observe that he did not play the ace of spades. Therefore...

(c) If one travels overseas, one must have a passport. She travelled overseas. Therefore...

# Part II
# Probability Theory

As discussed in the previous chapter, any discussion of Statistics requires a prior investigation of probability theory. The following chapters provide a brief introduction to that theory. Each topic discussed will correspond to some statistical procedure discussed later in the book.

The concept of a probability is quite a complex one. These complexities are not discussed here: we will be satisfied with a straightforward intuitive concept of probability as in some sense meaning a long-term frequency. For example, we would say when flipping a coin that the probability of a head is 1/2 if, in an infinitely long sequence of flips of the coin, a head will turn up half the time.

# Chapter 2
# Events

## 2.1 What Are Events?

We start by considering events and, later, the probabilities of events. An event is something which either will or will not occur when a certain experiment, field survey, etc. is performed. For example, an event might be "a head turns up when we flip this coin". Once the coin has been flipped, that event either did or did not occur. In a more serious example, an event might be "in a clinical trial, 3874 of the people given the proposed new medicine were cured of the illness of interest".

## 2.2 Notation

We denote events by upper-case letters at the beginning of the alphabet: $A, B, C, \ldots$, as well as the special notation $\phi$ defined below. It is also sometimes convenient to use the notation $A_1, A_2, \ldots$ when several similar events are involved.

## 2.3 Derived Events: Complements, Unions and Intersections of Events

(i) The event "the event $A$ did not occur" is said to be the *complement* of the event $A$ and is denoted $A^c$.

(ii) The event "both $A$ and $B$ occur in the same experiment" is said to be the *intersection* of the events $A$ and $B$. This event is denoted $A \cap B$. It sometimes happens that two events cannot both occur in the same experiment. For example, if a die is rolled once and the event $C$ is "on that roll, 5 turned up" and the event $D$ is "on that roll, 3 turned up", then $C$ and $D$ cannot both occur

© The Author(s), under exclusive license to Springer Nature Switzerland AG 2023
W. J. Ewens, K. Brumberg, *Introductory Statistics for Data Analysis*,
https://doi.org/10.1007/978-3-031-28189-1_2

on that roll of the die. In this case, the intersection event $C \cap D$ is said to be an empty, or impossible, event. Any impossible event is denoted by the special notation $\phi$ mentioned above: $\phi$ is the Greek letter "phi".

(iii) The event "either $A$ occurs or $B$ occurs or both events occur in the same experiment" is said to be the *union* of the events $A$ and $B$. This event is denoted $A \cup B$.

The complement of an event, the union of two events, and the intersection of two events are called "derived" events—they are derived from one event or more events. Examples of unions, intersections and complements of events are given in the problems.

## 2.4   Mutually Exclusive Events

The events $A$ and $B$ are said to be "mutually exclusive" if they cannot both occur in the same experiment. The events $C$ and $D$ discussed in item (ii) of Sect. 2.3 are mutually exclusive: they cannot both occur for any given roll of the die. The following example will be discussed often later. If a coin is flipped twice, the two events "head on first flip, tail on second flip" and "tail on first flip, head on second flip" are also mutually exclusive: they cannot both happen on the same two flips of the coin. The intersection of two mutually exclusive events is the impossible event $\phi$.

## 2.5   Problems

**2.1** A die is to be rolled once. Let $A$ be the event "3 or 6 turns up" and $B$ the event "3, 4 or 5 turns up". Describe in words (such as $x$ or $y$ or $z$ turns up) the events (a) $A^c$, (b) $B^c$, (c) $A \cup B$ and (d) $A \cap B$. Are $A$ and $B$ mutually exclusive events?

**2.2** You observe songbirds with long or short tails and orange or yellow beaks. Event $L$ is when a bird has a long tail, and event $O$ is when a bird has an orange beak. Describe in words (a) $L \cup O$, (b) $L \cap O$, (c) $L^C \cap O$, and (d) $L^C \cup O^C$.

**2.3** Describe why the complement of the event $A \cup B$ is the intersection of the events $A^c$ and $B^c$.

# Chapter 3
# Probabilities of Events

We write the probability that the event $A$ occurs in some given experiment, field survey, etc. as Prob($A$), the probability that the event $B$ occurs in this same experiment or field survey as Prob($B$), and so on. From now on, we take the word "experiment" to include field surveys, etc., and for convenience will often omit the expressions "in some given experiment" and "in the same experiment". In this section we will only consider those probability calculations that will be relevant to the statistical theory discussed later.

## 3.1 Probabilities of Derived Events

(i) *The probability of the complement of an event.* The total probability of all possible outcomes is always equal to 1. Since an event and its complement contain all possible outcomes,

$$\text{Prob}(A^c) = 1 - \text{Prob}(A). \qquad (3.1)$$

(ii) *The probability of the intersection of two events.* The probability of the intersection of the events $A$ and $B$, that is, the probability that both the event $A$ and the event $B$ occur in the same experiment, is denoted Prob($A \cap B$). The calculation of this probability is sometimes difficult. If $A \cap B$ is an impossible event, Prob($A \cap B$) = Prob($\phi$) = 0.

(iii) *The probability of the union of two events.* The probability of the union of the events $A$ and $B$, that is, the probability that either the event $A$ occurs, or the event $B$ occurs, or both the events $A$ and $B$ occur in the same experiment, is denoted Prob($A \cup B$). This probability is given by

$$\text{Prob}(A \cup B) = \text{Prob}(A) + \text{Prob}(B) - \text{Prob}(A \cap B). \qquad (3.2)$$

© The Author(s), under exclusive license to Springer Nature Switzerland AG 2023
W. J. Ewens, K. Brumberg, *Introductory Statistics for Data Analysis*,
https://doi.org/10.1007/978-3-031-28189-1_3

If $A$ and $B$ are mutually exclusive events, they cannot both occur in the same experiment, and their intersection is the empty event $\phi$ and has probability 0. In this case, (3.2) becomes

$$\text{Prob}(A \cup B) = \text{Prob}(A) + \text{Prob}(B). \qquad (3.3)$$

*Generalization.* If an event $G$ will happen if one of several mutually exclusive events happens in some experiment, the probability that $G$ will happen is the sum of the probabilities of the various ways that it can happen. That is, Eq. (3.3) can be generalized as follows: If the event $G$ occurs in some experiment if and only if one of the mutually exclusive events $A$, $B$, ..., $F$ occurs in that experiment, then

$$\text{Prob}(G) = \text{Prob}(A) + \text{Prob}(B) + \cdots + \text{Prob}(F). \qquad (3.4)$$

*Example* Suppose that an experiment consists of flipping a fair coin three times. We define the event $G$ as the event "heads turns up exactly twice in these three flips in this experiment". Suppose that $A$ is the event "in this experiment, two heads appear in the order HHT", that $B$ is the event "in this experiment two heads appear in the order HTH", and that $C$ is the event "in this experiment two heads appear in the order THH". Then $A$, $B$ and $C$ are mutually exclusive events and $G$ is the event that one of the events $A$, $B$ and $C$ occurs. Then from (3.4),

$$\text{Prob}(G) = \text{Prob}(A) + \text{Prob}(B) + \text{Prob}(C). \qquad (3.5)$$

To find $\text{Prob}(G)$ in this example we have to find $\text{Prob}(A)$, $\text{Prob}(B)$ and $\text{Prob}(C)$. This brings us to the concept of the *independence* of events.

## 3.2   Independence of Two Events

Two events $A_1$ and $A_2$ are said to be *independent* if and only if

$$\text{Prob}\,(A_1 \cap A_2) = \text{Prob}(A_1) \times \text{Prob}(A_2). \qquad (3.6)$$

In words, two events $A_1$ and $A_2$ are said to be *independent* if and only if the probability that they both occur in the same experiment is the probability that $A_1$ occurs in this experiment multiplied by the probability that $A_2$ occurs in this experiment. The intuitive meaning of independence of events is that the occurrence of one of the events does not change the probability that the other event occurs. Examples of independent (and also dependent) events will be given in the problems.

One has to be careful when considering the independence of more than two events. The events $A_1$, $A_2$, ..., $A_m$ are independent if and only if all of the following requirements are met:

$$\text{Prob}(A_i \cap A_j) = \text{Prob}(A_i) \times \text{Prob}(A_j) \text{ for all } (i, j), \ i \neq j,$$

$$\text{Prob}(A_i \cap A_j \cap A_k) = \text{Prob}(A_i) \times \text{Prob}(A_j)$$

$$\times \text{Prob}(A_k) \text{ for all } (i, j, k), \ i \neq j \neq k,$$

$$\vdots$$

$$\text{Prob}(A_1 \cap A_2 \cap \cdots \cap A_m) = \text{Prob}(A_1) \times \text{Prob}(A_2) \times \cdots \times \text{Prob}(A_m).$$

The fact that all of these requirements are needed is illustrated by following simple example. A fair die is to be rolled twice. The event $A_1$ is the event "an odd number will turn up on roll 1", the event $A_2$ is the event "an odd number will turn up on roll 2", and the event $A_3$ is the event "the sum of the two numbers to turn up is an odd number". It is easy to show that $\text{Prob}(A_i \cap A_j) = \text{Prob}(A_i) \times \text{Prob}(A_j)$ for all $(i, j), i \neq j$. However, since $\text{Prob}(A_1) = \text{Prob}(A_2) = \text{Prob}(A_3) = \frac{1}{2}$, whereas $\text{Prob}(A_1 \cap A_2 \cap A_3) = 0$, the three events are not independent. In other words, pairwise independence of a collection of events does not automatically imply independence of all the events.

Very often in practice we *assume* that two or more events are independent from experience or common sense. For example, we reasonably believe that the results of different flips of a coin are independent. This means that in the case of flipping a fair coin three times as discussed in the example at the end of the previous section, and with the events $A$, $B$ and $C$ as defined in that example, $\text{Prob}(A) = \text{Prob}(\text{head on flip 1}) \times \text{Prob}(\text{head on flip 2}) \times \text{Prob}(\text{tail on flip 3})$. From the requirements of the independence of more than two events, this is

$$\frac{1}{2} \times \frac{1}{2} \times \frac{1}{2} = \frac{1}{8}.$$

By the same reasoning, $\text{Prob}(B) = \frac{1}{8}$ and $\text{Prob}(C) = \frac{1}{8}$. The events $A$, $B$ and $C$ are mutually exclusive, since no two of them can both occur on the same three flips of the coin, so that from Eq. (3.5),

$$\text{Prob}(G) = \frac{1}{8} + \frac{1}{8} + \frac{1}{8} = \frac{3}{8}.$$

In some situations, the independence of two events can be found from some given information. For example, suppose that we know that a certain six-sided die is fair. The die is to be rolled once. Let $A$ be the event that an even number turns up and $B$ be the event that 1 or 2 turns up. From this information $\text{Prob}(A) = \frac{1}{2}$ and $\text{Prob}(B) = \frac{1}{3}$. Further, the event $A \cap B$ is the event that 2 turns up, and the probability of this is $\text{Prob}(A \cap B) = \frac{1}{6}$. Since $\frac{1}{6} = \frac{1}{2} \times \frac{1}{3}$, Eq. (3.6) shows that $A$

and $B$ are independent. In intuitive terms, if we are given that 1 or 2 turned up, the probability that an even number turns up (that is, 2 and not 1 turns up) is $\frac{1}{2}$, and this is the same probability for an even number turning up if we were not given the information that 1 or 2 turned up.

## 3.3   Conditional Probabilities

Suppose that a fair coin is flipped twice. Suppose that we are told that at least one head appeared. What is the probability that both flips gave heads? The quick intuitive answer is usually either $\frac{1}{2}$ or $\frac{1}{4}$. However, neither of these answers is correct. The correct answer is $\frac{1}{3}$. Deriving the correct answer to this question is an example of a *conditional probability* calculation. We want to find the probability that both flips gave heads under the condition that least one flip gave heads. Conditional probabilities are often needed in Statistics so we next discuss their calculation.

Suppose that $A$ and $B$ are two events and that $0 < \text{Prob}(B) < 1$. The *conditional* probability that the event $A$ occurs, given that the event $B$ has occurred, denoted by $\text{Prob}(A \mid B)$, is

$$\text{Prob}(A \mid B) = \frac{\text{Prob}(A \cap B)}{\text{Prob}(B)}. \tag{3.7}$$

This is a crucial formula. It must always be used when calculating conditional probabilities. Intuition is usually a very poor guide when calculating conditional probabilities.

The coin-flipping probability $\frac{1}{3}$ mentioned above is found from (3.7) as follows. Suppose that $A$ is the event that both flips gave heads and $B$ is the event that at least one flip gave heads. The intersection event $A \cap B$ is the event that both flips gave heads and also that there was at least one head, which is the same as the event that both flips gave heads. This has probability $\frac{1}{4}$. The event $B$, that there was at least one head, is the union of three mutually exclusive events: "head on both flips", "head on first flip, tail on second flip", and "tail on first flip, head on second flip". Each of these has probability $\frac{1}{4}$, so from (3.5), the probability of $B$ is $\frac{3}{4}$. Inserting these values in (3.7) we get

$$\text{Prob}(A \mid B) = (1/4)/(3/4) = 1/3. \tag{3.8}$$

Another way of seeing this result is that initially there are four equally likely possibilities: HH, HT, TH, TT. However, we are told that one of the three possibilities HH, HT and TH actually did occur, so that the probability that this was HH is 1/3.

As stated above, statistical operations depend on probabilities, and the take-home message from this and other examples is that probability calculations are often counter-intuitive. Take care when doing them!

## 3.4   Conditional Probabilities and Mutually Exclusive Events

Suppose that the events $A$ and $B$ are mutually exclusive. Then $\text{Prob}(A \cap B) = 0$, and Eq. (3.7) shows that $\text{Prob}(A|B) = 0$. This corresponds to the fact that if $A$ and $B$ cannot both happen in the same experiment and we are told that $B$ has occurred, then it is impossible that $A$ occurred.

## 3.5   Conditional Probabilities and Independence

Suppose that $A$ and $B$ are independent events, so that from Eq. (3.6), $\text{Prob}(A \cap B)$ $= \text{Prob}(A) \times \text{Prob}(B)$. Then from Eq. (3.7),

$$\text{Prob}(A \mid B) = \frac{\text{Prob}(A) \times \text{Prob}(B)}{\text{Prob}(B)} = \text{Prob}(A). \tag{3.9}$$

This implies that the information that $B$ has occurred has not changed the probability that $A$ will occur. This is perhaps a more natural concept of independence than the condition given in Eq. (3.6). Examples illustrating conditional probabilities will be given in the problems.

A flow-chart of the "events" part of the book is given on the following page to show the various topics covered in perspective.

## Flowchart: Events

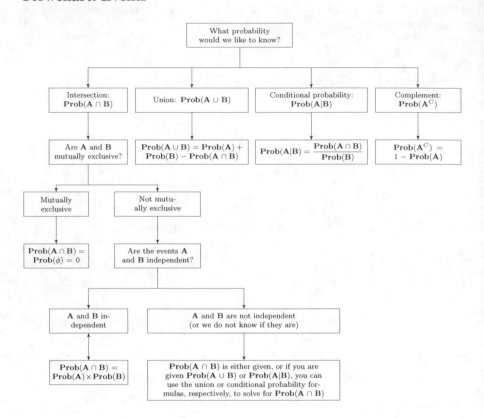

## 3.6   Problems

**3.1**   A fair die is to be rolled once. The event $A$ is: "an odd number turns up" and the event $B$ is: "a 2 or a 3 turns up".

(a)   Calculate (i) Prob($A$), (ii) Prob($B$), (iii) Prob($A \cup B$), (iv) Prob($A \cap B$).
(b)   Are $A$ and $B$ independent events?

**3.2**   This problem also refers to the events $A$ and $B$ in Problem 3.1. Suppose now that the die is unfair, and that the probability that the number $j$ turns up is $j/21$, ($j = 1, 2, \ldots, 6$). (That is, the probability that 1 turns up is 1/21, the probability that 2 turns up is 2/21, the probability that 3 turns up is 3/21, the probability that 4 turns up is 4/21, the probability that 5 turns up is 5/21 and the probability that 6 turns up is 6/21.)

(a)   Calculate (i) Prob($A$), (ii) Prob($B$), (iii) Prob($A \cap B$), (iv) Prob($A \cup B$).
(b)   Are $A$ and $B$ independent events?

**3.3**   A fair die is to be rolled once. D is the event that an even number turns up. E is the event that a 1, 2, or 3 turns up. Calculate (a) Prob($D$), (b) Prob($D \cap E$), (c) Prob($D \cup E$).

**3.4**  There is a generalization of the formula (3.2) for the probability of the union of two events $A$ and $B$. This is, that if $A$, $B$ and $C$ are three events,

$$\text{Prob}(A \cup B \cup C) = \text{Prob}(A) + \text{Prob}(B) + \text{Prob}(C) - \text{Prob}(A \cap B)$$

$$- \text{Prob}(A \cap C) - \text{Prob}(B \cap C) + \text{Prob}(A \cap B \cap C). \qquad (3.10)$$

Suppose that a die is fair, that the events $A$ and $B$ are as given in Problem 3.1, and the event $C$ is "a 3 or a 6 turns up". Calculate $\text{Prob}(A \cup B \cup C)$ (a) directly, by working out what the event $A \cup B \cup C$ is, and (b) by calculating the right-hand side in Eq. (3.10) and check that your two answers agree.

**3.5**  A fair die is to be rolled twice. It is assumed that the numbers turning up on the two rolls are independent. That is, if the event $A$ is: "the number turning up on the first roll is $x$" and the event $B$ is: "the number turning up on the second roll is $y$," then it is assumed that the events $A$ and $B$ are independent for all choices of $x$ and $y$.

By considering all the possible outcomes and their probabilities, consider the possible outcomes of the two rolls to find the probability (a) that the sum of the two numbers is 2, (b) that the sum of the two numbers is 3, (c) that the sum of the two numbers is 4.

**3.6**  Let $C$ be the event that an undergraduate chosen at random is female and $L$ be the event that a student chosen at random is left-handed. If the events $C$ and $L$ are independent, and $\text{Prob}(C) = 0.63$, $\text{Prob}(L) = 0.10$, (a) Find $\text{Prob}(C \cap L)$, (b) $\text{Prob}(C \cup L)$.

**3.7**  Referring to the songbirds in Problem 2.2, suppose now that $\text{Prob}(L) = 0.3$ and $\text{Prob}(O) = 0.6$.

(a)  Assuming that the events $L$ and $O$ are independent, find (i) $\text{Prob}(L \cap O)$, (ii) $\text{Prob}(L \cup O)$, (iii) $\text{Prob}(L^C \cap O)$, and (iv) $\text{Prob}(L^C \cup O^C)$.
(b)  Keep the same probabilities for $L$ and $O$, but now do not assume independence and let $\text{Prob}(L \cup O) = 0.64$. Find $\text{Prob}(L \cap O)$ and from this assess whether L and O are dependent or independent.
(c)  Use $\text{Prob}(L \cap O)$ you calculated in part (b) of the problem to find $\text{Prob}(L|O)$ and $\text{Prob}(O|L)$. How would you use these to check for independence instead?

**3.8**  Show that if $A$ and $B$ are independent events, then $A^c$ and $B^c$ are also independent events.
Hint: To do this, you have to show that $\text{Prob}(A^c \cap B^c) = \text{Prob}(A^c) \times \text{Prob}(B^c)$. You should start out by using the fact (which you may take as given or refer to Problem 2.3) that $\text{Prob}(A^c \cap B^c) = 1 - \text{Prob}(A \cup B)$, and then use a formula given in Eq. (3.2) for $\text{Prob}(A \cup B)$ and also the fact that $A$ and $B$ are independent.

**3.9**  Women over the age of 50 are advised to have a mammogram every 2 years to test for breast cancer. Women whose mammogram is positive then have a further test (a biopsy). It is important to work out various probabilities with respect to the mammogram part of this procedure. This problem is about this situation.

Let $A$ be the event (for any woman): "her mammogram is positive". Let $B$ be the event (for any woman): "she has breast cancer".

(a)  In words, what does the event $A^c$ mean?
(b)  In words, what does the event $B^c$ mean?
(c)  In words, what do the probabilities $\text{Prob}(B|A)$ and $\text{Prob}(B|A^c)$ mean?
(d)  What would it mean in terms of the usefulness of a mammogram if the probabilities $\text{Prob}(B|A)$ and $\text{Prob}(B|A^c)$ were equal?

# Chapter 4
# Probability: One Discrete Random Variable

## 4.1 Random Variables

In this section we define some terms that will be used often. We often adopt the coin flipping example as an illustration, but the corresponding definitions for other examples are easy to imagine.

If we plan to flip a coin 2000 times tomorrow, then today the number of heads that we will get tomorrow is unknown to us. This number is therefore a "random variable". The concept of a random variable is perhaps the most important one in all of probability theory. We now give the formal definition of a discrete random variable.

**Definition** A discrete random variable is a conceptual and numerical quantity that, in some future experiment involving chance, or randomness, will take one value from some discrete set of possible values. In some cases the respective probabilities of the members of this set of possible values are known and in other cases they are unknown.

The words "conceptual", "numerical" and "discrete" in this definition need further discussion. A random variable is conceptual because it is something that is only in our mind. For example, if we plan to flip a coin 2000 times tomorrow, the number of heads that we will get tomorrow is, today, only a concept of our minds. No specific number of heads has yet arisen. A random variable is required to be numerical because we will later do mathematical computations involving random variables. A discrete random variable can only take one of a discrete set of numbers (often restricted to the numbers 0, 1, 2, ... ). The number of heads that we will get tomorrow when we flip a coin 2000 times is therefore a discrete random variable: it can only take one of the discrete set of values $\{0, 1, \ldots, 2000\}$.

In practice, a random variable is either discrete or continuous. By contrast with a discrete random variable, a continuous random variable can take any value in some continuous interval of values. For example, the height of an individual whom we will

© The Author(s), under exclusive license to Springer Nature Switzerland AG 2023

W. J. Ewens, K. Brumberg, *Introductory Statistics for Data Analysis*, https://doi.org/10.1007/978-3-031-28189-1_4

randomly choose tomorrow is a continuous random variable: it can take any value in some interval of values. The mathematical theory for discrete random variables differs from that for continuous random variables—for continuous random variables we need calculus. Continuous random variables will be considered in a later section, but an understanding of calculus is not needed in this book.

Why is the concept of a random variable, either discrete or continuous, so important? As emphasized in Chap. 1, statistical operations depend on probability calculations, and probabilities relate to random variables. For example, it will be shown in Sect. 4.5 that it is possible to calculate the probability that tomorrow we will get $x$ or more heads from 2000 flips of a fair coin, for any number $x$. This probability calculation relates to the random variable "the number of heads that we will get tomorrow". Suppose that in the coin-flipping example mentioned above, we wish to assess whether the coin is fair. If tomorrow we flip the coin 2000 times and get 1087 heads, we cannot make any inference as to whether the coin is fair unless we have in hand the probability calculation of a fair coin giving 1087 or more heads. The take-home message is that statistical inferences depend on probability calculations, and these calculations often refer to discrete random variables. Therefore the probability theory relating to a discrete random variable is essential to Statistics.

## 4.2   Random Variables and Data

The concept of a discrete random variable is in contrast to what we mean by the word "data". By "data" we mean the observed value of a random variable once some experiment has been performed. In the coin example of the previous section, suppose that tomorrow has now come and we have flipped the coin 2000 times. The "data" is the observed number of heads that we did actually get, for example 1087. It is an "after the experiment" concept. It is the observed value of a random variable once the "experiment" of flipping the coin has been carried out.

It is crucial to distinguish between the "before the experiment" concept of a random variable and the "after the experiment" concept of data. In practice, we will often analyze experiments *after* they have occurred, but we will still need to consider random variables. In doing so, we will always put ourselves in the position of the experimenter *before* the data has been gathered, so that we can think of random variables as future concepts, whether or not the experiment has already taken place.

To assist us with keeping clear the distinction between random variables and data, and following the standard notational convention, a random variable is always denoted by an upper-case Roman letter near the end of the alphabet. We therefore use the upper-case letters $X$, $Y$ and $Z$ (and sometimes other upper-case letters) in this book to denote random variables. In the coin example, we might denote the random variable number of heads we will get tomorrow by $X$.

The notation for the "after the experiment" data value is the corresponding lower case letter. So if today we denote by $X$ the number of heads that we will get tomorrow when we flip the coin, then tomorrow, after we have flipped the coin, we would denote the number of heads that we did get by the corresponding lower-case letter $x$. Thus it makes sense, after the coin has been flipped 2000 times, to say "$x = 1087$". This simply states that after we flipped the coin 2000 times, we observed that heads turned up 1087 times. It does not make sense before the coin is flipped to say $X = 1087$. This statement "does not compute".

There are therefore two notational conventions: upper-case Roman letters for random variables, the corresponding lower-case Roman letters for data. We will later use a third notational convention (Greek letters) for "parameters". Parameters will be defined later.

We shall not consider data until later, when we turn to the Statistics part of this book. For the moment, we consider only random variables and the probability theory associated with them.

## 4.3   The Probability Distribution of a Discrete Random Variable

There are various ways in which one can present the probability distribution of a discrete random variable. The first is the "tableau" method. In this method, we give a list of all the possible values that the random variable (denoted here by $X$) can take, together with their respective probabilities. If there are $k$ possible values of $X$, these are denoted by $v_1, v_2, \ldots, v_k$, written in increasing order so that $v_1 < v_2 < \ldots < v_k$. If these values have respective probabilities $\text{Prob}(v_1)$, $\text{Prob}(v_2)$, $\ldots$, $\text{Prob}(v_k)$, the probability distribution of $X$ when written in the "tableau" form is

$$
\begin{array}{c|cccc}
\text{Possible values of } X & v_1 & v_2 & \ldots & v_k \\
\hline
\text{Respective probabilities} & \text{Prob}(v_1) & \text{Prob}(v_2) & \ldots & \text{Prob}(v_k)
\end{array}
\tag{4.1}
$$

The expression "$\text{Prob}(v_j)$" in (4.1) is a shorthand for the statement that "the probability, before the experiment is performed, that the eventually observed data value corresponding to the random variable $X$ will be $v_j$". These probabilities might be known or might be unknown. This shorthand is used later in this book. Examples of the tableau method of describing a probability distribution are given below in (4.2) and (4.3). In (4.2) the probabilities are known and in (4.3) they are unknown if the value of $\theta$ is unknown.

The *support* of a discrete random variable is the set of possible values that it can take. In the notation given in (4.1), the support of the random variable $X$ is the set of values $\{v_1, v_2, \ldots, v_k\}$. In both (4.2) and (4.3) the support is $\{0, 1, 2\}$.

The link between the notation "$\text{Prob}(v_j)$" and the notation for probabilities of events is that we think of "$\text{Prob}(v_j)$" as the probability of the event "after the experiment has been conducted, the observed value of the 'before the experiment' random variable $X$ will be $v_j$".

In the coin flipping case, if we know that the coin is fair, the probability distribution of $X$, the (conceptual) number of heads that we will get on two flips of the coin, is found as follows. The possible values of $X$ are 0, 1 and 2. We will get 0 heads if both flips give tails, and since the outcomes of the two flips are assumed to be independent, as discussed in Sect. 3.2, the probability of this is $(0.5) \times (0.5) = 0.25$. We can get 1 head in two ways: head on the first flip and tail on the second, and tail on the first flip and head on the second. These events are mutually exclusive, and each has probability 0.25. Thus the total probability of getting exactly 1 head is 0.5. The probability of 2 heads is $(0.5) \times (0.5) = 0.25$. This leads to the following probability distribution:

$$\begin{array}{c|ccc} \text{Possible values of } X & 0 & 1 & 2 \\ \hline \text{Respective probabilities} & 0.25 & 0.50 & 0.25 \end{array} \tag{4.2}$$

This tableau states that $\text{Prob}(0) = 0.25$, $\text{Prob}(1) = 0.5$, $\text{Prob}(2) = 0.25$.

In this fair coin example above, the probabilities for the possible values 0, 1 and 2 are known. In other situations, these probabilities might be unknown. In these situations we denote the probability of getting a head on any flip by $\theta$, which is the Greek letter "theta". The discussion below covers both cases, that is both when the numerical value of $\theta$ is known and when it is unknown to us. We continue to define $X$ as the number of heads that we get on two flips of the coin, and the possible values of $X$ are still 0, 1 and 2. We will get 0 heads if both flips give tails, and since the outcomes of the two flips are independent, the probability of this event is $(1 - \theta) \times (1 - \theta) = (1 - \theta)^2$. As above, we can get 1 head in two ways: head on the first flip and tail on the second, and tail on the first flip and head on the second. These events are mutually exclusive, and each has probability $\theta(1 - \theta)$. Thus the probability of getting exactly one head is $2\theta(1 - \theta)$. The probability of getting two heads is $\theta \times \theta = \theta^2$. This leads to the following probability distribution:

$$\begin{array}{c|ccc} \text{Possible values of } X & 0 & 1 & 2 \\ \hline \text{Respective probabilities} & (1 - \theta)^2 & 2\theta(1 - \theta) & \theta^2 \end{array} \tag{4.3}$$

In other words,

$$\text{Prob}(0) = (1 - \theta)^2, \quad \text{Prob}(1) = 2\theta(1 - \theta), \quad \text{Prob}(2) = \theta^2. \tag{4.4}$$

Even though the numerical value of $\theta$ might be unknown to us, so that we do not know the numerical values of any of the probabilities in (4.3), the probability distribution (4.3) is still useful. In this distribution, $\theta$ is a so-called *parameter*: these are discussed extensively below. The probability distribution (4.3), or equivalently (4.4), can be generalized to the case of an arbitrary number of flips of the coin—see (4.5) below. The probability distribution (4.2) is thus a special case of the probability distribution (4.3), corresponding to the value $\theta = \frac{1}{2}$.

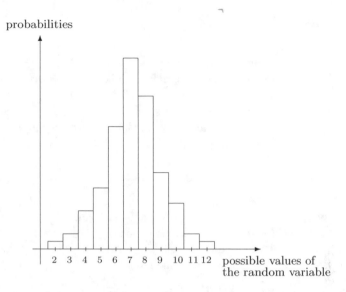

**Fig. 4.1**  A discrete probability distribution for the sum of two numbers to turn up on a biased die

In cases such as (4.2), where numerical values of all probabilities are known (in contrast to (4.3) where the numerical values of the probabilities are unknown if the numerical value of $\theta$ is unknown), a probability distribution can be presented graphically. This form of presentation has a visual appeal. An example is given in Fig. 4.1. In this example, the random variable is the sum of the two numbers to turn up on two rolls of a biased die, where the probabilities for the numbers 1, 2, 3, 4, 5 and 6 turning up on any roll are known. On the horizontal axis we write the possible values of the random variable (2, 3, ..., 12, as shown in the graph), and on the vertical axis we draw rectangles whose various heights indicate the probabilities of these various possible values.

Suppose that a given coin is fair. Although it is possible in principle to construct either a tableau or graphical presentation of a probability distribution of the number $X$ of heads to arise, this might not be easy in practice. For example, if we plan to flip a fair coin 1,000,000 times, it would be impractical in practice to list the probabilities of 0, 1, 2, ..., 1,000,000 heads or to draw a graph of these probabilities. In this case, we use a mathematical formula: an example is given in (4.5) below.

It is not always possible even in principle to give a graphical presentation of a probability distribution. For example, the probabilities given in (4.3) depend on the value of $\theta$, and therefore the general shape of the distribution differs, often substantially, from one value of $\theta$ to another. Thus it is not possible to draw a unique graph of the probability distribution (4.3) that applies for all values of the parameter $\theta$. This leads us to consider the concept of a parameter in more detail.

## 4.4    Parameters

The quantity $\theta$ introduced in the previous section is called a "parameter". A parameter is some constant whose numerical value is either known or (more often in practice) unknown to us. For example, in a clinical trial the probability that a proposed new medicine cures a patient of some illness is unknown, and thus this probability is regarded as a parameter. (If we did know this probability, there would be no need to conduct the clinical trial.) Other examples of parameters are given later.

When the numerical value of a parameter is unknown, large parts of Statistics consist of:

 (i)  Using data to estimate the numerical value of a parameter.
 (ii) Using data to get some idea of the precision of our estimate of a parameter (sometimes called finding the "margin of error").
(iii)  Using data to test hypotheses about the numerical value of a parameter.

We shall consider these three activities later in this book. In the clinical trial example, if $\theta$ is the (unknown) probability that the proposed new medicine cures a patient, these would be

 (i)  Estimating the numerical value of the parameter $\theta$.
 (ii) Using data to get some idea of the precision of our estimate of $\theta$.
(iii)  Using data to test hypotheses about the numerical value of this parameter, for example testing the hypothesis that $\theta = 0.8$.

As a notational convention in this book, we always use Greek letters (for example $\theta$) to denote parameters. Unfortunately statistical convention implies that Greek symbols are sometimes used to denote quantities that are not parameters. We have already seen one example of this with the empty event $\phi$. There will be two more cases later in this book when Greek letters are used for quantities other than parameters due to statistical convention; it will be pointed out when this occurs.

## 4.5    The Binomial Distribution

There are many important discrete probability distributions that arise often in the applications of probability theory and Statistics to real-world problems. Each of these distributions is appropriate under some set of requirements specific to that distribution. In this section, we focus on one of the most important of these distributions, namely the binomial distribution, and start by listing the requirements for it to be appropriate.

The binomial distribution arises if, and only if, all four of the following requirements hold.

(i)  First, we plan to conduct some fixed number of trials. By "fixed" we mean fixed in advance, and not, for example, determined by the outcomes of the trials as they occur. We always denote this number by $n$.

(ii)  Second, there must be exactly two possible outcomes on each trial. The two outcomes are often called, for convenience, "success" and "failure". For example, we might regard getting a head on the flip of a coin as a success and a tail as a failure, or the proposed new medicine curing a patient a "success" and not curing a patient a "failure".

(iii)  Third, the various trials must be independent—the outcome of any trial must not affect the outcome of any other trial.

(iv)  Finally, the probability of success, which we always denotes by $\theta$, must be the same on all trials.

One must be careful when using a binomial distribution to ensure that all four of these conditions hold. We reasonably believe that they hold when flipping a coin, but there are many situations in practice where they do not hold. For example, when rolling a die, there are six possible values for the number turning up, not two. If in baseball we call hitting a home run a success, then different players on a team will almost certainly have different probabilities of a success. If a proposed new medicine is given to twins, the outcomes (cured or not cured) might not be independent because of the genetic similarity of the twins.

For now we assume that the four requirements (i)–(iv) hold. The random variable of interest is the total number $X$ of successes in the $n$ trials. If the numerical value of $\theta$ is unknown, the probability distribution of $X$ cannot be given by a graph. It is best given by the binomial distribution formula

$$\text{Prob}(X = x) = \binom{n}{x}\theta^x(1 - \theta)^{n-x}, \quad x = 0, 1, 2, \ldots, n. \tag{4.5}$$

This compact formula presentation provides an example of the third method of describing a probability distribution, that is, by a mathematical formula.

In the formula (4.5), $\theta$ is called the parameter, and $n$ is called the index, of the binomial distribution. The support of $X$ is $\{0, 1, \ldots, n\}$.

The binomial coefficient $\binom{n}{x}$ in this formula is often spoken as "$n$ choose $x$" and is equal to the number of different orderings in which $x$ successes can arise in the $n$ trials. It is calculated from the formula

$$\binom{n}{x} = \frac{n!}{x! \times (n - x)!},$$

where for $x \geq 1$, we define $x! = x \times (x - 1) \times (x - 2) \times \cdots \times 3 \times 2 \times 1$ and for $x = 0$ we define $0! = 1$.

As an example, $\binom{4}{2} = \frac{4!}{2! \times (4-2)!} = \frac{24}{2 \times 2} = 6$. Thus there are six orderings in which we can get two successes from four trials. If we denote S for success and F for failure, these are SSFF, SFSF, SFFS, FSSF, FSFS, FFSS.

The word "choose" originates from another interpretation of $\binom{n}{x}$, namely, it is the number of ways of choosing a committee of $x$ people from a group of $n$ people. This is discussed in Problem 4.8.

***Proof of the Binomial Formula (4.5)*** We first consider the expression $\theta^x(1 - \theta)^{n-x}$ arising in (4.5). The probability of first obtaining $x$ successes and then obtaining $n - x$ failures (in that specific order) is $\theta \times \theta \times \cdots \times \theta \times (1 - \theta) \times (1 - \theta) \times \cdots \times (1 - \theta)$, where $\theta$ occurs $x$ times in the product and $(1 - \theta)$ occurs $n - x$ times. This is $\theta^x(1 - \theta)^{n-x}$. The probability of first obtaining $n - x$ failures and then obtaining $x$ successes (in that specific order) is $(1 - \theta) \times (1 - \theta) \times \cdots \times (1 - \theta) \times \theta \times \theta \times \cdots \times \theta$, where $\theta$ again occurs $x$ times in the product and $(1 - \theta)$ occurs $n - x$ times. This is also $\theta^x(1 - \theta)^{n-x}$ after rearranging the terms in the product. Indeed the probability of obtaining $x$ successes and $(n - x)$ failures in *any* specified order is $\theta^x(1 - \theta)^{n-x}$, since $\theta$ will occur exactly $x$ times and $(1 - \theta)$ will occur exactly $n - x$ times in finding the probability of $x$ successes and $(n - x)$ failures in any specified order.

Because the events corresponding to different orderings are mutually exclusive, and there are $\binom{n}{x}$ orderings by definition, Eq. (3.4) shows that the overall probability of $x$ successes from $n$ trials is $\binom{n}{x}\theta^x(1 - \theta)^{n-x}$, which is the binomial probability given in (4.5).

*Example* If $\theta = 0.4$, the probability of getting $x = 2$ successes from $n = 6$ trials is

$$\text{Prob}(2) = \binom{6}{2}(0.4)^2(0.6)^4 = 15 \times 0.16 \times 0.1296 = 0.31104. \tag{4.6}$$

We can use R to do this calculation explicitly as well using the function `choose()` where n is the number of trials and k is the number of successes: `choose(n = 6, k = 2) * 0.4^2 * 0.6^4`. We can also use the built in function `dbinom()` in R for finding binomial probabilities where x is the number of successes, `size` is the number of trials, and `prob` is the probability of success $\theta$: `dbinom(x = 2, size = 6, prob = 0.4)`.

Chart 1, the chart of binomial probabilities provided at the back of the book, gives 0.3110 for this probability. This occurs because the probabilities in the binomial chart are accurate only to four decimal places.

The case $n = 1$ deserves explicit discussion. The particular case of the binomial distribution when $n = 1$ is called the *Bernoulli distribution*. The random variable $X$, the number of successes, can only assume the values 0 (with probability $1 - \theta$) or 1 (with probability $\theta$). The various properties that will be given for the binomial distribution apply equally for the Bernoulli distribution by putting $n = 1$.

The case $n = 2$ also deserves explicit discussion. The factor 2 in (4.4) is an example of a binomial coefficient, reflecting the fact that there are two orderings (success followed by failure and failure followed by success) in which we can obtain one success and one failure in two trials. This is also given by the binomial calculation $\binom{2}{1} = \frac{2!}{1! \times (2-1)!} = \frac{2}{1 \times 1} = 2$.

The following examples involve some cases where the binomial distribution applies and some cases where it does not apply.

*Example 4.5.1*

(a) Suppose that the probability that a man is left-handed is 0.1 and the probability that a woman is left-handed is also 0.1. In a group consisting of two men and two women, what is the probability that there is exactly one left-handed person?

Since the probabilities of being left-handed are the same for men and women, the four requirements for a binomial distribution apply and the required probability is $\binom{4}{1}(0.1)^1(0.9)^3 = 0.2916$.

(b) Suppose now that the probability that a man is left-handed is 0.1 and the probability that a woman is left-handed is 0.08. In a group consisting of two men and two women, what is the probability that there is exactly one left-handed person?

Since the probabilities of being left-handed are not the same for men and women, the answer can only be found by applying one binomial distribution for men and another for women. The details are as follows.

The event "exactly one left-handed person" is the union of two mutually exclusive events, namely "exactly one man is left-handed, neither of the two women is left-handed" and "neither of the two men is left-handed, exactly one of the two women is left-handed". Using two different binomial distributions, one for men and one for women, together with the probability formula for independent events and also for the union of two mutually exclusive events, the required probability is

$$\binom{2}{1}(0.1)^1(0.9)^1 \times \binom{2}{0}(0.08)^0(0.92)^2 + \binom{2}{0}(0.1)^0(0.9)^2$$

$$\times \binom{2}{1}(0.08)^1(0.92)^1 = 0.26204544.$$

(c) The result of part (a) of this question can be found by using the (unnecessarily complicated) method employed in part (b) of finding the answer by using two binomial calculations. The event "exactly one left-handed person" is the union of two mutually exclusive events, as described in part (b). Using the same binomial distributions for both men and for women, together with the probability formula for independent events and also for the union of two mutually exclusive events, the required probability is

$$\binom{2}{1}(0.1)^1(0.9)^1 \times \binom{2}{0}(0.1)^0(0.9)^2 + \binom{2}{0}(0.1)^0(0.9)^2$$

$$\times \binom{2}{1}(0.1)^1(0.9)^1 = 0.2916.$$

This agrees with the simpler calculation given above.

*Example 4.5.2* You have to carry two eggs home from a shop. There are two methods by which this can be done. Under Method 1, each egg is carried in its own basket. Basket 1 is dropped, and the egg in it is broken, with probability $\theta$. Independently of this, Basket 2 is dropped, and the egg in it is broken, also with probability $\theta$. Because of the independence assumption, the number of broken eggs has a binomial distribution with index $n = 2$ and parameter $\theta$. Under Method 2, both eggs are put in the same basket. This basket is dropped with probability $\theta$ (the same numerical value as in Method 1) and if the basket is dropped, both eggs are broken. Under this second method, the number of broken eggs does not have a binomial distribution because the independence assumption does not hold: if one egg is broken, then the other egg is also broken. If one egg is not broken, the other egg is not broken. The number $X$ of broken eggs has the following probability distribution for Method 2:

$$
\begin{array}{c|ccc}
\text{Possible values of } X & 0 & 1 & 2 \\
\hline
\text{Respective probabilities} & 1 - \theta & 0 & \theta
\end{array}
\tag{4.7}
$$

We will see later what this means concerning the expression "don't put all your eggs in one basket".

*Example 4.5.3 (The "Hat-Check" Problem)* Suppose that two men go to a restaurant and leave their hats at the hat-check desk. After they finish their meal, the hat-check clerk returns the hats at random to the two men. Let $X$ be the number of men (0, 1 or 2) who get their correct hat. We call it a success for each man if he gets his correct hat and let $X$ be the total number of successes. Then $X$ does not have a binomial distribution. The reason for this is that the binomial requirement of independence does not hold—if the first man gets his correct hat then the second man must also get his correct hat and if the first man gets the incorrect hat then the second man also gets the incorrect hat. The probability distribution of $X$ is

$$
\begin{array}{c|ccc}
\text{Possible values of } X & 0 & 1 & 2 \\
\hline
\text{Respective probabilities} & 0.5 & 0 & 0.5
\end{array}
\tag{4.8}
$$

## 4.6  The Hypergeometric Distribution

Although the binomial distribution is discussed frequently in this book, there are of course many other discrete probability distributions which arise when the requirements for the binomial distribution to hold are not met. In this section, we introduce one such distribution using a simple example.

Suppose that an urn contains $r$ red marbles and $b$ blue marbles, the total number $r + b$ of marbles being denoted by $n$. A total of $d$ marbles is drawn from the urn ($1 \leq d \leq n$) at random and *without* replacement. The number $d$ of marbles drawn is fixed in advance. The number $X$ of red marbles taken out is then a random variable and our aim is to find its probability distribution.

Before considering this distribution, called the hypergeometric distribution, we observe that it is *not* the binomial distribution. There is a dependence in the outcomes of the successive draws from the urn because we do not replace the drawn marble after each draw. If, for example, many red marbles happen to have been drawn initially, this somewhat decreases the probability that on the next draw a red marble is drawn compared to the situation where few red marbles were drawn initially. Thus two of the requirements for the binomial distribution to hold, independence and equal success probabilities, are not satisfied.

Before discussing the probability distribution of $X$, it is necessary first to consider the support of $X$, and doing this is not straightforward. If more than $b$ marbles are taken from the urn, then we will draw at least $d - b$ red marbles. By definition, $X$ can never exceed the number $r$ of red marbles initially in the urn or the number $d$ of marbles taken from the urn. These considerations show that the support of $X$ is $\{\ell, \ell + 1, \ldots, h\}$, where $\ell$ is the maximum of 0 and $d - b$ and $h$ is the minimum of $r$ and $d$. For example, if $r = 10$, $b = 10$ and $d = 6$, then $\ell = 0$ since it is possible that all six marbles drawn are blue and $h = 6$ because it is also possible that all six marbles drawn are red. If, however, $d = 16$, then $\ell = 6$ since at least six of the marbles drawn out must be red because only ten blue marbles exist and we draw sixteen marbles. Next, $h = 10$, since even though we will draw 16 marbles, only ten red marbles exist.

For any number $x$ in its support, the random variable $X$ has the following *hypergeometric* distribution:

$$\text{Prob}(X = x) = \frac{\binom{r}{x}\binom{b}{d-x}}{\binom{n}{d}}. \tag{4.9}$$

**Proof** The proof follows the general lines of the proof of the binomial distribution formula (4.5). We first find the probability of first drawing $x$ red marbles and then $d - x$ blue marbles (in that specific order). This is

$$\frac{r}{n} \times \frac{r-1}{n-1} \times \cdots \times \frac{r-x+1}{n-x+1} \times \frac{b}{n-x} \times \frac{b-1}{n-x-1} \times \cdots \times \frac{b-d+x+1}{n-d+1}. \tag{4.10}$$

Using the fact that for any numbers $u$ and $v$ with $u > v$, $u \times (u-1) \times \cdots \times (u-v+1)$ can be written as $\frac{u!}{(u-v)!}$, this probability can be written as

$$\left( \frac{r!}{(r-x)!} \times \frac{b}{(b-d+x)!} \right) \bigg/ \left( \frac{n!}{(n-d)!} \right) = \frac{r!\, b!\, (n-d)!}{(r-x)!\, (b-d+x)!\, n!}. \tag{4.11}$$

The probability of first drawing $d - x$ blue marbles and then $x$ red marbles (in that specific order) is

$$\frac{b}{n} \times \frac{b-1}{n-1} \times \cdots \times \frac{b-d+x+1}{n-d+x+1} \times \frac{r}{n-d+x} \times \frac{r-1}{n-d+x-1} \times \cdots \times \frac{r-x+1}{n-d+1},$$

and this is identical to the expression in (4.10) since the order of multiplication can be interchanged. More generally, the probability of drawing $x$ red marbles and $d - x$ blue marbles in *any* specified order is also equal to the expression in (4.10) since all that changes is the order of terms in the numerator.

From this, the required probability is the expression given in (4.11) multiplied by the number of orders in which $x$ red marbles and $d - x$ blue marbles can be drawn, equal to $\binom{d}{x}$ or equivalently $\binom{d}{d-x}$, as specifying the draws with red marbles will determine the draws with blue marbles and vice versa. We then have

$$\frac{r! \, b! \, (n-d)!}{(r-x)! \, (b-d+x)! \, n!} \times \frac{d!}{x! \, (d-x)!}. \tag{4.12}$$

Rearranging terms, we have $\dfrac{r!}{x! \, (r-x)!} \times \dfrac{b!}{(d-x)! \, (b-d+x)!} \times \dfrac{d! \, (n-d)!}{n!}$,

which can also be written as $\dfrac{\binom{r}{x}\binom{b}{d-x}}{\binom{n}{d}}$, as given in (4.9).

*Example* The hypergeometric distribution arises in various versions of a lottery. The following is a typical example. A contestant selects six numbers without replacement from the set $\{1, 2, \ldots, 45\}$. The lottery administrators choose six numbers (the "winning" numbers) at random from the same set, and the contestant wins the lottery if all six numbers that she chooses are the winning numbers. By analogy with the marbles example, the probability that the contestant wins the lottery is the same as the probability that all six red marbles are drawn at random from a bag containing 45 marbles, 6 of which are red and 39 are blue. This probability is

$$\frac{\binom{6}{6}\binom{39}{0}}{\binom{45}{6}} = \frac{1}{\binom{45}{6}} \approx 0.00000012. \tag{4.13}$$

Suppose next that the contestant also wins the lottery if she chooses five of the six winning numbers. The probability of this event is

$$\frac{\binom{6}{5}\binom{39}{1}}{\binom{45}{6}} = \frac{234}{\binom{45}{6}} \approx 0.00002873. \tag{4.14}$$

The overall probability of winning the lottery is then the sum of the two values in (4.13) and (4.14), that is about 0.00002885.

In R, to simultaneously obtain the hypergeometric probabilities of choosing 5 and 6 correct numbers, we use the dhyper() function, which takes arguments x, m, n, k. These correspond to $x$, $r$, $b$, $d$ in our notation: dhyper(x = 5:6, m = 6, n = 39, k = 6). To find the probability of choosing 5 or 6 correct numbers, equivalent to getting *more than* 4 correct numbers, we can use the phyper() function with the new arguments q = 4 and lower.tail = FALSE: phyper(q = 4, m = 6, n = 39, k = 6, lower.tail = FALSE).

The hypergeometric distribution also arises in the situation described in the following paragraphs, and in Sect. 10.2 we shall see the relevance of this new situation to statistical operations.

Suppose that we plan to conduct two experiments, both involving a binomial random variable. The number of successes in Experiment 1, namely $X_1$, has a binomial distribution with index $r$ and parameter $\theta$. The number of successes in Experiment 2, namely $X_2$, has a binomial distribution with index $b$ and also with parameter $\theta$. We denote $r + b$ by $n$. The outcomes of the two experiments are independent events. Suppose that you are given that after the two experiments have been completed, the total number of successes is $d$. Given this information, what is $\text{Prob}(X_1 = x)$?

The required probability is a conditional probability (we are given the event that the total number of successes is $d$). This implies that we have to use the conditional probability formula (3.7), repeated here for convenience.

$$\text{Prob}(A \mid B) = \frac{\text{Prob}(A \cap B)}{\text{Prob}(B)}. \tag{4.15}$$

In terms of the notation in (4.15), the event that we are given is $B$, that the total number of successes is $d$. The denominator in the right-hand side of Eq. (4.15) is $\text{Prob}(B)$, and we find this by conceptually amalgamating the two experiments, so that we now consider $n = r + b$ trials, where the probability of success on each trial is $\theta$. The probability of $d$ successes in these $n$ trials is given by the binomial probability formula

$$\binom{n}{d} \theta^d (1 - \theta)^{n-d}. \tag{4.16}$$

We now have to find the numerator in (4.15). We define the event $A$ as "$x$ successes in Experiment 1". The intersection event $(A \cap B)$ involved in the numerator of (4.15) is the event "$x$ successes in Experiment 1, $d$ successes in total". The probability of this is not easy to evaluate directly, since the events $A$ and $B$ are not independent. However, the intersection event $(A \cap B)$ is also the intersection of the two events "$x$ successes in Experiment 1, $d - x$ successes in Experiment 2". These two events *are* independent, so that from (3.6) and (4.5), the probability that they both occur is

$$\binom{r}{x}\theta^x(1-\theta)^{r-x} \times \binom{b}{d-x}\theta^{d-x}(1-\theta)^{b-d+x} = \binom{r}{x}\binom{b}{d-x}\theta^d(1-\theta)^{n-d}.$$

$$(4.17)$$

The probability that we want is the ratio of the probabilities in (4.17) and (4.16). In this ratio, the factor $\theta^d(1-\theta)^{n-d}$ cancels out and we are left with

$$\text{Prob}(A \mid B) = \frac{\binom{r}{x}\binom{b}{d-x}}{\binom{n}{d}}. \qquad (4.18)$$

This is precisely the hypergeometric probability (4.9). Given that in both trials combined there were $d$ successes, the probability that $x$ of these successes arose from Experiment 1 is given by (4.18). Although this calculation might seem unnecessarily complicated, we shall see that it is relevant to the statistical operations discussed in Sect. 10.2.

## 4.7   The Mean of a Discrete Random Variable

The mean of a random variable is often confused with the concept of an average, and it is important to keep a clear distinction between the two concepts. There is much confusion between the respective meanings of the words "mean" and "average". So for this book we use a very precise definition: the mean of the discrete random variable $X$ whose probability distribution is given in tableau form in (4.1) is defined as

$$v_1\text{Prob}(v_1) + v_2\text{Prob}(v_2) + \cdots + v_k\text{Prob}(v_k). \qquad (4.19)$$

That is, the mean of a discrete random variable is the smallest possible value that the random variable can take multiplied by the probability of that value, plus the next to smallest possible value that the random variable can take multiplied by the probability of that value, and so on, and finally, plus the largest possible value that the random variable can take multiplied by the probability of that value. In more mathematical shorthand "sigma" notation, the mean is

$$\sum_{i=1}^{k} v_i\text{Prob}(v_i), \qquad (4.20)$$

the summation being over all possible values $v_1, v_2, \ldots, v_k$ that the random variable $X$ can take. We call the expression (4.19), or equivalently the expression (4.20), the "long" formula for a mean. It always gives the correct value for the mean of any discrete random variable $X$.

*Example 4.7.1 (Die Roll)* As another example of the calculation of a mean, consider the number $X$ to turn up when a die is rolled once. Then $X$ is a random variable with possible values 1, 2, 3, 4, 5 and 6. If the die is fair, each of these values has probability $\frac{1}{6}$. Thus the probability distribution of $X$, given in tableau form, is

$$
\begin{array}{l|cccccc}
\text{Possible values of } X & 1 & 2 & 3 & 4 & 5 & 6 \\
\hline
\text{Respective probabilities} & \frac{1}{6} & \frac{1}{6} & \frac{1}{6} & \frac{1}{6} & \frac{1}{6} & \frac{1}{6}
\end{array}
\tag{4.21}
$$

In this case, the mean of $X$ is found from the long formula (4.19) to be

$$
1 \times \frac{1}{6} + 2 \times \frac{1}{6} + 3 \times \frac{1}{6} + 4 \times \frac{1}{6} + 5 \times \frac{1}{6} + 6 \times \frac{1}{6} = 3.5.
\tag{4.22}
$$

Suppose on the other hand that the die is unfair, and that the probability distribution of $X$ is:

$$
\begin{array}{l|cccccc}
\text{Possible values of } X & 1 & 2 & 3 & 4 & 5 & 6 \\
\hline
\text{Respective probabilities} & 0.15 & 0.25 & 0.10 & 0.15 & 0.30 & 0.05
\end{array}
\tag{4.23}
$$

In this case, the mean of $X$ is found from the long formula (4.19) to be

$$
1 \times 0.15 + 2 \times 0.25 + 3 \times 0.10 + 4 \times 0.15 + 5 \times 0.30 + 6 \times 0.05 = 3.35.
\tag{4.24}
$$

*Example 4.7.2 (Hat-Check)* Another example of the calculation of a mean derives from the hat-check example given at the end of Sect. 4.5. From the probability distribution (4.8), the mean of $X$ is $0 \times 0.5 + 1 \times 0 + 2 \times 0.5 = 1$. This is not a realizable value for the number of men getting their correct hats, and in general a mean is often not a realizable value for a random variable.

*Example 4.7.3 (Binomial)* As an important example, the mean of a random variable having the binomial distribution (4.5) is found from (4.5) and (4.19) to be

$$
0 \times \binom{n}{0} \theta^0 (1-\theta)^{n-0} + 1 \times \binom{n}{1} \theta^1 (1-\theta)^{n-1} + \ldots + n \times \binom{n}{n} \theta^n (1-\theta)^{n-n}.
\tag{4.25}
$$

Using the shorthand "sigma" notation, this is

$$
\sum_{x=0}^{n} x \binom{n}{x} \theta^x (1 - \theta)^{n-x}.
\tag{4.26}
$$

The binomial long formula expression in (4.25) can be shown, after some algebra, to simplify to $n\theta$. We call the expression $n\theta$ the "short" formula for the mean of the binomial distribution. It is the first of the short formulas to be discussed in this book. It is so important that we display it explicitly:

If $X$ is a random variable having a binomial distribution with index $n$ and parameter $\theta$, then

$$\text{the mean of the binomial random variable } X = n\theta. \qquad (4.27)$$

In the case of a random variable $X$ having the Bernoulli distribution, the mean is found by putting $n = 1$ in (4.27), yielding a mean of $\theta$. This result can also be found from the fact that the possible values of a Bernoulli random variable are 0 and 1, with respective probabilities $1 - \theta$ and $\theta$, so the mean of a random variable having the Bernoulli distribution as found from (4.19) is $0 \times (1 - \theta) + 1 \times \theta = \theta$. We will see later how the binomial mean $n\theta$ can be found from this Bernoulli distribution mean.

If a short formula for a mean is available, it is more convenient than the long formula. For example, in the case of a random variable having the binomial distribution, it is much easier to calculate $n\theta$ than the expression in (4.25) if the numerical values of $n$ and $\theta$ are given.

As another example, the probabilities listed in (4.4) are a particular case (for $n = 2$) of the binomial probabilities as given in (4.5). We can check the short formula (4.27) for the mean in the case $n = 2$ by using the probabilities in (4.4) and the long formula (4.19) for a mean. The long formula gives

$$\text{mean} = 0 \times (1-\theta)^2 + 1 \times \{2\theta(1-\theta)\} + 2 \times \theta^2 = 2\theta - 2\theta^2 + 2\theta^2 = 2\theta, \qquad (4.28)$$

and this agrees with (4.27) for the case $n = 2$.

*Example 4.7.4 (Hypergeometric)* Another important case for which we do have a short formula arises for the mean of the hypergeometric random variable. With some algebra it can be shown from Eq. (4.9) that the mean of the hypergeometric random variable $X$ defined in Sect. 4.6 is as given in Eq. (4.29) below:

$$\text{the mean of the hypergeometric random variable } X = \frac{dr}{n}. \qquad (4.29)$$

It is interesting to consider the relation of this mean to the value that would be obtained if sampling were done *with* replacement, that is, if once a marble were drawn from the urn and its color noted, the marble were replaced in the urn before the next draw. In this case, all the requirements for the binomial distribution apply, and the probability that a red marble appears on any draw is $\frac{r}{n}$. The binomial distribution formula shows that the mean of the number of red marbles drawn is $\frac{dr}{n}$. The mean number of red marbles drawn in both cases is the same, namely $\frac{dr}{n}$. We will see in the next section how these two distributions differ.

For probability distributions other than the binomial and hypergeometric distributions, it is not always the case that a convenient short formula exists. When this is so, the mean has to be calculated using the long formula (4.19).

*Example 4.7.5 (Eggs)* The "eggs" example at the end of Sect. 4.5 provides an illustration of this. Under Method 1 the number of broken eggs has a binomial distribution with index $n = 2$ and parameter $\theta$. Then from (4.27) the mean number of broken eggs is $2\theta$. There is no short formula for the mean number of broken eggs under Method 2 and we have to use the long formula (4.19) and the probabilities in (4.7). These give a mean of $0 \times (1 - \theta) + 2 \times \theta = 2\theta$ for the number of broken eggs under Method 2. Thus the mean number of broken eggs is the same under both methods. This did not arise because the binomial distribution applies for both methods, since it does not apply for Method 2. The means just happen to be the same for both methods. So the expression "don't put all your eggs into one basket" does not relate to the mean number of broken eggs. We will see in the next section where it comes from.

*Notes Concerning the Mean of a Discrete Random Variable*

(i) The expression "the mean of the probability distribution of a discrete random variable" is often used instead of "the mean of a discrete random variable". These expressions are equivalent: sometimes it is more natural or convenient to use one expression and at other times it is more natural or convenient to use the other expression.

(ii) The Greek letter "mu", $\mu$, is always used for a mean in this book and is a reserved notation: in Statistics and probability theory, the symbol $\mu$ rarely, if ever, denotes anything other than a mean.

(iii) In many practical situations the mean $\mu$ of a discrete random variable $X$ is unknown to us because we do not know the numerical values of the probabilities of the possible values of the random variable involved. That is to say $\mu$ is often a parameter, and this is why we use Greek notation for it. As an example, if in the binomial distribution case we do not know the numerical value of the parameter $\theta$, then we do not know the numerical value of the mean $\mu \, (= n\theta)$ of that distribution.

(iv) The mean of a probability distribution is its center of gravity, its "knife-edge balance point". This implies that if a probability distribution is symmetric about some point, that point is the mean of the corresponding random variable.

(v) Estimating the numerical value of a mean and testing hypotheses about the numerical value of a mean are perhaps the most important of statistical operations. Different $t$ tests, to be discussed later in this book, provide important and frequently used examples of tests of hypotheses about means.

(vi) The word "average" is *not* an alternative for the word "mean", and has a quite different interpretation from that of "mean". This distinction will be discussed often in this book.

## 4.8   The Variance of a Discrete Random Variable

A quantity of importance equal to that of the mean of a random variable is its *variance*. The variance (always denoted by $\sigma^2$, where $\sigma$ is the Greek letter "sigma") of the discrete random variable $X$ whose probability distribution is given in (4.1) is defined by

$$\sigma^2 = (v_1 - \mu)^2 \text{Prob}(v_1) + (v_2 - \mu)^2 \text{Prob}(v_2) + \ldots + (v_k - \mu)^2 \text{Prob}(v_k). \quad (4.30)$$

In a more mathematical notation, we write this as

$$\sigma^2 = \sum_{i=1}^{k} (v_i - \mu)^2 \text{Prob}(v_i), \quad (4.31)$$

the summation being taken over all possible values of the random variable $X$. We call the expression (4.30), or equivalently the expression (4.31), the long formula for the variance of the random variable $X$.

*Example 4.8.1 (Fair Die)*  In the case of a fair die, we have already calculated (in (4.22)) the mean of the random variable $X$, the random number to turn up on a roll of the die, to be 3.5. Application of (4.30) shows that the variance $\sigma^2$ of $X$ is

$$(1 - 3.5)^2 \times \frac{1}{6} + (2 - 3.5)^2 \times \frac{1}{6} + (3 - 3.5)^2 \times \frac{1}{6} + (4 - 3.5)^2$$

$$\times \frac{1}{6} + (5 - 3.5)^2 \times \frac{1}{6} + (6 - 3.5)^2 \times \frac{1}{6} = \frac{35}{12}. \quad (4.32)$$

As we saw with the mean, the long formula for the variance always gives the correct answer. However, in some cases the calculation simplifies to a short formula.

*Example 4.8.2 (Binomial)*  As an important example, for the binomial distribution (4.5), the long formula (4.30) can be shown, after some algebra, to simplify to $n\theta(1 - \theta)$. This is so important that we display it explicitly: if $X$ has a binomial distribution with index $n$, parameter $\theta$, then

$$\text{variance of the binomial random variable } X = n\theta(1 - \theta). \quad (4.33)$$

This short formula is used frequently in Statistics. This short formula applies *only* for the binomial distribution.

The variance of a Bernoulli random variable $X$ with parameter $\theta$ can be found from (4.31) to be $(0 - \theta)^2(1 - \theta) + (1 - \theta)^2\theta = \theta(1 - \theta)$, and this agrees with the value found from (4.33) upon setting $n = 1$.

*Example 4.8.3 (Hypergeometric)*  Another important case for which we do have a short formula is the variance for a hypergeometric random variable. With some algebra it can be shown from Eq. (4.9) that the variance of the hypergeometric random variable $X$ defined in Sect. 4.6 is as given in Eq. (4.34) below:

$$\text{variance of the hypergeometric random variable } X = \frac{dr(n-r)(n-d)}{n^2(n-1)}.$$

$$(4.34)$$

It is interesting to consider the relation of this variance to the value that would be obtained if sampling were done *with* replacement, that is, if once a marble were drawn from the urn and its color noted, the marble were replaced in the urn before the next draw. In this case, all the requirements for the binomial distribution apply, and the probability that a red marble appears on any draw is $\frac{r}{n}$. The binomial distribution formulas show that the variance of the number of red marbles drawn is $\frac{dr(n-r)}{n^2}$. The variances of the number of red marbles drawn differ by the multiplicative factor $\frac{n-d}{n-1}$, and it is instructive to consider the effects of this factor.

When $d = 1$, the two variance formulas are identical, and this is so since if only one marble is drawn from the urn, the replacement policy is immaterial. In all other situations, the variance in the hypergeometric case is less than that in the binomial case, indicating a higher level of predictability for the number of red marbles drawn when sampling is without replacement compared to the case when sampling is with replacement. In the extreme case, if $d = n$, so that all the marbles are drawn from the urn, the variance of the number of red marbles drawn in the hypergeometric case is zero, and this is so since in this case the number of red marbles drawn, namely $r$, is completely predictable.

*Notes on the Variance of a Discrete Random Variable*

(i) The expression "the variance of the probability distribution of a discrete random variable" is often used instead of "the variance of a discrete random variable". These expressions are equivalent: sometimes it is more natural or convenient to use one expression and at other times it is more natural or convenient to use the other expression.

(ii) The variance has the standard notation $\sigma^2$, as anticipated above. The notation $\sigma^2$ is a reserved notation for a variance, and the symbol $\sigma^2$ is rarely, if ever, used for anything other than a variance in Statistics and probability theory.

(iii) A quantity that is often more useful than the variance of a probability distribution is the *standard deviation*. This is defined as the positive square root of the variance, and (naturally enough) is denoted by $\sigma$. It must be calculated by first calculating the variance.

(iv) The variance, like the mean, is often unknown to us. This is why we denote it by a Greek letter.

(v) A formula equivalent to (4.30) is

$$\sigma^2 = v_1^2 \text{Prob}(v_1) + v_2^2 \text{Prob}(v_2) + \ldots + v_k^2 \text{Prob}(v_k) - \mu^2.$$

$$(4.35)$$

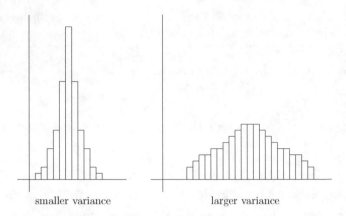

smaller variance                                larger variance

**Fig. 4.2** A comparison of two variances

In more mathematical terms this alternative formula is

$$\sigma^2 = \sum_{i=1}^{k} v_i^2 \text{Prob}(v_i) - \mu^2, \tag{4.36}$$

the summation being taken over all possible values of the random variable $X$. This alternative formula often leads to easier computations than does the formula in (4.30).

As an example of the use of this alternative variance formula, the variance of a binomial random variable with index 2 and parameter $\theta$ is

$$0^2 \times (1 - \theta)^2 + 1^2 \times 2\theta(1 - \theta) + 2^2 \times \theta^2 - (2\theta)^2 = 2\theta(1 - \theta), \tag{4.37}$$

and this agrees with (4.33) for the case $n = 2$.

(vi) The variance is a measure of the dispersion of the probability distribution of the random variable around its mean—see Fig. 4.2. A random variable with a small variance is likely to take a value close to its mean. The value taken by a random variable with a large variance is less predictable.

The "eggs" example discussed in the previous two sections provides an interesting comparison of two variances. It was shown above that the mean number of broken eggs is the same under both Method 1 and Method 2. Under Method 1, the number of broken eggs has a binomial distribution and, as shown in Eq. (4.37), has variance $2\theta(1 - \theta)$. There is no short formula for the variance of the number of broken eggs under Method 2 and we have to use the tableau (4.7) and the long formula (4.35). These give the value

$$0^2 \times (1 - \theta) + 2^2 \times \theta - (2\theta)^2 = 4\theta - 4\theta^2 = 4\theta(1 - \theta)$$

for the variance of the number of broken eggs under Method 2. This variance is twice that for the number of broken eggs under Method 1. Thus the expression "don't put all your eggs into one basket" is motivated by the **variance** of the number of broken eggs and not by the **mean** number of broken eggs. The number of broken eggs is less predictable under Method 2 than under Method 1, and this is apparently why we are advised not to put all our eggs in one basket.

A flow-chart of the "means and variances" part of this book is given below to show the various topics covered in perspective. Note that proportions and their relevant formulas have not been covered yet and will be covered in Sect. 5.6.

## Flowchart: Means and Variances of a Single Random Variable, $X$ or $P$

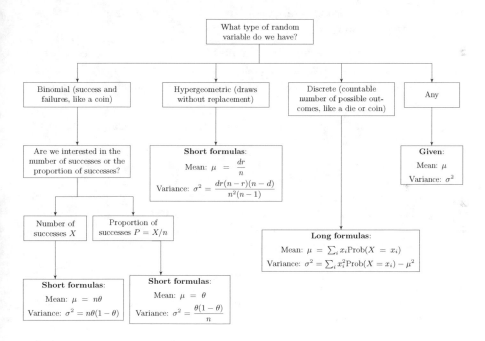

## 4.9   Problems

**4.1** Suppose that a fair die is to be rolled twice. In Problem 3.5, you found the probabilities that the sum of the two numbers to appear will be (a) 2, (b) 3, (c) 4. Now extend the reasoning that you used in that problem to find the probabilities that this sum takes the respective values $5, 6, \ldots, 12$. Then write down in tableau form the probability that the sum of the two numbers, which we denote $T_2$, is (a) 2, (b) 3, ..., (k) 12.

Note. Present all your probability calculations in this problem in *exact* form, that is, in the form $a/b$, where $a$ and $b$ are integers, with no rounding or approximations involved in your calculations. Also, use the *same* value of the denominator $b$, namely 36, for *all* the probabilities that you calculate. (This helps with later calculations.) (For example, write the probability that $T_2 = 3$ as $\frac{2}{36}$ and the probability that $T_2 = 4$ as $\frac{3}{36}$.)

**4.2 (Continuation from Problem 4.1)** We define the (random variable) average ($\bar{X}$) of the two numbers to turn up on the two rolls as $\bar{X} = T_2/2$. Use your answer to Problem 4.1 to write down in tableau form the probability distribution of $\bar{X}$. That is, write down all possible values of $\bar{X}$ and their associated probabilities.

Hint. The probabilities can be found quickly from the probabilities for $T_2$ by noting, for example, that if $T_2 = 7$, then $\bar{X} = \frac{7}{2}$. Thus Prob($\bar{X} = \frac{7}{2}$) = Prob($T_2 = 7$).

**4.3** Write down the probability distribution in tableau form for the number of heads that appear in two coin flips where the probability of a head is 0.4.

**4.4** A coin is to be flipped five times. Write down all possible orders in which exactly three heads arise. Then calculate 5!, 3! and 2! and then from these calculate $\binom{5}{3}$. Check that you get the same number of orders as you found by considering all possibilities.

**4.5** Use the formula $\binom{n}{x}$ or R to find the number of orders of getting three heads from seven flips of a coin.

**4.6** A fair coin is to be flipped seven times. We assume that the results of the various flips are independent of each other. What is the probability of getting three heads and four tails in the specific order HHHTTTT? What is the probability of getting three heads and four tails in the specific order HTHTTHT? What is the probability of getting three heads and four tails in the specific order THHTTHT? Use your answers and your answer to Problem 4.5 to find the probability of getting three heads in seven flips of a fair coin.

**4.7** Suppose that in the binomial distribution, $n = 2$, $\theta > 0$, and the probability of exactly two successes is the same as the probability of exactly one success. What is the value of $\theta$?

**4.8** The definition of $\binom{n}{x}$ as a number of orders is not the original one. The original derivation of the word "choose" is that $\binom{n}{x}$ is the number of ways of choosing a committee of $x$ people from a group of $n$ people. (Although these two definitions of $\binom{n}{x}$ might at first appear to be unrelated, we will see that they are equivalent.) This question and the following one relate to the "choosing" definition.

Given a group of four people, namely A (= Ashley), B (= Bobbi), C (= Corina), D (= Daniel), the calculation of $\binom{4}{2} = 6$ shows that there are six committees of size 2 that can be formed from these four people. Write down what all of these six committees are. (For example, one committee is AC.)

**4.9** Given the group of seven people, namely A (= Anusha), B (= Brian), C (= Chuyun), D (= Dylan, E (= Esha), F (= Fatima) and G (= Giselle), write down all possible committees of three people from this group of seven people. (For example, one possible committee is ADF). Check that the total number of possible committees is the same as the number that you calculated in Problem 4.5.

**4.10** The definition of $\binom{n}{x}$ shows that $\binom{n}{x}$ is equal to $\binom{n}{n-x}$. Thinking of the choice of $x$ people from a group of $n$ people, can you explain why $\binom{n}{x}$ is equal to $\binom{n}{n-x}$ without using any mathematics?

**4.11** Use the binomial chart to find the probability that $X = 7$ where $X$ has a binomial distribution with $n = 12$ and $\theta = 0.7$. Check your answer using the binomial distribution formula (4.5).

**4.12** The random variable $X$ has a binomial distribution with index $n = 10$ and parameter $\theta = 0.4$. Use R, the binomial chart, or the binomial probability formula (4.5) to find (a) the probability that $X = 5$, (b) the probability that $X$ is either 3, 4, 5 or 6, (c) the probability that $X$ is 5 or fewer.

**4.13** You plan to flip a coin (probability of head $\theta = 0.4$ on each flip) three times in the morning and also three times in the afternoon. You are interested in the probability of the event $A$, that in the entire day you get exactly four heads. This probability can be calculated in two ways:

Method 1. The event $A$ can occur in three mutually exclusive ways, one head in the morning and three in the afternoon, two heads in the morning and two heads in the afternoon, or three heads in the morning and one in the afternoon. Calculate the probabilities of $x$ heads from three flips for various relevant values of $x$, from this calculate the probabilities of each of these three mutually exclusive events, and by addition calculate the probability of the event $A$.

Method 2. Think of the morning and afternoon flips together as comprising six flips of the coin, and then directly calculate the probability of getting exactly four heads.

Calculate the probability of exactly four heads by both methods and check that your answers agree. Note: To check that both methods give exactly the same probability, do not use the binomial chart, which is accurate only to four decimal places, but use exact calculations without any rounding.

**4.14** With reference to Problem 4.13, suppose now that you plan to flip a coin (probability of head $\theta_1 = 0.4$ on each flip) three times in the morning and a different coin (probability of head $\theta_2 = 0.6$ on each flip) three times in the afternoon. Can the calculation of the probability of getting four heads in total be done by Method 1? Can it be done by Method 2? (Do not do any calculations. Just say "yes" or "no" to each question and give the reason for your answer.)

**4.15** Find the mean of the random variable described by the following probability tableau:

| Possible values | 1 | 2 | 3 | 4 | 5 | 6 |
|---|---|---|---|---|---|---|
| Probabilities | 0.1 | 0.3 | 0.1 | 0.4 | 0.05 | 0.05 |

**4.16** Find the variance of the random variable having the probability distribution given in Problem 4.15.

**4.17**

(a) Use binomial probabilities as given in the binomial distribution chart, or from R, together with the long formula for the mean of a random variable (4.19) to compute the mean of a random variable having a binomial distribution with index 3 and parameter 0.5.
(b) The short formula for the mean of a binomial random variable with index $n$ and parameter $\theta$ is $n\theta$. Use this formula to compute the mean of a random variable having a binomial distribution with index 3 and parameter 0.5.
(c) Check that answers to part (a) and part (b) of this problem agree.

**4.18**

(a) Use the alternative long formula for the variance of a random variable (4.35), together with probability values given in the binomial distribution chart, to compute the variance of a random variable having a binomial distribution with index 3 and parameter 0.5.
(b) The short formula for the variance of a random variable having a binomial distribution with index $n$ and parameter $\theta$ is $n\theta(1 - \theta)$. Use this formula to compute the variance of a random variable having a binomial distribution with index 3 and parameter 0.5. Does your answer agree with that found in part (a) of this question?

**4.19 (This Question Involves Algebra, Not Numerical Calculation. Your Answer Will Be a Function of $\theta$)** This question refers to the case of $n = 2$ binomial trials, where the probability of success on each trial is $\theta$. Use the long formula for the mean of a random variable, together with the probabilities (4.3) for the probabilities of 0, 1 and 2 successes, to show that the mean number of successes is identical to that given by the short formula value, namely $2\theta$.

**4.20** The medicine that we are currently using to cure some illness cures a patient with probability 0.9. We plan a clinical trial testing a proposed new medicine, in which we will give this proposed new medicine to 5000 people. The number $X$ of people who will be cured in the clinical trial is a random variable which we assume has a binomial distribution. If the new medicine has the same cure probability (0.9) as the current one, what is the mean of $X$? What is the variance of $X$?

**4.21**

(a) An urn contains five red marbles and six blue marbles. Four marbles are to be drawn from the urn at random and without replacement. Let $X$ be the (random) number of red marbles drawn from the urn. Find the support of $X$.

(b) Using the hypergeometric probability formula (4.9) or R, find the probability of every possible value of $X$ in its support. (Note: calculate these probabilities *exactly*, that is in the form $a/b$, where $a$ and $b$ are whole numbers. It is convenient to use a common denominator $b$ for all the calculations.) Check that these probabilities sum exactly to 1.

(c) Now find the mean and variance of $X$ using the long formulas (4.19) and (4.30) respectively, and check that these agree with the values given by the short formulas in (4.29) and (4.34).

**4.22**

(a) An urn contains five red marbles and three blue marbles. Four marbles are to be drawn from the urn at random and without replacement. Let $X$ be the (random) number of red marbles drawn from the urn. Find the support of $X$.

(b) Using the hypergeometric probability formula (4.9) or R, find the probability of every possible value of $X$ in its support. Check that these probabilities sum exactly to 1.

(c) Now find the mean and variance of $X$ using the long formulas (4.19) and (4.30) respectively, and check that these agree with the values given by the short formulas in (4.29) and (4.34).

**4.23** Suppose that in the urns example $d = n - 1$. (That is, all but one of the marbles are taken out of the urn.) Find the (two) possible values of $X$, the number of red marbles taken from the urn. Then find the mean and variance of $X$ using the long formulas for a mean and a variance, and check that the values that you obtain agree with those found from Eqs. (4.29) and (4.29).

**4.24** This problem is a variant of the lottery example in Sect. 4.6. Suppose that a contestant selects six numbers from the set $\{1, 2, \ldots, 40\}$ and wins the lottery if all six numbers chosen are the winning numbers.

(a) What is the probability that the contestant wins the lottery?

(b) Suppose that the contestant wins the lottery if she chooses at least five of the six winning numbers. What is the probability that the contestant wins the lottery?

# Chapter 5
# Many Random Variables

## 5.1 Introduction

Almost every application of statistical methods requires the analysis of many observations, that is many data values. For example, if a psychologist plans an experiment to assess the effects of sleep deprivation on the time needed to answer the questions in a questionnaire, she would want to test a reasonably large number of people in order to get reliable results. Before this experiment is performed, the various times that the people in the experiment will need to answer the questions are all random variables.

This introduces the concept of the "sample size". If the psychologist tested 100 people in the sleep deprivation example, we say that the sample size is 100. Different sample sizes arise in different experiments, and in this book we will always denote a sample size by $n$ (or, if there are two samples, by $m$ for one sample and $n$ for the other sample).

In line with the approach in this book, the theory given below for many random variables will often be discussed in terms of simple examples, for instance the rolling of a die, but now with many rolls of the die and not just one. The number of times that the die is to be rolled is therefore denoted by $n$.

The die example illustrates an important point, namely the distinction between $n$ and $k$. As just described, $n$ is the sample size: in the die case, it is the number of times that we plan to roll the die. By contrast, the notation $k$ used earlier is the number of possible values for the discrete random variable of interest. In the die case, $k = 6$: there are six possible numbers that could turn up on any one roll of the die. The number 6 is fixed by the six-sided nature of the die. By contrast, the number $n$ of times that the die is rolled is at the choice of the experimenter.

© The Author(s), under exclusive license to Springer Nature Switzerland AG 2023
W. J. Ewens, K. Brumberg, *Introductory Statistics for Data Analysis*,
https://doi.org/10.1007/978-3-031-28189-1_5

## 5.2  Notation

Since we are now considering many random variables, the notation "$X$" for one single random variable is no longer sufficient. We therefore denote the first random variable by $X_1$, the second by $X_2$, and so on. As an example, suppose as above that we plan to roll the die $n = 1000$ times. We would then denote the (random) number that will turn up on the first roll of the die by $X_1$, the (random) number that will turn up on the second roll of the die by $X_2$, ..., the (random) number that will turn up on roll 1000 of the die by $X_{1000}$.

Correspondingly, we need a separate notation for the actual observed numbers that did turn up once the die was rolled $n$ times. We denote these by $x_1, x_2, \ldots, x_n$. Thus it makes sense to say, after the die was rolled $n$ times, that "$x_{68} = 4$", meaning that on the 68th roll of the die, a 4 turned up. It does not make sense to say "$X_{68} = 4$": this statement "does not compute". Before we roll the die, or if we think about such a time, we do not know what number will turn up on the 68th roll of the die. This number is a random variable.

To assess whether we can reasonably assume that the die is fair, we will not only use the data values $x_1, x_2, \ldots, x_n$, but also the probability theory relating to the $n$ random variables $X_1, X_2, \ldots, X_n$. This is why both concepts, the concept of data and the concept of random variables, are necessary, and also why it is necessary to distinguish between them. The relationship between them will be discussed extensively in this book.

Similarly, in the sleep deprivation experiment of Sect. 5.1, it makes sense after the experiment is completed to say $x_{21} = 18$. This means that it took the twenty-first person in the sample 18 min to do the test. It does not make sense to say "$X_{21} = 18$": this statement "does not compute". Before we do the experiment, we do not know how long it will take the twenty-first person to do the test. That length of time, before the experiment, is a random variable.

It is important to distinguish between $X_1$ and $v_1$, and also between $x_1$ and $v_1$. $X_1$ is a random variable: in the die example, it is the random number that will turn up on the first roll of the die. It is a concept of our mind referring to the time before the die is rolled. $v_1$ is the smallest possible value that the random variable can take: in the case of a die, this is $v_1 = 1$. Finally, $x_1$ is the number that turns up on the first roll of the die once that roll has occurred. If, for example, the number 4 did turn up on the first roll of the die, then $x_1 = 4$.

## 5.3  Independently and Identically Distributed Random Variables

The die example introduces two important concepts. First, we would reasonably assume that the random variables $X_1, X_2, \ldots, X_n$, the numbers that will turn up on the $n$ rolls of the die, all have the same probability distribution, since it is the same die that is being rolled each time. For example, we would reasonably assume that the probability that 3 will turn up on roll 77, whatever it might be, is the same as the probability that 3 will turn up on roll 144. Second, we would also reasonably assume that the various random variables $X_1, X_2, \ldots, X_n$ are all independent of each other. That is, we would reasonably assume that the value of any one of these would not affect the value of any other one. For example, we reasonably believe that whatever number that will turn up on roll 77 has no influence on the number that will turn up on roll 144.

Random variables which are independent of each other, and which all have the same probability distribution, are said to be *iid* (independently and identically distributed). The *iid* concept is often discussed and used in this book.

The assumptions that the various random variables $X_1, X_2, \ldots, X_n$ are all independent of each other, and that they all have the same probability distribution, are often made in the application of statistical methods. However, in areas such as psychology, medicine and biology that are obviously more scientifically important and complex than rolling a die, the assumption of identically and independently distributed random variables might not be reasonable. Thus if twin sisters were used in the sleep deprivation example, the times that they take to complete the questionnaire might not be independent, since we might expect them to be quite similar because of the common environment and genetic make-up of the twins. If the people in the experiment were not all of the same age, it might not be reasonable to assume that the times needed are identically distributed—people of different ages might tend to need different amounts of time to do the test. Thus, in practice, care must often be exercised and common sense used when applying the theory of *iid* random variables, and the *iid* assumption might not be easy to justify.

Another practical consideration is that the people involved in experiments such as the sleep deprivation example must be volunteers who are made aware in advance of the full details of the experiment and then are still willing to be involved in the experiment. This is an ethical concern. In this book we focus on theory, but we do not underestimate the importance of ethical and other practical concerns.

## 5.4 The Mean and Variance of a Sum and of an Average

Given $n$ random variables $X_1, X_2, \ldots, X_n$, two very important *derived* random variables are their sum, or total, denoted by $T$, defined by

$$T = X_1 + X_2 + \cdots + X_n,\tag{5.1}$$

and their average, denoted by $\bar{X}$, defined by

$$\bar{X} = \frac{X_1 + X_2 + \cdots + X_n}{n} = \frac{T}{n}.\tag{5.2}$$

Since both $T$ and $\bar{X}$ are functions of the random variables $X_1, X_2, \ldots, X_n$, they are themselves *random variables*. For example, in the die-rolling case, we do not know, before we roll the die, what the sum or the average of the $n$ numbers that will turn up will be. This is why we use upper-case letters for the sum and the average of random variables.

As a matter of notation, $T$ and $\bar{X}$ are often written as $T_n$ and $\bar{X}_n$ to emphasize that these are respectively the sum and the average of $n$ random variables. However, the notation $\bar{X}_n$ might be confused with the notation $X_n$ for the $n$th random variable, so we often simply use the notation $\bar{X}$ and $T$, using $T_n$ if the sample size $n$ is to be emphasized.

The probability distribution of a sum and an average can be quite complicated. For example, the probability distribution of the sum of the numbers to turn up on 100 rolls of a fair die is quite difficult to calculate. Despite this, the mean and variance of a sum and of an average of $iid$ random variables must be related in some way to the mean and the variance of each of $X_1, X_2, \ldots, X_n$. The general theory of many random variables shows that if $X_1, X_2, \ldots, X_n$ are $iid$, with common mean $\mu$ and common variance $\sigma^2$, then the mean and the variance of the random variable $T$ are, respectively,

$$\text{mean of } T = n\mu, \quad \text{variance of } T = n\sigma^2, \tag{5.3}$$

and the mean and the variance of the random variable $\bar{X}$ are, respectively,

$$\text{mean of } \bar{X} = \mu, \quad \text{variance of } \bar{X} = \frac{\sigma^2}{n}. \tag{5.4}$$

These are are important short formulas and we shall refer to them often.

It is crucial to remember that a mean and an average are two entirely different concepts. A mean is a parameter, that is, some constant number whose value is often unknown to us. For example, with an unfair die for which the respective probabilities Prob(1), ..., Prob(6) for the number to turn up on any roll are all unknown, the mean $\mu$ of the number to turn up, namely $1 \times$ Prob(1) $+ \cdots + 6 \times$ Prob(6), is unknown. It is a parameter.

By contrast, the average $\bar{X}$ as defined above is a random variable. It is a "before we do our experiment and get our data" concept. It has a probability distribution and thus has a mean and a variance, as illustrated in (5.4) for the $iid$ case. Thus in the case of rolling a fair die, it makes sense to replace Eq. (5.4) by the statement "the mean of the average of the numbers to turn up on $n$ rolls of a fair die is 3.5". If we conflated the meanings of the words "mean" and "average", this statement would make no sense.

There is also a second concept of an average, and this is now exemplified in the die-rolling example. This is the actual average $\bar{x}$ of the numbers that actually turned up once the $n$ rolls were completed. This is a number that can be calculated from the numbers that did turn up, for example 3.38. This can be thought of as the realized value of the random variable $\bar{X}$ once the experiment of rolling the die $n$ times has taken place. Thus the statement "$\bar{x} = 3.38$" makes sense, but the statement "$\bar{X} = 3.38$" does not: it "does not compute". We discuss $\bar{x}$ extensively in the Statistics part of this book.

Thus there are three related concepts: first a mean (a parameter), second a "before the experiment" average $\bar{X}$ (a random variable, and a concept of probability theory), and third an "after the experiment" average $\bar{x}$ (a number calculated from data, and a concept of Statistics). They are all important and must not be confused with each other. Thus it is *never* correct to say things like: $\bar{x} = \mu$, $\bar{X} = \mu$ or $\bar{x} = \bar{X}$. These statements "do not compute".

Why do we need all three concepts? Suppose that we wish to estimate a mean $\mu$ (the first concept). Given our data after we have done our experiment, we would perhaps naturally estimate $\mu$ by $\bar{x}$ (the third concept). How precise $\bar{x}$ is as an estimate of $\mu$ depends on the properties of the random variable $\bar{X}$ (the second concept), in particular its mean and variance. This is one of the reasons why we have to spend time considering the properties of a random variable, in particular its mean and variance.

*Example* Suppose that we plan to roll a fair die 1000 times. Define $X_1$ as the (random) number that will turn up on roll $1, \ldots, X_{1000}$ as the (random) number that will turn up on roll 1000. We know that each $X_i$ has mean 3.5 and variance 35/12, as given by (4.24) and (4.32), and thus the standard deviation of each $X$ is $\sqrt{(35/12)}$, or about 1.708. The second equation in (5.4) then shows us that if the die is to be rolled 1000 times, the variance of $\bar{X}$ is 35/12,000, so that the standard deviation of $\bar{X}$ is $\sqrt{(35/12,000)}$, or approximately 0.0540. This small standard deviation implies that once we roll the die 1000 times, it is very likely that the observed average $\bar{x}$ of the numbers that actually turned up will be very close to 3.5.

More specifically, we will see later that if the die is fair, the probability that the observed average $\bar{x}$ will be between 3.392 and 3.608 is about 0.95. This statement is one of probability theory. It is an implication, or deduction. As shown later, it is derived from the mean 3.5 and the standard deviation $\sqrt{35/12,000}$ of the random variable $\bar{X}$. It could not be made without these random variable concepts.

Although it is premature to discuss Statistics now, the following is an example of a statistical induction, or inference, corresponding to the calculations in the previous paragraph. We have now rolled the die 1000 times, and the observed average $\bar{x}$ of the 1000 numbers that turned up was 3.324. This is outside the interval 3.392 to 3.608 calculated above, and is thus unlikely to arise if the die is fair. Therefore we have good evidence that the die is not fair. This claim is an act of Statistics. It is an inference, or induction. More importantly, it could not have been made without the probability theory calculation given above.

We will later make many statistical inferences, each of which will be based, as is the one given above, on whatever is the relevant corresponding probability theory calculation corresponding to some random variable.

Equation (5.4) implies that the standard deviation of the random variable $\bar{X}$ is $\sigma/\sqrt{n}$. The standard deviation of an average is sometimes called "the standard error of the mean". This terminology can be confusing. To be pedantic, it should be "the standard deviation of the random variable average $\bar{X}$". However, many textbooks, research papers, and statistical packages use this terminology.

## 5.5  The Mean and the Variance of a Difference

In the particular case $n = 2$, two further equations are important. If $X_1$ and $X_2$ are $iid$ random variables, each having mean $\mu$ and variance $\sigma^2$, and we define the random variable $D$ by $D = X_1 - X_2$ (think of $D$ standing for "difference") then

$$\text{mean of } D = 0, \quad \text{variance of } D = 2\sigma^2. \tag{5.5}$$

These are also short formulas and we shall refer to them several times, especially when making comparison studies. Statistical procedures often address questions like: "given our data, do we have significant evidence of a difference between the mean blood pressure for men and the mean blood pressure for women?" Formulas like (5.5) are useful in addressing questions like this.

There are two important generalizations of the formulas in (5.5) to the case where $X_1$ and $X_2$ are independent random variables but not identically distributed random variables. Suppose that $X_1$ and $X_2$ have respective means $\mu_1$ and $\mu_2$ and respective variances $\sigma_1^2$ and $\sigma_2^2$. Then

$$\text{mean of } D = \mu_1 - \mu_2, \quad \text{variance of } D = \sigma_1^2 + \sigma_2^2. \tag{5.6}$$

These two short formulas are used often in Statistics. The formulas in (5.5) are special cases of these formulas.

As we shall see later in the Statistics part of the book, we are often interested in the difference between two averages. Let $X_{11}, X_{12}, \ldots, X_{1n}$ be $n$ $iid$ random variables, each with mean $\mu_1$ and variance $\sigma_1^2$, and let $X_{21}, X_{22}, \ldots, X_{2m}$ be $m$ $iid$ random variables, each with mean $\mu_2$ and variance $\sigma_2^2$. We assume also that each $X_{1i}, i = 1, 2, \ldots n$ is independent of each $X_{2j}, j = 1, 2, \ldots, m$. Define $\bar{X}_1$ and $\bar{X}_2$ by

$$\bar{X}_1 = \frac{X_{11} + X_{12} + \cdots + X_{1n}}{n}, \qquad \bar{X}_2 = \frac{X_{21} + X_{22} + \cdots + X_{2m}}{m}.$$

Then

$$\text{mean  of } \bar{X}_1 - \bar{X}_2 = \mu_1 - \mu_2, \quad \text{variance  of } \bar{X}_1 - \bar{X}_2 = \frac{\sigma_1^2}{n} + \frac{\sigma_2^2}{m}. \tag{5.7}$$

## 5.6   The Proportion of Successes in $n$ Binomial Trials

The random variable in the binomial distribution is the *number* of successes in $n$ binomial trials, with probability distribution given in (4.5). In some applications, it is necessary to consider instead the *proportion* of successes in these trials (more exactly, the proportion of trials leading to success). Here is an example which shows why a consideration of proportions is necessary.

Suppose that we wish to test whether the probability that a middle-schooler gets less than the recommended amount of sleep for their age is equal to that of a high-schooler. Suppose that to test this, we get the following data:

|                   | sleep-deprived | well-rested | total |
|-------------------|:--------------:|:-----------:|:-----:|
| middle-schoolers  | 173            | 127         | 300   |
| high-schoolers    | 135            | 65          | 200   |
| total             | 308            | 192         | 500   |

It makes no sense to compare the numbers 173 and 135 since the number of middle-schoolers in the sample differs from the number of high-schoolers in the sample. However, it does make sense to compare the proportions 173/300 and 135/200. Because of this, the procedure for testing whether there is a difference between middle and high-schoolers getting enough sleep has to be carried out using proportions. We now establish some of the relevant background probability theory for proportions.

If $X$ is the (random) number of successes to occur in $n$ binomial trials, then the proportion of successes is $X/n$, which we denote by $P$. Since $X$ is a discrete random variable, $P$ is also a discrete random variable, and its possible values can be found directly from the possible values of $X$, and are $0, \frac{1}{n}, \frac{2}{n}, ..., \frac{(n-1)}{n}, 1$.

The random variable $P$ has a probability distribution which can be found from the binomial distribution (4.5), since for any value of $x$ the probability that the observed proportion of successes is $p = x/n$ is the same as the probability that the observed number of successes is $x$. That is, from (4.5), the probability distribution of $P$ is given by

$$\text{Prob}\,(P = p) = \binom{n}{np} \theta^{np}(1-\theta)^{n(1-p)}, \quad p = 0, \frac{1}{n}, \frac{2}{n}, ..., 1. \tag{5.8}$$

Because $P$ is a random variable, it has a mean and variance. These can be found from Eq. (5.8), and are found after some algebra to be

$$\text{mean of } P = \theta, \quad \text{variance of } P = \theta(1-\theta)/n. \tag{5.9}$$

These equations bear a similarity to the formulas for the mean and variance of an average given in (5.4). They are important short formulas.

A special case of (5.6) is the following. Let $P_1$ be the proportion of successes in $n$ binomial trials where the probability of success on each trial is $\theta_1$, and $P_2$ be the proportion of successes in $m$ different binomial trials where the probability of success on each trial is $\theta_2$. $P_1$ and $P_2$ are independent of each other, and if $D$ is defined as $D = P_1 - P_2$,

$$\text{mean of } D = \theta_1 - \theta_2, \quad \text{variance of } D = \frac{\theta_1(1 - \theta_1)}{n} + \frac{\theta_2(1 - \theta_2)}{m}. \tag{5.10}$$

In the important particular cases where $\theta_1 = \theta_2 = \theta$, Eq. (5.10) become

$$\text{mean of } D = 0, \quad \text{variance of } D = \frac{\theta(1 - \theta)}{n} + \frac{\theta(1 - \theta)}{m} = \frac{n + m}{nm}\theta(1 - \theta). \tag{5.11}$$

As the example and the data values above indicate, when testing for the equality of two binomial parameters, it is often necessary in Statistics to operate via the *proportion of trials* giving success rather than by the *number* of trials giving success. It will also be necessary to consider the difference between these two proportions. In this testing procedure the formulas in (5.10) and (5.11) will be important.

A flow-chart of the "sums, averages and differences" part of the book is given below to show the various topics covered in perspective.

## Flowchart: Sums, Averages, and Differences of Random Variables

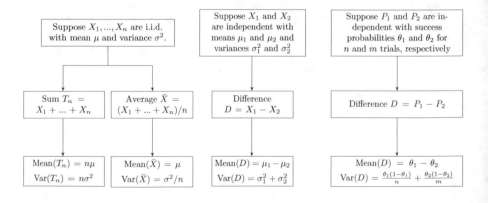

## 5.7 Problems

Note. It is important that you present all your probability calculations in *exact* form, that is, in the form $a/b$, where $a$ and $b$ are integers (i.e. whole numbers), with no rounding or approximations involved in your calculations. In particular, it is important that you do **not** present your probability answers in decimal form such as $0.wxyz$. Using decimals usually involves rounding or an approximation, and it is essential in these questions that all the probability calculations be exact. Also, in your probability calculations, it is convenient to use the *same* value of the denominator $b$ for **all** the probabilities that you calculate in any given question. (The value of $b$ might be different in different questions.)

**5.1**

(a) In Problem 4.1, the probability distribution of $T_2$ $(= X_1 + X_2)$, the sum of the two numbers to turn up on two rolls of a fair die, was found in "tableau" form. From the answer to that problem, use the relevant long formulas (4.19) and (4.30) or (4.35) to find (i) the mean and (ii) the variance of $T_2$.

(b) Can you find an interesting relation between the mean of $T_2$ and the mean of $X_1$? Can you find an interesting relation between the variance of $T_2$ and the variance of $X_1$?

**5.2**

(a) In Problem 4.2, the probability distribution of $\bar{X} = \frac{1}{2}(X_1 + X_2)$ was found in "tableau" form. From the answer to that problem, use the relevant long formulas (4.19) and (4.30) or (4.35) to find (i) the mean and (ii) the variance of $\bar{X}$. (Hint: For finding the variance of $\bar{X}$ it is convenient to use the "alternative" variance formula (4.35).)

(b) Can you find an interesting relation between the mean of $\bar{X}$ and the mean of $X_1$? Can you find an interesting relation between the variance of $\bar{X}$ and the variance of $X_1$?

**5.3** The mean and variance of $X_1$, the random number to turn up on one roll of the die, are respectively given in (4.22) and (4.32). Use this mean and this variance, together with the relevant short formulas to:

(a) Find quickly the mean and variance of $T_2$ in Problem 5.1 above using formula (5.3). Do your answers agree with those that you found in Problem 5.1? Were they easier to calculate using the short formulas than they were in Problem 5.1?

(b) Find quickly the mean and variance of $\bar{X}$ in Problem 5.2 above using formula (5.4) in the notes. Do your answers agree with those that you found in Problem 5.2? Were they easier to calculate using the short formulas than they were in Problem 5.2?

**5.4** The answer to Problem 4.1 gives the probability distribution of $T_2$, the sum of the two numbers to turn up on two rolls of a fair die. The reasoning used to find this distribution can be extended to find the probability distribution of $T_4$, the sum of the four numbers to turn up on four rolls of a fair die. This probability distribution is given below.

| Possible values of $T_4$ | 4 | 5 | 6 | 7 | 8 | 9 | 10 | 11 | 12 | 13 | 14 |
|---|---|---|---|---|---|---|---|---|---|---|---|
| Probabilities | $\frac{1}{1296}$ | $\frac{4}{1296}$ | $\frac{10}{1296}$ | $\frac{20}{1296}$ | $\frac{35}{1296}$ | $\frac{56}{1296}$ | $\frac{80}{1296}$ | $\frac{104}{1296}$ | $\frac{125}{1296}$ | $\frac{140}{1296}$ | $\frac{146}{1296}$ |

| Possible values of $T_4$ | 15 | 16 | 17 | 18 | 19 | 20 | 21 | 22 | 23 | 24 |
|---|---|---|---|---|---|---|---|---|---|---|
| Probabilities | $\frac{140}{1296}$ | $\frac{125}{1296}$ | $\frac{104}{1296}$ | $\frac{80}{1296}$ | $\frac{56}{1296}$ | $\frac{35}{1296}$ | $\frac{20}{1296}$ | $\frac{10}{1296}$ | $\frac{4}{1296}$ | $\frac{1}{1296}$ |

Use the values in the tableau, together with the long formulas for a mean and a variance, to find the mean and variance of $T_4$. (Use Eq. (4.19) to calculate the mean of $T_4$, and use either (4.30) or (4.35), whichever you prefer, to calculate the variance of $T_4$.)

Note: Your answer for the mean should simplify to a whole number. Present your answer for the variance as a fraction, that is in the form $a/b$, where $a$ and $b$ are whole numbers (i.e. integers), not decimals. Simplify this fraction so that $b$ is as small as possible.

**5.5** The mean and variance of $X_1$, the random number to turn up on one roll of the die, are given in Eqs. (4.22) and (4.32). Use this mean and this variance, together with the relevant short formulas (5.3), to find quickly the mean and variance of $T_4$. Do your answers agree with those that you found in Problem 5.4? Were they easier to calculate using the short formulas than they were in 5.4?

**5.6**

(a) Use the tableau given in Problem 5.4 to write down (in tableau form) the probability distribution of $\bar{X}$, defined as $\bar{X} = \frac{T_4}{4}$.

   Hint. As an example, Prob($\bar{X} = \frac{11}{4}$) is the same as Prob($T_4 = 11$).

(b) Use the values in the tableau that you found in part (i) of this question, together with the long formulas for a mean and a variance, to find the mean and variance of $\bar{X}$. (Use Eq. (4.19) to calculate the mean, and use either (4.30) or (4.35), whichever you prefer, to calculate the variance of $\bar{X}$.)

(c) The mean and variance of $X_1$, the random number to turn up on one roll of the die, are given in Eqs. (4.22) and (4.32). Use this mean and this variance, together with the relevant short formulas (5.4) to find quickly the mean and variance of $\bar{X}$. Do your answers agree with those that you found in part (b) of this question? Were they easier to calculate using the short formulas than they were in part (b) of this question?

**5.7** A fair die is to be rolled 2000 times tomorrow. Define $T_{2000}$ as the sum of the 2000 numbers that will turn up tomorrow and $\bar{X}_{2000}$ as the average of the 2000 numbers that will turn up tomorrow. These are both random variables.

(a) Use Eq. (5.3) to find the mean and variance of $T_{2000}$.
(b) Use Eq. (5.4) to find the mean and variance of $\bar{X}_{2000}$.

**5.8** A fair die is to be rolled 4000 times tomorrow. Define $T_{4000}$ as the sum of the 4000 numbers that will turn up tomorrow and $\bar{X}_{4000}$ as the average of the 4000 numbers that turn up tomorrow. These are both random variables.

(a) Use Eq. (5.3) to find the mean and variance of $T_{4000}$.
(b) Use Eq. (5.4) to find the mean and variance of $\bar{X}_{4000}$.

**5.9** A fair die is to be rolled 6000 times tomorrow. Define $T_{6000}$ as the sum of the 6000 numbers that turn up tomorrow and $\bar{X}_{6000}$ as the average of the 6000 numbers that turn up tomorrow. These are both random variables.

(a) Use Eq. (5.3) to find the mean and variance of $T_{6000}$.
(b) Use Eq. (5.4) to find the mean and variance of $\bar{X}_{6000}$.

NOTE. This and the two previous problems make it clear that the expression "mean of an average" makes sense. In all three cases, the average of the numbers that will turn up tomorrow is a random variable. It therefore has a probability distribution and hence has a mean.

**5.10** Do the respective means of $\bar{X}_{2000}$, $\bar{X}_{4000}$ and $\bar{X}_{6000}$ in Problem 5.7, Problem 5.8 and Problem 5.9 "make sense"? Given the respective variances of $\bar{X}_{2000}$, $\bar{X}_{4000}$ and $\bar{X}_{6000}$ in Problems 5.7, 5.8 and 5.9, what can you say about the likely values of the sample averages $\bar{x}_{2000}$, $\bar{x}_{4000}$ and $\bar{x}_{6000}$ as the number of rolls increases from 2000 to 4000 to 6000?

**5.11**

(a) We plan to roll a fair die twice. Let $X_1$ be the number that will turn up on the first roll of the die and $X_2$ be the number that will turn up on the second roll of the die. We define $D$ by $D = X_1 - X_2$. Since both $X_1$ and $X_2$ are random variables, then $D$ is also a random variable, and some of the possible values of $D$ are negative.

Find and write down in "tableau" form the probability distribution $D$. That is, write down a table showing all the possible values of $D$, together with their associated probabilities.

Hint. This will involve some tedious work, using however nothing more than "common sense". For example, the number that will turn up on the first roll minus the number that will turn up on the second roll will equal $-2$ if and only if one of the four following mutually exclusive events occur:

  (i) the number that will turn up on the first roll is 1 and the number that will turn up on the second roll is 3 (probability 1/36),
 (ii) the number that will turn up on the first roll is 2 and the number that will turn up on the second roll is 4 (probability 1/36),
(iii) the number that will turn up on the first roll is 3 and the number that will turn up on the second roll is 5 (probability 1/36),
 (iv) the number that will turn up on the first roll is 4 and the number that will turn up on the second roll is 6 (probability 1/36).

Therefore Prob($D = -2$) = 4/36. Probabilities for other possible values of $D$ are found similarly.

Although the probability 4/36 found above simplifies to 1/9, it is best, for the purposes of part (b) of this question below, to leave this probability in the form 4/36 and to leave all other probabilities that you calculate in the form $a/36$, where $a$ is a whole number.

(b) Use your tableau and the relevant long formulas to find the mean and variance of $D$. Use (4.19) for the mean, and whichever of the two alternative long formulas (4.30) and (4.35) that you prefer, for the variance of $D$.

(c) Use the numerical values given in Eqs. (4.22) and (4.32) for the mean and variance of $X_1$ and of $X_2$, together with the short formulas (5.5), to find the mean and the variance of $D$. Do your values agree with the values that you found in part (b) of this question? Which calculations, using the long formulas or using the short formulas in Eq. (5.5), were the easier ones to use?

**5.12** Let $X$ be a random variable with mean 7 and variance 16. Let $Y$ be a random variable with 10 and variance 9. What is (i) the mean and (ii) variance of $D = X - Y$?

**5.13** Suppose that the blood pressure of a diabetic taken at random is a random variable with mean 125 and variance 25 (and thus standard deviation 5). Suppose also that the blood pressure of a non-diabetic taken at random is a random variable with mean 118 and variance 36 (and thus standard deviation 6). We are interested in investigating further the difference in blood pressure between diabetics and non-diabetics. For this purpose we plan to take a sample of 100 diabetics and 144 non-diabetics, calculate the average blood pressure of the diabetics in the sample and the average blood pressure of the non-diabetics in the sample and then calculate the difference between these two averages (diabetic average—non-diabetic average). Before we take this sample, this difference is a random variable, which we denote by $D$. Find the mean and variance of $D$.

**5.14** Let $P_1$ be the *proportion* of successes in 300 binomial trials, where the probability of success on each trial is $\theta$. The numerical value of $\theta$ is unknown. Let $P_2$ be the *proportion* of successes in 200 binomial trials, where the probability of success on each trial is also $\theta$. Define $D$ by $D = P_1 - P_2$. Then $D$ is a random variable. Find the mean and variance of $D$. (Your answer for the variance will be a function of $\theta$.)

**5.15** Let $P_1$ be the proportion of successes in 300 binomial trials, where the probability of success on each trial is 0.4. Let $P_2$ be the proportion of successes in 200 binomial trials, where the probability of success on each trial is 0.3. Define $D$ by $D = P_1 - P_2$. Then $D$ is a random variable. Find the mean of $D$ and variance of $D$. Hint: Use the equations in (5.10).

**5.16** Rashmi and Logan each have a fair coin. Rashmi and Logan plan to independently flip their coins twice and four times, respectively. They each record the proportion of their flips giving heads. Before the coins are flipped, these two proportions, respectively denoted by $U$ and $V$, are random variables.

(a) Find the probability distribution for $U$ and the probability distribution of $V$.
(b) From these distributions or the short formulas (5.9), find the mean and variance of $U$ and the mean and variance of $V$.
(c) From the probability distributions of $U$ and of $V$, find the probability distribution of $D$, where $D$ is defined by $D = U - V$. (This will require considering all possible combinations of $U$ and $V$ values to find all possible values of $D$.)
(d) Use this probability distribution of $D$ to find the mean and variance of $D$.
(e) Check that the values of the mean and the variance of $D$ which you calculated in part (d) of this question agree with those found using an appropriate set of short formulas. (You can use the formulas in (5.6) along with the means and variances found in part (b), the formulas in (5.10), or the formulas in (5.11).)

**5.17** Let $P_1$ be the proportion of successes in 10 binomial trials with probability of success equal to 0.5. Let $P_2$ be the proportion of successes in 15 binomial trials with probability of success equal to 0.3. Find the mean and variance of $D = P_1 - P_2$.

# Chapter 6
# Continuous Random Variables

## 6.1 Definition

Some random variables by their nature are discrete, such as the number of heads in 2000 flips of a coin. Other random variables, by contrast, are by their nature continuous. Continuous random variables can take any value in some continuous interval of values. Measurements such as the height and blood pressure of a randomly chosen person are of this type. The interval from $\ell$ to $h$, written $(\ell, h)$, is the *support* of the continuous random variable $X$: $X$ can take any value between the lowest value $\ell$ and the highest value $h$. Sometimes $\ell = -\infty$ and $h = +\infty$, which means that $X$ can take any value.

We use the same notation for continuous random variables as we do for discrete random variables, so that we denote a continuous random variable in upper case, for example by $X$, $Y$ and $Z$.

The definition of a continuous random variable is similar to, but not identical to, that for a discrete random variable. It is as follows.

**Definition** A continuous random variable is a conceptual numerical quantity which in some future experiment will take some value in a continuous interval of values.

The words "conceptual" and "numerical" arise for the same reasons as those given for discrete random variables as discussed in Sect. 4.1.

Probabilities for continuous random variables are not allocated to specific values, but rather they are allocated to some continuous interval of values. The probability that a continuous random variable takes some specified numerical value is zero.

One way to think about this notion is by considering how many possible values there are for a continuous random variable. Even if the support of the random variable is a short interval, perhaps between 10 and 11 inches, there are an infinite number of possible values. By adding more precision, or decimal points, to the values, we can always consider more possible values (if not, then the random variable is actually discrete by definition). If each of the infinite possible values had

© The Author(s), under exclusive license to Springer Nature Switzerland AG 2023
W. J. Ewens, K. Brumberg, *Introductory Statistics for Data Analysis*,
https://doi.org/10.1007/978-3-031-28189-1_6

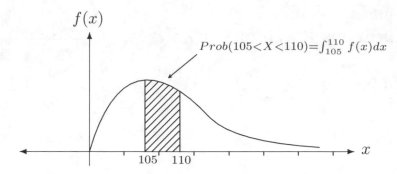

**Fig. 6.1** Shaded area = Prob($105 < X < 110$)

an associated probability, the total probability would also be infinite. However, the total probability must always sum to 1. Thus each individual value has no probability of occurring.

Another way to think about this concept is due to measurement precision. Suppose we take a measurement of 10.5 inches. This is only accurate to a certain level of precision. A ruler has markings at every 1/8th of an inch, so we might say something is 10.5 inches because it is closer to the marking for 10.5 than for 10.375. We are not really sure that the measurement is exactly 10.5 inches. Rather, we are sure that it is between 10.375 and 10.5. Thus it makes sense to assign a probability to this interval of possibilities, rather than to the precise value 10.5 alone.

Probabilities for continuous random variables are allocated in the following way. Every continuous random variable $X$ has an associated *density function* $f(x)$. The density function $f(x)$ is the continuous random variable analogue of a discrete random variable probability distribution such as (4.5). This density function can be drawn as a graph in the $(x, f(x))$ plane; for an example, see the curve in Fig. 6.1. The probability that the random variable $X$ takes a value in some given interval $a$ to $b$ is the shaded area under this curve between $a$ and $b$: an example is given in Fig. 6.1, with $a = 105, b = 110$.

In practice, we would usually not know what this probability is since we would usually not know the precise mathematical form of this density function. In this sense, a density function is like the probabilities in a discrete probability distribution.

We now give a concrete example. Suppose that we are doing research on the blood pressure of a person having some given medical condition and plan to take one person with this condition and measure that person's blood pressure. At this stage, we are conceptualizing about this blood pressure, so it is a continuous random variable because (a) it is continuous (it can take any value in a continuous interval of values), and (b) it is a random variable, as we do not know in advance of choosing the person what its value will be. Because it is a random variable, we denote it in upper case, for example as $X$. We can conceptualize a density function for $X$ such as that shown in Fig. 6.1. The shaded area is then the probability that the blood pressure of the person chosen at random is between 105 and 110.

From a calculus point of view, the probability that the observed value of a random variable $X$ having density function $f(x)$ will take a value between $a$ and $b$ is obtained by integrating its density function over the support $(a, b)$, so that

$$\text{Prob}(a < X < b) = \int_a^b f(x)\, dx. \tag{6.1}$$

This is just the area under the density function between $a$ and $b$ as shown above the density function $f(x)$ in Fig. 6.1. However, we will never carry out any mathematical integration procedures in this book.

The interpretation to be put on the left-hand side in (6.1) and in the caption to Fig. 6.1 is that it is a shorthand for the probability that, when the experiment is carried out, the observed value $x$ of the random variable $X$ will take a value between $a$ and $b$.

Because the probability that a continuous random variable takes some specified numerical value is zero, the three probabilities $\text{Prob}(a \le X < b)$, $\text{Prob}(a < X \le b)$, and $\text{Prob}(a \le X \le b)$ are also given by the right-hand side in (6.1).

As a particular case of Eq. (6.1),

$$\int_\ell^h f(x)\, dx = 1. \tag{6.2}$$

This equation simply states that a random variable must take some value in its support, that is, in its interval of possible values.

## 6.2   The Mean and Variance of a Continuous Random Variable

As we will not be calculating integrals in this book, we will not be able to calculate means and variances of continuous random variables directly from their probability density functions, as we did for discrete random variables with their probability distributions. However, it is useful to see how the formulas for continuous random variables parallel those for discrete random variables.

The mean $\mu$ and variance $\sigma^2$ of a continuous random variable $X$ having support $(\ell, h)$ and density function $f(x)$ are defined respectively by

$$\mu = \int_\ell^h x f(x) dx \tag{6.3}$$

and

$$\sigma^2 = \int_\ell^h (x - \mu)^2 f(x) dx. \tag{6.4}$$

These definitions are the natural analogues of the corresponding definitions (4.19) and (4.30) for a discrete random variable, with summations replaced by integrations.

A formula for $\sigma^2$ equivalent to that in Eq. (6.4), and which which is parallel to Eq. (4.35) for discrete random variables, is

$$\sigma^2 = \int_\ell^h x^2 f(x) dx - \mu^2. \tag{6.5}$$

The general properties for the mean and variance of a continuous random variable parallel those for a discrete random variable. In particular, we always denote a mean by $\mu$ and a variance by $\sigma^2$, as indicated above. The mean is the "center of gravity" of the density function $f(x)$ and the variance is a measure of the dispersion of the density function around the mean.


## 6.3   The Normal Distribution

There are many continuous probability distributions relevant to statistical operations. The most important one of these is the normal, or Gaussian, distribution. It is defined as follows.

The (continuous) random variable $X$ has a *normal*, or *Gaussian*, distribution if its support is $(-\infty, \infty)$ and its density function $f(x)$ is given by the formula

$$f(x) = \frac{1}{\sqrt{2\pi}\sigma} e^{-\frac{(x-\mu)^2}{2\sigma^2}}, \qquad -\infty < x < +\infty. \tag{6.6}$$

The shape of this density function is the well-known bell-shaped curve. Here $\pi$ (the Greek letter "pi") is the well-known geometrical concept having a numerical value of about 3.1416 and $e$ is the equally important exponential constant having a numerical value of about 2.7183. The mean of this normal distribution is $\mu$ and its variance is $\sigma^2$, and these parameters are built into the functional form of the distribution, as (6.6) shows. Note that the support of $X$ runs from minus infinity to plus infinity, so that any interval of values of $X$ is possible.

As stated above, the probability that a continuous random variable takes a value between $a$ and $b$ is defined by a calculus operation, which gives the area under the density function of the random variable between $a$ and $b$. Thus, for example, the probability that a random variable having a normal distribution with mean 6 and variance 16 takes a value between 5 and 8 is

$$\int_5^8 \frac{1}{\sqrt{2\pi}\sqrt{16}} e^{-\frac{(x-6)^2}{32}} dx. \tag{6.7}$$

Amazingly, the processes of calculus are unable to evaluate the integral in (6.7): it is just "too hard". This indicates an interesting limit as to what mathematics can do. This, however, does not mean that there is no numerical value to this integral. There is a numerical value, but it cannot be found by the processes of calculus. We will see later how to find a very accurate approximate value for this integral in a chart or in R.

There is a whole family of normal distributions, each member of the family corresponding to some pair of $(\mu, \sigma^2)$ values. The case $\mu = 6$ and $\sigma^2 = 16$ just considered is an example of one member of this family. However, probability charts are available only for one particular member of this family, namely the normal distribution for which $\mu = 0$ and $\sigma^2 = 1$. This is sometimes called the *standardized normal* distribution, for reasons which will appear shortly. A graph of this specific normal distribution density function is shown in Fig. 6.2 below, and the "bell-shaped" form of the distribution is apparent.

A random variable having a normal distribution with mean 0 and variance 1 is often denoted by $Z$, and in this book, this notation is reserved for this random variable. Often some random variable has a probability distribution very close to a normal distribution with mean 0 and variance 1. Such a random variable will be typically denoted by "$Z$", the quotation signs indicating "approximately

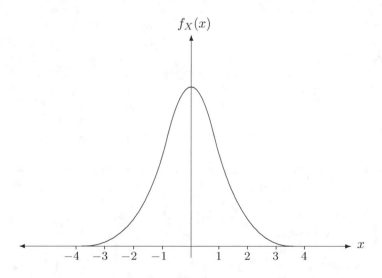

**Fig. 6.2**  The density function for the standard normal distribution with $\mu = 0, \sigma = 1$

a $Z$ random variable", implying that its probability distribution is approximately a normal distribution with mean 0 and variance 1.

The formula (6.6) shows that the probability that the random variable $Z$ takes a value less than some chosen number $z$ is

$$\int_{-\infty}^{z} \frac{1}{\sqrt{2\pi}} e^{-x^2/2} dx. \tag{6.8}$$

As noted above, this integration cannot be performed by the processes of calculus. However, very accurate approximations can be found for this probability by the use of numerical methods. From these numerical approximations, a chart giving numerical values for this probability for various values of $z$ between $-3.49$ and $3.49$ can be constructed. Two charts, Chart 2 for for negative values of $z$ and Chart 3 for positive values of $z$, are given in the Charts section of this book. We use both the expression "normal distribution chart" and the expression "the Z chart" for this set of charts, using the second expression to emphasize that it relates to the random variable $Z$. The values in the charts are accurate to four decimal places. For values of $z$ greater than 3.49, we approximate the value of the expression in (6.8) by 1. For values of $z$ less than $-3.49$, we approximate the value of the expression in (6.8) by 0.

Computers have now all but replaced charts and it is possible to evaluate approximate probabilities such as those given below by a computer package such as R, as seen below.

Here are several examples of the use of the Z chart and of R. First, Chart 3 shows that the probability that the random variable $Z$ takes a value less than 0.5, that is, between minus infinity and 0.5, is 0.6915. Second, Chart 2 shows that the probability that a $Z$ takes a value less than $-1.73$, that is, between minus infinity and $-1.73$, is 0.0418. Although these are approximate probabilities, they are accurate to four decimal places and thus we will typically use "=" when using values from the chart as opposed to "≈".

In R, we use the pnorm() function, which by default gives "less than" probabilities and takes the value of interest as the q argument. For the examples in the previous paragraph, we would use pnorm(q = 0.5) and pnorm(q = -1.73).

We often have to find "greater than" probabilities. The event "$Z > 1.44$" is the complement of the event "$Z \leq 1.44$", so from Eq. (3.1), its probability is $1 - 0.9251 = 0.0749$. Similarly, the probability of the event $Z > -1.44$ is $1 - 0.0749 = 0.9251$.

In R, we can apply the same logic as from the chart with 1 - pnorm(q = 1.44), or we can specify a second argument lower.tail = FALSE to reverse the direction of the calculation: pnorm(q = 1.44, lower.tail = FALSE).

We often have to calculate "between" probabilities. For example, the probability that a $Z$ takes a value between $-1.73$ and $+0.5$ is the probability that $Z$ is less than $+0.5$ minus the probability that $Z$ is less than $-1.73$. This is $0.6915 - 0.0418 = 0.6497$. Similarly, the probability that a $Z$ takes a value between 1.23 and 2.46 is $0.9931 - 0.8907 = 0.1024$.

In R, we apply the same logic with pnorm(q = 0.5) - pnorm(q = -1.73) and pnorm(q = 2.46) - pnorm(q = 1.23).

*A Note on Interpolation* Suppose that one wishes to calculate the probability that $Z$ takes a value less than 1.643. The value 1.643 does not appear on the normal distribution chart. For this book, a sufficiently good approximation is to calculate either the probability that $Z$ takes a value less than 1.64 (0.9495) or the probability that $Z$ takes a value less than 1.65 (0.9505). To be more accurate, we could use a standard linear interpolation formula and arrive at the value 0.9498. An example of linear interpolation is given in the following section.

## 6.4 The Standardization Procedure

Why is there a probability chart for only one member of the normal distribution family, that is, the member of the family with mean 0 and variance 1? The answer to this question is given by the implications of the following theorem.

**Theorem** *Suppose that a random variable $X$ has the normal distribution (6.6), that is, with arbitrary mean $\mu$ and arbitrary variance $\sigma^2$. Then the "standardized" random variable $(X - \mu)/\sigma$ has a normal distribution with mean 0, variance 1.*

*In line with a convention adopted above, we will call such a standardized random variable $Z$. That is, we can write $(X - \mu)/\sigma = Z$. This standardization procedure is used very frequently to find probabilities involving a random variable having a normal distribution with any given mean and any given variance.*

*Example 6.4.1* If $X$ is a random variable having a normal distribution with mean 6 and variance 16 (and thus standard deviation 4), Prob(7 < X < 10) can be found by standardizing and creating a $Z$ statistic:

$$\text{Prob}(7 < X < 10) = \text{Prob}\left(\frac{7-6}{4} < \frac{X-6}{4} < \frac{10-6}{4}\right)$$

$$= \text{Prob}(0.25 < Z < 1), \tag{6.9}$$

and this probability is found from the normal distribution chart to be $0.8413 - 0.5987 = 0.2426$. One can think of this activity as "creating a $Z$ and then using the $Z$ chart".

*Example 6.4.2* Suppose that $X$ is a random variable having a normal distribution with mean 6 and variance 20 (and thus standard deviation $\sqrt{20} \approx 4.4721$) and we wish to find Prob($X < 10$). The standardization procedure gives

$$\text{Prob}(X < 10) = \text{Prob}\left(\frac{X-6}{\sqrt{20}} < \frac{10-6}{\sqrt{20}}\right) \approx \text{Prob}(Z < 0.8944). \tag{6.10}$$

This probability is not given by the Z chart, and situations such as this arise often as a result of the standardization procedure. The convention taken in this book is that since 0.8944 is closer to 0.89 than it is to 0.90, a sufficiently accurate approximation to the required probability is Prob($Z \leq 0.89$) = 0.8133.

A more accurate approximation, provided by the process of linear interpolation, is $0.56 \times$ Prob($Z \leq 0.89$) $+ 0.44 \times$ Prob($Z \leq 0.90$) $\approx 0.814444$. To six decimal place accuracy, the required probability is known to be 0.814453, and clearly the approximation found by linear interpolation is very accurate and is better than that given by the approximate procedure described above. Despite this, the approximate procedure described above is followed in this book unless a more accurate approximation is desired.

In R, we can apply the same rounding as used in the Z chart, yielding `pnorm(q = 0.89)`, or we can calculate the more accurate `pnorm(q = 0.8944)` with no additional effort. We could be even more accurate by eliminating the rounding step by doing `pnorm(q = (10-6)/sqrt(20))`. This will be as accurate as R's level of precision. Note that the calculations in this book are primarily done via the Z chart and so your answers may differ slightly if you choose to use more precision.

In R, we can also forgo the standardization procedure entirely, letting R do the work for us. To do this, we give the original value of interest as well as two additional arguments, `mean` and `sd`. In this case: `pnorm(q = 10, mean = 6, sd = sqrt(20))`. However, the standardization procedure is essential to much of the theory that follows and thus it is important to understand it even when using a computer package.

## 6.5  Numbers that Are Seen Often in Statistics

The following probabilities, slightly more accurate than those that can be found in Charts 2 and 3, are all used often in Statistics and thus stated in this section.

First, we have

$$\text{Prob}(Z \leq +1.645) = 0.95. \tag{6.11}$$

Derived from this using the probability of the complement and the symmetry of the normal distribution, we have

$$\text{Prob}(Z \geq +1.645) = 0.05, \tag{6.12}$$

$$\text{Prob}(Z \leq -1.645) = 0.05, \tag{6.13}$$

$$\text{Prob}(Z \geq -1.645) = 0.95. \tag{6.14}$$

Another important result is that

$$\text{Prob}(-1.960 \leq Z \leq +1.960) = 0.95. \tag{6.15}$$

Again, using properties of the complement and the symmetry of the normal distribution, we also have

$$\text{Prob}(Z \leq -1.960) + \text{Prob}(Z \geq +1.960) = 0.05, \tag{6.16}$$

$$\text{Prob}(Z \geq +1.960) = 0.025, \tag{6.17}$$

$$\text{Prob}(Z \leq -1.960) = 0.025. \tag{6.18}$$

Another useful calculation is

$$\text{Prob}(Z \leq -2.326) = 0.01. \tag{6.19}$$

$$\text{Prob}(Z \geq +2.326) = 0.01. \tag{6.20}$$

The final important calculation is

$$\text{Prob}(Z \leq -2.576) = 0.005, \tag{6.21}$$

$$\text{Prob}(Z \geq +2.576) = 0.005, \tag{6.22}$$

$$\text{Prob}(Z \leq -2.576) + \text{Prob}(Z \geq +2.576) = 0.01, \tag{6.23}$$

$$\text{Prob}(-2.576 \leq Z \leq +2.576) = 0.99. \tag{6.24}$$

The numbers 1.645, 1.960, 2.326 and 2.576 arise very often in statistical procedures, as we will see later. They are therefore worth remembering or bookmarking.

If $X$ is a random variable having a normal distribution with mean $\mu$ and variance $\sigma^2$, the standardization procedure shows that $(X - \mu)/\sigma$ has a normal distribution with mean 0 and variance 1. Equation (6.15) then shows that

$$\text{Prob}\left(-1.96 < \frac{X - \mu}{\sigma} < +1.96\right) = 0.95. \tag{6.25}$$

This implies after some algebraic manipulation that

$$\text{Prob}(\mu - 1.96\sigma < X < \mu + 1.96\sigma) = 0.95. \tag{6.26}$$

This result is used often in Statistics.

A convenient approximation is derived from Eq. (6.26) by replacing 1.96 by 2. This is

$$\text{Prob}(\mu - 2\sigma < X < \mu + 2\sigma) \approx 0.95. \tag{6.27}$$

Similarly, replacing $Z$ by $\frac{X-\mu}{\sigma}$ in (6.24) shows after some algebraic manipulation that

$$\text{Prob}(\mu - 2.576\sigma < X < \mu + 2.576\sigma) = 0.99. \tag{6.28}$$

This result is also used often in Statistics.

## 6.6   Using the Normal Distribution Chart in Reverse

So far, we have been given a number, or perhaps two numbers, and asked to find a probability. For example, if $X$ has a normal distribution with some mean 6 and some variance 16, we have found the probability $\text{Prob}(7 \leq X \leq 10)$ to be 0.2426 from the calculations in (6.9). In this section, we consider the situation where we are given a probability and are asked to find a number corresponding to that probability. Here are two examples which are similar to those we will use later in Statistics.

*Example 6.6.1* Suppose that $X$ has a normal distribution with mean 10 and variance 25. Find the number $a$ such that $\text{Prob}(X \leq a) = 0.05$.
   To answer this question we first carry out a standardization procedure to get

$$\text{Prob}\left(\frac{X-10}{5} \leq \frac{a-10}{5}\right) = 0.05, \tag{6.29}$$

that is,

$$\text{Prob}\left(Z \leq \frac{a-10}{5}\right) = 0.05. \tag{6.30}$$

But, from the Z chart or from Eq. (6.13),

$$\text{Prob}(Z \leq -1.645) = 0.05. \tag{6.31}$$

Therefore $\frac{a-10}{5} = -1.645$, so that $a = 1.775$.
   In R, we can run the following to get the same answer, parallel with the "un-standardizing" done in the last line above: qnorm(p = 0.05) * 5 + 10. Or, more simply, we can run qnorm(p = 0.05, mean = 10, sd = 5), removing the need for standardizing or un-standardizing.

*Example 6.6.2* Suppose that $X$ has a normal distribution with mean 200 and variance 100. We want to find the number $b$ such that $\text{Prob}(X \geq b) = 0.01$. To find this probability, we first carry out a standardization procedure to get

$$\text{Prob}\left(\frac{X - 200}{10} \geq \frac{b - 200}{10}\right) = 0.01. \qquad (6.32)$$

This gives

$$\text{Prob}\left(Z \geq \frac{b - 200}{10}\right) = 0.01. \qquad (6.33)$$

But from the Z chart or from Eq. (6.20),

$$\text{Prob}(Z \geq 2.326) = 0.01. \qquad (6.34)$$

Therefore $\frac{b-200}{10} = 2.326$, so that $b = 223.26$.

In R, we can run the following to get the same answer (with no need to standardize first):

`qnorm(p = 0.01, mean = 200, sd = 10, lower.tail = FALSE)`.

The numbers $-1.645$ and $+2.326$ are both displayed in the previous section, in Eqs. (6.13) and (6.20) respectively.

These numbers can also be found in R by running `qnorm(p = 0.05)` and `qnorm(p = 0.01, lower.tail = FALSE)`.

## 6.7 Sums, Averages and Differences of Independent Normal Random Variables

An important property of independent random variables $X_1, X_2, \ldots, X_n$, each of which has a normal distribution, is that their sum $T$, their average $\bar{X}$ and the difference $D$ between any two of them also have normal distributions. Thus in the important case where $X_1, X_2, \ldots, X_n$ are *iid*, each having a normal distribution with mean $\mu$ and variance $\sigma^2$, it follows that $T$, $\bar{X}$ and $D$ each have a normal distribution with means and variances as given respectively in Eqs. (5.3), (5.4) and (5.5).

We now give an example of the use of this result. Suppose that we know that the height of a woman chosen at random is a random variable having a normal distribution with mean 67 inches, variance 4 (inches squared), and thus standard deviation 2 inches. We wish to find the probability that the height $X$ of a woman chosen at random will be between 66 and 68 inches. That is, we wish to calculate

$$\text{Prob}(66 \leq X \leq 68).$$

The standardizing procedure shows that this probability is

$$\text{Prob}\left(\frac{66-67}{2} \leq \frac{X-67}{2} \leq \frac{68-67}{2}\right),$$

or

$$\text{Prob}\left(-\frac{1}{2} \leq Z \leq +\frac{1}{2}\right).$$

The $Z$ chart shows that this probability is $0.6915 - 0.3085 = 0.3830$.

Next, we find the probability that the average $\bar{X}$ of the heights of 4 women chosen at random will be between 66 and 68 inches. From Eq. (5.4), this average has a normal distribution with mean 67 and variance $4/4 = 1$. The standardizing procedure shows that Prob$(66 \leq \bar{X} \leq 68)$ is

$$\text{Prob}\left(\frac{66-67}{1} \leq \frac{\bar{X}-67}{1} \leq \frac{68-67}{1}\right),$$

or

$$\text{Prob}(-1 \leq Z \leq 1).$$

The $Z$ chart shows that this probability is $0.6826$.

Finally, we find the probability that the average of the heights of 16 women chosen at random will be between 66 and 68 inches. For this case, Eq. (5.4) show that the mean of $\bar{X}$ is 67 and the variance of $\bar{X}$ is $\frac{4}{16} = 0.25$. Thus the standard deviation of $\bar{X}$ is 0.5. Proceeding as above, the desired probability is

$$\text{Prob}\left(\frac{66-67}{0.5} \leq \frac{\bar{X}-67}{0.5} \leq \frac{68-67}{0.5}\right),$$

or

$$\text{Prob}(-2 \leq Z \leq 2).$$

The $Z$ chart shows that this probability is $0.9544$.

These calculations show that it becomes increasing likely that the average will be close to the mean (of 67) as the sample size increases. This result accords with common sense, but the formula for the variance of an average allows us to make precise calculations concerning this phenomenon.

If $X_1, X_2, ..., X_n$ are $iid$ random variables each having a normal distribution with mean $\mu$ and variance $\sigma^2$, so that $\bar{X}$ has a normal distribution with mean $\mu$

and variance $\sigma^2/n$, then plugging this mean and variance of the average $\bar{X}$ into Eq. (6.26) shows that

$$\text{Prob}\left(\mu - 1.96\frac{\sigma}{\sqrt{n}} \leq \bar{X} \leq \mu + 1.96\frac{\sigma}{\sqrt{n}}\right) = 0.95. \tag{6.35}$$

A convenient rule of thumb approximation deriving from Eq. (6.35) is

$$\text{Prob}\left(\mu - 2\frac{\sigma}{\sqrt{n}} \leq \bar{X} \leq \mu + 2\frac{\sigma}{\sqrt{n}}\right) \approx 0.95. \tag{6.36}$$

Another form of calculation relates to differences of random variables each having a normal distribution. This is now illustrated by some examples.

*Example 6.7.1* Suppose that $X_1$ has a normal distribution with mean 56 and variance 16 and $X_2$ has a normal distribution with mean 54 and variance 9. What is the probability that $X_1 \geq X_2$?

This sort of question is answered by considering the difference $D = X_1 - X_2$. To say that $X_1 \geq X_2$ is the same as saying $D \geq 0$. To find the probability that $D \geq 0$, we first have to find the mean and variance of $D$. The equations in (5.6) show that the mean of $D$ is $56 - 54 = 2$ and the variance of $D$ is $16 + 9 = 25$. Thus the standard deviation of $D$ is 5. A standardization procedure then shows that

$$\text{Prob}(D \geq 0) = \text{Prob}\left(\frac{D-2}{5} \geq \frac{0-2}{5}\right) = \text{Prob}(Z \geq -0.4) = 0.6554.$$

*Example 6.7.2* This is a more colorful example. Suppose that the height $X_1$ of a Dutchman taken at random has a normal distribution with mean 73 and standard deviation 4, and the height $X_2$ of an American man taken at random has a normal distribution with mean 69 and standard deviation 3. (All measurements are in inches.) What is the probability that the height of a Dutchman taken at random is greater than or equal to the height of an American man taken at random? That is, what is $\text{Prob}(X_1 \geq X_2)$?

We proceed as in Example 6.7.1, defining $D$ as $X_1 - X_2$. The mean of $D$ is 4 and the variance of $D$ is $16 + 9 = 25$, so the standard deviation of $D$ is $\sqrt{25} = 5$. A standardization procedure shows that

$$\text{Prob}(D \geq 0) = \text{Prob}\left(\frac{D-4}{5} = \frac{0-4}{5}\right) = \text{Prob}(Z \geq -0.8) = 0.7881.$$

*Example 6.7.3* Suppose that the *iid* random variables $X_{11}, X_{12}, X_{13}$ and $X_{14}$ are the heights of four Dutchmen taken at random, each having a normal distribution with mean 73 and standard deviation 4 (as in Example 6.7.2) and the *iid* random variables $X_{21}, X_{22}, X_{23}$ and $X_{24}$ are the heights of four American men taken at random, each having a normal distribution with mean 69 and standard deviation 3 (as in Example 6.7.2). We define $\bar{X}_1$ and $\bar{X}_2$ by

$$\bar{X}_1 = \frac{X_{11} + X_{12} + X_{13} + X_{14}}{4} \quad \text{and} \quad \bar{X}_2 = \frac{X_{21} + X_{22} + X_{23} + X_{24}}{4}.$$

What is the probability that $\bar{X}_1 \geq \bar{X}_2$?

To answer this question, we have to do three things. We first have to find the mean and variance of $\bar{X}_1$ and also the mean and variance of $\bar{X}_2$. Second, from these, we have to find the mean and variance of $D = \bar{X}_1 - \bar{X}_2$. Finally, we have to find Prob($D \geq 0$) by doing a standardization procedure.

The mean and variance of $\bar{X}_1$ are found from Eq. (5.4) and the fact that $X_{11}, X_{12}, X_{13}$ and $X_{14}$ each have a normal distribution with mean 73 and variance 16. From these facts, we see that the mean of $\bar{X}_1$ is 73 and the variance of $\bar{X}_1$ is $\frac{16}{4} = 4$. Similarly, the mean of $\bar{X}_2$ is 69 and the variance of $\bar{X}_2$ is $\frac{9}{4} = 2.25$.

From these facts and Eq. (5.6), the mean of $D$ is 4 and the variance of $D$ is $\frac{25}{4} = 6.25$. Thus the standard deviation of $D$ is $\sqrt{6.25} = 2.5$.

Finally,

$$\text{Prob}(D \geq 0) = \text{Prob}\left(\frac{D-4}{2.5} \geq \frac{0-4}{2.5}\right) = \text{Prob}(Z \geq -1.6) = 0.9452.$$

This probability exceeds that found in Example 6.7.2. This eventually derives from the fact that the variances for the averages in Example 6.7.3 are smaller than the variances for the individuals in Example 6.7.2.

*Example 6.7.4* Examples 6.7.2 and 6.7.3 show that if there are $n$ Dutchmen in the sample and $n$ American men in the sample, and $D = \bar{X}_1 - \bar{X}_2$, where $\bar{X}_1$ is the average of the heights of the Dutchmen in the sample and $\bar{X}_2$ is the average of the heights of the American men in the sample, the mean of $D$ is 4 and the variance of $D$ is $\frac{25}{n}$, so that

$$\text{Prob}(D \geq 0) = \text{Prob}\left(Z \geq \frac{-4}{\sqrt{25/n}}\right).$$

If $n = 20$, this is approximately Prob($Z \geq -3.5777$) $\approx 0.9998$. It is now almost certain that the average of the heights of the Dutchmen will exceed the average of the heights of the American men.

## 6.8  The Central Limit Theorem

An important property of an average and of a sum of several random variables derives from the so-called *Central Limit Theorem* (CLT). Part of this extremely important theorem states that if the random variables $X_1, X_2, \ldots, X_n$ are *iid*, then no matter what the probability distribution of these random variables might be, the average $\bar{X} = (X_1 + X_2 + \cdots + X_n)/n$ and the sum $T = X_1 + X_2 + \cdots + X_n$ both have approximately a normal distribution. Further, this approximation becomes increasingly accurate the larger $n$ is.

This is an astonishing result and the Central Limit Theorem is one of the most important theorems in all of mathematics. For the purposes of this book, its importance lies in its practical implications. Many statistical procedures use either sums or averages, so that the Central Limit Theorem is important in practice. Thus, for example, even if the $iid$ random variables $X_1, \ldots, X_n$, each having mean $\mu$ and variance $\sigma^2$, do not have a normal distribution, the random variable $\bar{X}$ should have close to a normal distribution if $n$ is large. Applying Eq. (6.35) to the random variable $\bar{X}$ gives

$$\text{Prob}\left(\mu - \frac{1.96\sigma}{\sqrt{n}} < \bar{X} < \mu + \frac{1.96\sigma}{\sqrt{n}} < \bar{X}\right) \approx 0.95, \tag{6.37}$$

when $n$ is large, even though the $iid$ random variables $X_1, \ldots, X_n$ do not have a normal distribution. Because $X_1, \ldots, X_n$ do not have a normal distribution, Eq. (6.37) is an approximation, unlike Eq. (6.35) where we had the average of $iid$ normal random variables.

There is no precise answer to the question of how large $n$ has to be for the approximation (6.37) to be sufficiently accurate for all practical purposes. A common rule of thumb is that $n$ should be at least 30. However, the accuracy depends on the extent to which the distribution of the random variables $X_1, \ldots, X_n$ differs from the normal distribution, and thus $n$ should be even larger if the data suggest that the distribution of $X_1, \ldots, X_n$ appears to be extremely different from the normal distribution.

We show in the next section that for discrete random variables $X_1, X_2, \ldots, X_n$, the approximation (6.37) can be quite accurate even for quite small values of $n$ if a continuity correction is used.

The Central Limit Theorem also has an important implication with respect to a random variable having a binomial distribution. Suppose that $X$ has a binomial distribution with index $n$ (the number of trials). If $X_1$ is the number of successes on trial 1 (either 0 or 1), $X_2$ is the number of successes on trial 2 (either 0 or 1), $\ldots, X_n$ is the number of successes on trial $n$ (either 0 or 1), then we can write the binomial $X$ as the sum $X = X_1 + X_2 + \cdots + X_n$. Therefore $X$ is the sum of $iid$ Bernoulli random variables, and thus from the Central Limit Theorem has approximately a normal distribution. Similarly, the proportion $P$ of successes in $n$ binomial trials is the average $\frac{1}{n}(X_1 + X_2 + \cdots + X_n)$ and thus has, to a very close approximation, a normal distribution. It can be shown in both cases that the approximation gets better as $n$ increases. This statement is rather imprecise since a random variable having a binomial distribution is discrete and a random variable having a normal distribution is continuous. A more precise statement is made in Sect. 6.9.

Applying the Central Limit Theorem to the binomial $X$ with index $n$ and parameter $\theta$, we can plug the binomial mean and standard deviation into Eq. (6.26) to get the approximation

$$\text{Prob}(n\theta - 1.96\sqrt{n\theta(1 - \theta)} < X < n\theta + 1.96\sqrt{n\theta(1 - \theta)}) \approx 0.95 \qquad (6.38)$$

Similarly if $P = X/n$ is the proportion of successes, then

$$\text{Prob}\left(\theta - 1.96\sqrt{\frac{\theta(1 - \theta)}{n}} < P < \theta + 1.96\sqrt{\frac{\theta(1 - \theta)}{n}}\right) \approx 0.95 \qquad (6.39)$$

A convenient rule of thumb approximation to (6.39) is

$$\text{Prob}\left(\theta - 2\sqrt{\frac{\theta(1 - \theta)}{n}} < P < \theta + 2\sqrt{\frac{\theta(1 - \theta)}{n}}\right) \approx 0.95. \qquad (6.40)$$

The importance of the Central Limit Theorem in the context of a binomial random variable or proportion derives from the fact that many statistical procedures deal with the number of successes in $n$ binomial trials and the proportion of successes in $n$ binomial trials. This means that the approximations (6.38), (6.39) and (6.40) are often used when carrying out statistical procedures.

## 6.9  Approximating Discrete Random Variable Probabilities Using the Normal Distribution

The Central Limit theorem implies that probabilities associated with sums and averages of discrete random variables, and random variables having the binomial distribution, can be approximated using the normal distribution. We consider here only the case of discrete random variables which can only take integer values.

The key fact is that we approximate the probability that an integer-valued discrete random variable $X$ takes the value $x$ by the probability that a random variable having a normal distribution with the same mean and variance of $X$ takes a value between $x - \frac{1}{2}$ and $x + \frac{1}{2}$. This implies that we approximate the probability that the discrete random variable takes a value in the set $\{a, a + 1, \cdots, b\}$ by the probability that a random variable having a normal distribution with the same mean and variance of $X$ takes a value between $a - \frac{1}{2}$ and $b + \frac{1}{2}$. The value $\frac{1}{2}$ is a so-called *continuity correction*.

### 6.9.1 The Binomial Case

We would not use the normal distribution to approximate binomial probabilities when $n$ is small, first because exact binomial probabilities are easy to calculate for small $n$ and second, because for small $n$ the normal approximation is not accurate. Despite this, we now calculate the normal distribution approximation to the probability that a binomial random variable with $n = 16$ and $\theta = \frac{1}{2}$ takes a value in the set $\{6, 7, 8, 9, 10\}$, first without and then with the continuity correction. The aim is to assess the benefit of a continuity correction.

The mean of the binomial random variable is 8 and the variance is 4, so without using a continuity correction, the normal distribution approximation is

$$\text{Prob}\left(\frac{6-8}{2} \leq Z \leq \frac{10-8}{2}\right) = \text{Prob}\,(-1 \leq Z \leq +1) = 0.6826.$$

If a continuity correction is used, the approximating probability is

$$\text{Prob}\left(\frac{5.5-8}{2} \leq Z \leq \frac{10.5-8}{2}\right) = \text{Prob}\,(-1.25 \leq Z \leq +1.25) = 0.7498.$$

The binomial chart shows that to four decimal place accuracy the true binomial probability is 0.7900. The approximation using the continuity correction, while not closely accurate, is clearly superior to the approximation that does not use the continuity correction.

The accuracy of the normal distribution approximation to the binomial increases as $n$ increases, and for large $n$ we are usually prepared to use equations such as (6.38) and (6.39). Thus in an example in Sect. 9.2.5 where $n = 5000$, we assume that the normal distribution approximation is sufficiently accurate, even without using a continuity correction.

### 6.9.2 The Die Example

From the probabilities given in Problem 5.4, if a fair die is to be rolled four times, the probability that the sum $T_4$ of the four numbers turning up takes a value from 12 to 16 inclusive is $\frac{125+140+145+140+125}{1296} \approx 0.5208$. The mean of $T_4$ is 14 and the variance of $T_4$ is $\frac{35}{3}$. The probability that a normal random variable with this mean and this variance takes a value between 12 and 16 is found to be about 0.4414, so that using a normal distribution to approximate the exact probability without using a continuity correction is not very accurate. A continuity-corrected approximation would find the probability that a normal random variable with this mean and this variance takes a value between 11.5 and 16.5, which is about 0.5346. While this is still not very accurate, it is nevertheless more accurate than the value found when a continuity correction is not used.

## 6.10  A Window Into Statistics

The normal distribution approximation to the binomial leads to a window into Statistics. It shows that *if* a newborn is equally likely to have brown eyes as not, then the probability is about 0.99 that in a well-conducted representative unbiased sample of 2500 newborns, the number of brown-eyed babies that we shall see will be between 1185 and 1315. This is a probability theory deduction, or implication, and uses many of the probability theory concepts described above. It is a probability theory "zig". It is made under the assumption that a newborn is equally likely to be brown-eyed as not. Suppose now that when we actually took a sample of 2500 newborns, we saw 1334 brown-eyed babies. This is outside what we might loosely call the "0.99 probability interval if a newborn is equally likely to have brown eyes as not", and we therefore have good evidence that it is *not* equally likely for a newborn to have brown eyes as not. This operation is a statistical induction, or inference. It is a statistical "zag", deriving from and corresponding to the probability theory "zig" deductive calculations leading to the values 1185 and 1315 and cannot be made without these probability theory calculations. We have now reached the point where we can use the probability theory results found above to carry out a variety of statistical applications.

A flow-chart of the "normal distribution" part of this book is given below to describe in perspective the various topics covered.

## Flowchart: Normal Random Variables and the CLT

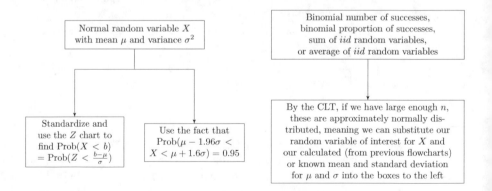

## 6.11  Problems

**6.1** The random variable $Z$ has a normal distribution with mean 0, variance 1. Find

(a) Prob$(-\infty < Z \le 1.32)$,
(b) Prob$(0 \le Z \le 1.32)$,
(c) Prob$(-0.44 \le Z \le 0)$,
(d) Prob$(0.62 \le Z \le 1.37)$,
(e) Prob$(Z \ge 1.17)$,
(f) Prob$(Z \ge -1.26)$.

**6.2**  The random variable $X$ has a normal distribution with mean 3, variance 4. Use the standardization procedure to standardize $X$ and then use the $Z$ chart or R to find

(a) Prob$(-\infty < X \le 4.14)$,
(b) Prob$(-\infty < X \le 2.24)$,
(c) Prob$(X \ge 3.68)$,
(d) Prob$(X \ge 2.56)$,
(e) Prob$(1.76 \le X \le 2.48)$,
(f) Prob$(3.66 \le X \le 4.42)$.

**6.3**  The random variable $Z$ has a normal distribution with mean 0, variance 1. Use the $Z$ chart in reverse or R to answer the following prompts.

(a) Given that Prob$(-\infty < Z \le a) = 0.7088$, find the value of $a$.
(b) Given that Prob$(-\infty < Z \le b) = 0.3336$, find the value of $b$.
(c) Given that Prob$(c \le Z \le +\infty) = 0.3372$, find the value of $c$.
(d) Given that Prob$(d \le Z \le +\infty) = 0.8485$, find the value of $d$.
(e) Given that Prob$(-e < Z < +e) = 0.3830$, find the value of $e$.

   Hint. Here you have to proceed in four steps. First, use the fact that for any number $m$,

$$\text{Prob}(0 \le Z \le m) = \frac{1}{2}\,\text{Prob}(-m \le Z \le +m).$$

(This follows from the symmetry of the $Z$ distribution around 0.) Second, from this, find Prob$(0 \le Z \le m)$. Third, then find

$$\text{Prob}(-\infty < Z \le m) \text{ as } \frac{1}{2} + \text{Prob}(0 \le Z \le m).$$

This follows from the fact (from the $Z$ chart) that Prob$(-\infty < Z \le 0) = \frac{1}{2}$. Fourth, having found Prob$(-\infty < Z \le m)$, you then find $m$ from the Z chart or from R.

(f) Given that Prob$(-f \le Z \le +f) = 0.3472$, find the value of $f$.

**6.4**  The random variable $X$ has a normal distribution with mean 3, variance 4.

(a) Given that Prob$(-\infty < X \le a) = 0.7088$, find the value of $a$.
(b) Given that Prob$(-\infty < X \le b) = 0.3336$, find the value of $b$.
(c) Given that Prob$(c \le X \le +\infty) = 0.3372$, find the value of $c$.

(d)  Given that $\mathrm{Prob}(d \leq X \leq +\infty) = 0.8485$, find the value of $d$.

**6.5**  The random variable $X$ has a normal distribution with mean 2, variance 25. Find

(a)  $\mathrm{Prob}(X > 5)$,
(b)  $\mathrm{Prob}(X < 1)$,
(c)  $\mathrm{Prob}(1 < X < 5)$,
(d)  the number $b$ such that $\mathrm{Prob}(X \leq b) = 0.5987$.

**6.6**  You are given that $X$ has a normal distribution with mean $\mu$ and variance $\sigma^2$, and also that

$$\mathrm{Prob}(\mu - k\sigma \leq X \leq \mu + k\sigma) = 0.5160.$$

Find the value of $k$.

**6.7**  $X$ and $Y$ are independent random variables, both having a normal distribution. $X$ has mean 5 and variance 3. $Y$ has mean 2 and variance 6. Find $\mathrm{Prob}(X > Y)$.

**6.8**  The weight $X_1$ of an adult female platypus taken at random has a normal distribution with mean 2.5 pounds and variance 0.36 (pounds squared) (and thus standard deviation of $\sqrt{0.36} = 0.6$ pounds).

(a)  Find $\mathrm{Prob}(X_1 \geq 3.0)$.
(b)  Suppose now that we consider the weights $X_1, X_2, X_3$ and $X_4$ of four adult female platypuses taken at random. Define $\bar{X}$ by $\bar{X} = \frac{1}{4}(X_1 + X_2 + X_3 + X_4)$. Find $\mathrm{Prob}(\bar{X} \geq 3.0)$.
(c)  Does the relation between your answers to (a) and (b) "make sense"? If so, why?

**6.9**  The weight of a muskrat taken at random has a normal distribution with mean 2.75 pounds and variance 0.625 (pounds squared), and thus standard deviation of 0.79 pounds.

(a)  Find the probability that the weight of a muskrat taken at random is less than 2 pounds.
(b)  Find the probability that the average of the weights of four muskrats taken at random is less than 2 pounds.
(c)  Does the relation between your answers to (a) and (b) "make sense"? If so, why?

**6.10 (Continuation from Problems 6.8 and 6.9)**

(a)  Find the probability that the weight of a muskrat taken at random exceeds the weight of a platypus taken at random.
(b)  Find the probability that the average weight of four muskrats taken at random exceeds the average weight of four platypuses taken at random.
(c)  Do the respective answers to (a) and (b) make sense?

**6.11**  Let $X_1, X_2, X_3, X_4, X_5$ be *iid* and normally distributed, each with mean 5 and variance 16.

(a)  Find Prob($\bar{X} > 6$) where $\bar{X} = (X_1 + X_2 + X_3 + X_4 + X_5)/5$.
(b)  Find Prob($T_5 > 30$), where $T_5 = X_1 + X_2 + X_3 + X_4 + X_5$.
(c)  Compare your answers to parts (a) and (b) of this problem.

**6.12**

(a)  A fair six-sided die is to be rolled 200 times. Use the Central Limit Theorem to calculate two numbers $a$ and $b$ such that the probability that the average $\bar{X}_{200}$ of the 200 numbers that turn up will lie between $a$ and $b$ is approximately 0.95.
(b)  As in part (a) of this question, but now the die is to be rolled 500 times. Use the Central Limit Theorem to calculate two numbers $c$ and $d$ such that the probability that the average $\bar{X}_{500}$ of the 500 numbers that turn up will lie between $c$ and $d$ is approximately 0.95.
(c)  As in part (a) of this question, but now the die is to be rolled 1000 times. Use the Central Limit Theorem to calculate two numbers $e$ and $f$ such that the probability that the average $\bar{X}_{1000}$ of the 1000 numbers that turn up will lie between $e$ and $f$ is approximately 0.95.
(d)  Do the difference between your answers in parts (a), (b) and (c) of this problem make sense?

**6.13**

(a)  A fair coin is to be flipped 500 times. Use Eq. (6.39) to calculate two numbers $a$ and $b$ such that the probability that the proportion $P$ of times that a head turns up will lie between $a$ and $b$ is approximately 0.95.
(b)  As in part (a) of this question, but now the coin is to be flipped 5000 times. Calculate two numbers $c$ and $d$ such that the probability that the proportion $P$ of times that a head turns up lies between $c$ and $d$ is approximately 0.95.
(c)  Comment on the difference between your answers in parts (a) and (b) of this question. That is, does the difference "make sense"?

**6.14**  Suppose that the mean weight of adult males is 160 pounds with a standard deviation of 8 pounds. Use Eq. (6.37) to

(a)  approximate the numbers $a$ and $b$ such that the probability that the average of the weights of 4 randomly chosen adult males taken at random is between $a$ and $b$ is approximately 0.95,
(b)  approximate the numbers $c$ and $d$ such that the probability that the average of the weights of 16 randomly chosen adult males taken at random is between $c$ and $d$ is approximately 0.95,
(c)  approximate the numbers $e$ and $f$ such that the probability that the average of the weights of 64 randomly chosen adult males taken at random is between $e$ and $f$ is approximately 0.95.

**6.15**  A coin was flipped 2000 times and we saw 1072 heads. Use the normal approximation to the binomial as justified by the Central Limit Theorem to find the approximate probability of getting 1072 or more heads **if the coin is fair.**

**6.16** A coin was flipped 500 times and we saw 260 heads and thus a proportion of $260/500 = 0.52$. Use the normal approximation to the binomial as justified by the Central Limit Theorem to find the approximate probability of getting a proportion of 0.52 or more of heads **if the coin is fair.**

**6.17** The random variable $X$ has a binomial distribution with index 20 and parameter 0.4. Find

(a) the probability as given by the binomial chart that $X$ takes a value from 7 to 12 inclusive,
(b) the normal distribution approximation to this probability without using a continuity correction,
(c) the normal distribution approximation to this probability using a continuity correction.
(d) Compare your results to parts (a)–(c).

**6.18** A fair die is to be rolled four times. The sum $T_4$ of the four numbers turning up has mean 14 and variance 35/3, and the probability that $T_4$ is either 13, 14 or 15 is $\frac{425}{1296} \approx 0.3279$ (see Sect. 6.9.2). Approximate this probability using the normal distribution

(a) not using a continuity correction,
(b) using a continuity correction.
(c) Comment on your results in parts (a) and (b).

# Part III
# Statistics

# Chapter 7
# Introduction

In this and the following chapters we discuss the applications to Statistics of the probability theory results discussed in previous chapters. So far, we have been contemplating the situation *before* some experiment is carried out, and therefore have been discussing random variables and their probability theory properties. *We now do our experiment, and wish to analyze the data that we obtained in it in the light of the probability theory introduced in the previous chapters.* In other words, we turn from deductive probability theory statements to inductive statistical procedures. These procedures cannot be carried out without the corresponding probability theory calculations and the deductive statements that are made from them.

The data arising from any experiment are thought of as the observed values of what were, before the experiment, random variables. If, before the experiment, we had been considering several random variables $X_1, X_2, \ldots, X_n$, we denote the actually observed value of these random variables, once the experiment has been carried out, by $x_1, x_2, \ldots, x_n$. These observed values are our *data*. For example, if an experiment consisted of the rolling of a die $n = 3$ times and after the experiment, we observe that a 5 turned up on the first roll and a 3 on both the second and third rolls, we would write $x_1 = 5, x_2 = 3, x_3 = 3$, and $(x_1, x_2, x_3)$ defined this way are our data. It does *not* make sense to say that $X_1 = 5, X_2 = 3, X_3 = 3$. Before the die is rolled, we do not know what numbers will turn up on the various rolls. At that stage, $X_1, X_2$ and $X_3$ are random variables, that is, they are just concepts of our mind.

The three main activities of Statistics as discussed in this book are using data to estimate of the numerical value of a parameter or the values of several parameters, assessing the accuracy of this estimate or these estimates, and testing hypotheses about the numerical value of a parameter or of several parameters. All of these activities are based on properties of the random variables corresponding to the data. We now consider each of these activities in turn.

© The Author(s), under exclusive license to Springer Nature Switzerland AG 2023
W. J. Ewens, K. Brumberg, *Introductory Statistics for Data Analysis*,
https://doi.org/10.1007/978-3-031-28189-1_7

# Chapter 8
# Estimation of a Parameter

## 8.1 Introduction

In some of the discussion in this book so far, the values of the various parameters entering the probability distributions considered were taken as being known. The fair coin distribution given in (4.2) is an example of this. However, in practice, the numerical values of parameters are usually unknown and must be estimated from data. This means that the fair coin example is not typical of a statistical situation. The real-life situation in research is that we do not know the relevant parameter. For example, we might be interested in $\mu$, the mean blood-sugar level of diabetics. To get some idea about what the value of this mean might be, we might take a sample of 1000 diabetics, measure the blood sugar reading for each of these 1000 people and use the data average $\bar{x}$ of these to estimate $\mu$. But in doing this, we are only estimating $\mu$ and not calculating it, since the data average $\bar{x}$ and the mean $\mu$ are two different concepts.

## 8.2 Estimating the Binomial Parameter $\theta$

### 8.2.1 Properties of Estimates and Estimators

We illustrate the general principles of estimation by considering the following questions. We have now conducted $n$ binomial trials, each having unknown probability $\theta$ of success on each trial, and have observed a proportion $p$ successes from these $n$ trials. What can we say about $\theta$? In particular, how should we estimate $\theta$? How precise can we expect the estimate to be?

If, after the experiment is conducted, the observed number of successes is $x$, the natural estimate of $\theta$ is $p\ (= x/n)$, the observed proportion of successes. What are the properties of this estimate? It is crucial to understand that the answers to

© The Author(s), under exclusive license to Springer Nature Switzerland AG 2023
W. J. Ewens, K. Brumberg, *Introductory Statistics for Data Analysis*,
https://doi.org/10.1007/978-3-031-28189-1_8

these questions depend on the properties of the random variable $P$, the (random) proportion of successes before we do the experiment. We know from Eq. (5.9) that the mean of $P$ is $\theta$ and that the variance of $P$ is $\theta(1 - \theta)/n$. What does this imply?

Since the random variable $P$ has a mean of $\theta$, the estimate $p$ of $\theta$, once we have done our experiment, is said to be an *unbiased* estimate of $\theta$. It is the result of a procedure that was "aiming at the right target". Correspondingly, the random variable $P$ is said to be an unbiased *estimator* of $\theta$. These are desirable properties, and therefore

$$\text{the estimate of } \theta \text{ is } p. \tag{8.1}$$

Note the two different words, *estimate* and *estimator*. One $(p)$ is a quantity calculated from data. The other $(P)$ is a random variable. These are both different from a third concept, namely $\theta$, the parameter which is being estimated. It is natural to ask why we have to consider the estimator $P$ of $\theta$, since the estimate $p$ is so natural. There are two reasons why one has to consider the estimator $P$. The first reason is the fact that the mean of $P$ is $\theta$ shows that $p$ is an unbiased estimate of $\theta$, as discussed above. The second reason is that in order to assess the accuracy of $p$ as an estimate of $\theta$, one has to consider the variance of $P$. We take up this matter in the next section.

## 8.2.2   The Precision of the Estimate of θ

Having found an estimate of a parameter, it is then important to find out how precise this estimate is. An estimate of a parameter without any indication of its precision is not of much value. The concept of precision is now illustrated in the binomial example discussed above.

We start with the approximate Eq. (6.39). We now turn this equation "inside-out" to get

$$\text{Prob}(P - 1.96\sqrt{\theta(1 - \theta)/n} < \theta < P + 1.96\sqrt{\theta(1 - \theta)/n}) \approx 0.95. \tag{8.2}$$

The reason why we derive Eq. (8.2) is that we want to find two numbers for which we are approximately 95% certain that $\theta$ is between the two numbers and deriving Eq. (8.2) is the first step in achieving this aim.

Suppose now that we have collected our data and have an observed value $p$ for the proportion of successes. From Eq. (8.2), a first attempt at finding an approximate 95% confidence interval for $\theta$ is

$$p - 1.96\sqrt{\theta(1 - \theta)/n} \quad \text{and} \quad p + 1.96\sqrt{\theta(1 - \theta)/n}. \tag{8.3}$$

We still have a problem. Since we do not know the value of $\theta$, we do not know the value of the expression $\sqrt{\theta(1 - \theta)/n}$ occurring twice in Eq. (8.3). However, at least we have an estimate of $\theta$, namely $p$. Since Eq. (8.3) is already an approximation, we make a further approximation and say that an approximate 95% confidence interval for $\theta$ is

$$p - 1.96\sqrt{\frac{p(1-p)}{n}} \quad \text{to} \quad p + 1.96\sqrt{\frac{p(1-p)}{n}}. \tag{8.4}$$

As an example, suppose that in $n = 1000$ binomial trials, we see 470 successes, so that $p = 0.47$. The lower bound in Eq. (8.4) is $0.47 - 1.96\sqrt{0.47 \times 0.53/1000} = 0.47 - 0.0309 = 0.4391$ and the upper bound is $0.47 + 1.96\sqrt{0.47 \times 0.53/1000} = 0.47 + 0.0309 = 0.5009$. We could then say "we estimate the value of $\theta$ to be 0.47, and we are (approximately) 95% certain that $\theta$ is between 0.4391 and 0.5009." In saying this, we have not only indicated our estimate of $\theta$, but we have also given some idea of the precision, or reliability, of that estimate.

*Notes on the Precision of the Estimate of $\theta$*

1. The interval 0.4391–0.5009 in the above example is usually called a "95% confidence interval for $\theta$". The interpretation of this statement is that we are approximately 95% certain that the true value of $\theta$ is within this interval. Thus the confidence interval gives us an idea of the precision of the estimate 0.47.
2. The precision of the estimate 0.47 as indicated by the confidence interval depends on the variance $\theta(1-\theta)/n$ of the random variable $P$. This is an example of why we have to consider random variables, their properties, and in particular their variances, before we carry out statistical operations.
3. We now consider two further approximations which lead to a simple approximate confidence interval. First, it is a mathematical fact that $p(1-p)$ can never exceed $\frac{1}{4}$, whatever the value of $p$. Further, for values of $p$ between 0.3 and 0.7, $p(1-p)$ is reasonably close to $\frac{1}{4}$. So, for these values of $p$, we can approximate $p(1-p)$ by $\frac{1}{4}$. Second, 1.96 is quite close to 2. These two approximations lead to the following approximate confidence interval for $\theta$:

$$p - 2\sqrt{\frac{1/4}{n}} \quad \text{to} \quad p + 2\sqrt{\frac{1/4}{n}}. \tag{8.5}$$

Since $\sqrt{1/4} = 1/2$, we arrive from the interval (8.5) at an equivalent and simpler approximate 95% confidence interval for $\theta$ as

$$p - \sqrt{1/n} \quad \text{to} \quad p + \sqrt{1/n}. \tag{8.6}$$

This confidence interval is quite easy to remember and may be used in place of interval (8.4) as a reasonable conservative approximation when $p$ is between 0.3 and 0.7. By "conservative", we mean wider than the interval given by (8.4). In the above numerical example, the interval (8.6) gives a slightly wider confidence interval (0.4384, 0.5016) than the interval (0.4391, 0.5009) given above.

4. What was the sample size? Suppose that a TV announcer says, before an election between two candidates Bauer and Lee, that a Gallup poll predicts that 52% of the voters will vote for Bauer, "with a margin of error of 3%". This "margin of error" in effect came from the approximate 95% confidence interval (8.4) or, more likely, from the interval (8.6). The "margin of error" is the "plus or minus" value $\sqrt{1/n}$ shown in the interval (8.6). So we can work out, from the interval (8.6), how many individuals were in the sample that led to the estimate 52%, or 0.52. All we have to do is to equate $\sqrt{1/n}$ with the "margin of error" 0.03. We find from this that $n = 1111$. (Probably their sample size was about 1000, and with this value the "margin of error" is $\sqrt{1/1000} = 0.0316$, and this was approximated by $0.03 = 3\%$.)

5. All of the above discussion relates to an approximate 95% confidence interval for $\theta$. To obtain a 99% confidence interval, we start by comparing Eq. (6.24) with Eq. (6.15). This comparison implies that to obtain an approximate 99% confidence interval for $\theta$, we have to replace the 1.96 in the interval (8.4) by 2.576. This implies that an (approximate) 99% confidence interval for $\theta$ is

$$p - 2.576\sqrt{p(1-p)/n} \quad \text{to} \quad p + 2.576\sqrt{p(1-p)/n}. \tag{8.7}$$

If $0.3 < p < 0.7$, we can approximate this confidence interval by

$$p - 1.288\sqrt{1/n} \quad \text{to} \quad p + 1.288\sqrt{1/n} \tag{8.8}$$

instead of the interval (8.7).

*Example* This example is from the field of medical research. Suppose that an entirely new medicine is proposed for curing some illness. Beforehand, we know nothing about the properties of this medicine, and in particular we do not know the probability $\theta$ that it will cure someone of the illness involved. Therefore, $\theta$ is a parameter. We want to carry out a clinical trial to estimate $\theta$ and to assess the precision of our estimate.

Suppose now that we have conducted this clinical trial and have given the new medicine to 10,000 people with the illness and of these, 8716 were cured. Then the *estimate* of $\theta$ is $p = 8716/10,000 = 0.8716$. Next, since we want to be very precise in a medical context, we might prefer to use a 99% confidence interval instead of a 95% confidence interval. Since $p$ is outside the interval (0.3, 0.7), we prefer to use the interval (8.7) instead of the interval (8.8). Since $2.576\sqrt{p(1-p)/n} = 0.0086$, the interval (8.7) leads to a confidence interval from 0.8630 to 0.8802. To the level of accuracy appropriate from the data, we would say that we estimate the probability of a cure with this proposed medicine to be 0.87 and are about 99% certain that this probability is between 0.86 and 0.88.

6. The lengths of both confidence intervals (8.6) and (8.8) are proportional to $1/\sqrt{n}$. This means that if we want to be twice as accurate, we need four times the sample size and that if we want to be three times as accurate, we need nine times

the sample size, and so on. This often implies that a very large (and possibly expensive) sample is needed to meet a required high level of accuracy.

7. Often in research publications, the result of an estimation procedure is written as something like: "estimate $\pm$ some measure of precision of the estimate". Thus the result in the medical example above might be written as something like: "$\theta = 0.87 \pm 0.01$." This can be misleading because, for example, it is not indicated if this is a 95% or a 99% confidence interval.

## 8.3  Estimating the Mean $\mu$

### 8.3.1  The Estimate of $\mu$

Suppose that we wish to estimate the mean blood sugar level $\mu$ of diabetics. We take a random sample of $n$ diabetics and measure their blood sugar levels, getting the observed data values $x_1, x_2, \ldots, x_n$. It is natural to estimate the mean $\mu$ by the average $\bar{x}$ of these data values. What are the properties of this estimate? To answer these questions, we have to zig-zag backwards and forwards between probability theory and Statistics.

We start with probability theory and first think of the situation before we got the data. We think of the data values $x_1, x_2, \ldots, x_n$ as the observed values of $n$ $iid$ random variables $X_1, X_2, \ldots, X_n$, all having some probability density function with mean $\mu$ and variance $\sigma^2$, where the values of both $\mu$ and $\sigma^2$ are unknown to us. (The $iid$ assumption is discussed in Sect. 5.3.) Our aim is to estimate $\mu$ from the data and to assess the precision of the estimate.

We first consider the average $\bar{X}$ of the random variables $X_1, X_2, \ldots, X_n$. Equation (5.4) shows that the mean of $\bar{X}$ is $\mu$, so that $\bar{X}$ is an unbiased estimator of $\mu$. Thus $\bar{x}$ is an unbiased estimate of $\mu$. It is also the natural estimate of $\mu$. Therefore

$$\text{the estimate of } \mu \text{ is } \bar{x}. \tag{8.9}$$

In this procedure there are three separate and different things involved: the estimator $\bar{X}$, the estimate $\bar{x}$, and the quantity $\mu$ that is being estimated. All three are important. The importance of $\bar{X}$ is discussed in the following section.

### 8.3.2  The Precision of the Estimate of $\mu$

It is just as important to assess how precise $\bar{x}$ is as an estimate of $\mu$ as it is to give the estimate itself. This precision depends on the variance of $\bar{X}$. We know from Eq. (5.4) that the variance of $\bar{X}$ is $\sigma^2/n$, and even though we do not know the value of $\sigma^2$, this result is still useful to us. Next, the Central Limit Theorem shows that the probability distribution of $\bar{X}$ is approximately normal when $n$ is large, so that to a good approximation, we can use normal distribution theory. These facts lead us to an approximate 95% and an approximate 99% confidence interval for $\mu$, as discussed below.

Suppose first that we know the numerical value of $\sigma^2$. (In practice it is very unlikely that we would know this, but we will remove this assumption soon.) The Central Limit Theorem and the properties of the normal distribution show that, for large $n$, the approximation (6.37), repeated here for convenience, holds:

$$\text{Prob}\left(\mu - \frac{1.96\sigma}{\sqrt{n}} < \bar{X} < \mu + \frac{1.96\sigma}{\sqrt{n}}\right) \approx 0.95. \tag{8.10}$$

The inequalities (8.10) can be written in the equivalent "turned inside-out" form

$$\text{Prob}\left(\bar{X} - \frac{1.96\sigma}{\sqrt{n}} < \mu < \bar{X} + \frac{1.96\sigma}{\sqrt{n}}\right) \approx 0.95. \tag{8.11}$$

This leads to an approximate 95% *confidence interval* for $\mu$, given the data values $x_1, x_2, \ldots, x_n$, as

$$\bar{x} - \frac{1.96\sigma}{\sqrt{n}} \quad \text{to} \quad \bar{x} + \frac{1.96\sigma}{\sqrt{n}}. \tag{8.12}$$

If we knew the numerical value of $\sigma$, this interval would be valuable in providing a measure of precision of the estimate $\bar{x}$ of $\mu$. To be told that the estimate of a mean is 14.7 and that it is approximately 95% likely that the mean is between 14.3 and 15.1 is far more useful information than being told only that the estimate of a mean is 14.7.

The main problem with the confidence interval (8.12) is that, in practice, the standard deviation $\sigma$ is almost certainly unknown, so that this confidence interval is not immediately applicable. However, it is possible to estimate $\sigma^2$ from the data values $x_1, x_2, \ldots, x_n$. The following result is given without proof: the unbiased estimate $s^2$ of $\sigma^2$ found from the data values $x_1, x_2, \ldots, x_n$ is

$$s^2 = \frac{x_1^2 + x_2^2 + \cdots + x_n^2 - n(\bar{x})^2}{n - 1}. \tag{8.13}$$

Then we estimate $\sigma$ by $s$, the square root of $s^2$.

This leads from the interval (8.12) to the following approximate 95% confidence interval for $\mu$:

$$\bar{x} - \frac{1.96s}{\sqrt{n}} \quad \text{to} \quad \bar{x} + \frac{1.96s}{\sqrt{n}}. \tag{8.14}$$

Similarly, Eq. (6.24) implies that an approximate 99% confidence interval for $\mu$ is

$$\bar{x} - \frac{2.576s}{\sqrt{n}} \quad \text{to} \quad \bar{x} + \frac{2.576s}{\sqrt{n}}. \tag{8.15}$$

Both confidence intervals (8.14) and (8.15) can be computed from the data. However, both are inexact since they take no account of the fact that they were obtained by replacing an unknown standard deviation $\sigma$ by the estimate $s$. This matter will be addressed in Sect. 13.6, where more precise confidence intervals are derived.

*Example* This example refers to the "full sun" data in Table (1.1). We wish to estimate $\mu$, the mean biomass in containers exposed to full sun and to find two limits between which we are approximately 95% certain that $\mu$ lies. We view these data values as the realized values of 11 *iid* random variables $X_1, \ldots, X_{11}$, each having mean $\mu$ and variance $\sigma^2$.

Given the data values in Table (1.1), we calculate the unbiased estimate of $\mu$ by the average $\bar{x}$, which is

$$\frac{1903 + 1935 + \cdots + 1714}{11} = 1877.6364. \tag{8.16}$$

In R, we can calculate the data average using the mean() function. However, we must remember this is only an *estimate* of the mean using the data average and not a calculation.

```
x <- c(1903, 1935, 1910, 2096, 2008, 1961, 2060, 1644, 1612,
  1811, 1714)
xbar <- mean(x)
xbar
```

To arrive at the approximate 95% confidence interval (8.14) for $\mu$, we first have to calculate $s^2$, the unbiased estimate of $\sigma^2$. This estimate is, from Eq. (8.13),

$$\frac{(1903)^2 + (1935)^2 + \cdots + (1714)^2 - 11(1877.6364)^2}{10} = 26,623.05 \tag{8.17}$$

Following interval (8.14), these calculations lead to an approximate 95% confidence interval for $\mu$ as

$$1877.64 - \frac{1.96\sqrt{26,623.05}}{\sqrt{11}} \quad \text{to} \quad 1877.64 + \frac{1.96\sqrt{26,623.05}}{\sqrt{11}}, \tag{8.18}$$

that is, from 1781.21 to 1974.06.

In R, we could have directly estimated $\sigma$ with sd() and arrived at the same answer:

```
s <- sd(x)
n <- length(x)
xbar - 1.96 * s / sqrt(n)
xbar + 1.96 * s / sqrt(n)
```

Since the various measured levels are rounded to whole numbers, it is not appropriate to be more accurate than this in our final statement, which is: "we estimate the mean biomass to be 1878 and we are about 95% certain that it is between 1781 and 1974."

The confidence interval deriving from (8.18) is sometimes written in the form $\mu = 1878 \pm 96$. This can be misleading because, for example, it is not indicated if this is a 95% or a 99% confidence interval. Also, it is not the best way to present the conclusion.

As stated below Eq. (8.15), any confidence interval deriving from Eq. (8.14) is inexact. Therefore, the confidence interval below (8.18) is inexact. A more exact confidence interval is given in Sect. 13.6.

*Notes on the Confidence Intervals (8.14) and (8.15)*

1. The fact that the standard deviation estimate $s$ occurs in both confidence intervals (8.14) and (8.15) shows that although these confidence intervals concern a mean, they cannot be calculated without considering the concepts of a variance and a standard deviation.
2. Why do we have $n - 1$ in the denominator of the formula (8.13) for $s^2$ and not $n$? This question leads to the concept of "degrees of freedom", which will be discussed later.
3. *The effect of changing the sample size.* Consider two investigators both interested in the blood sugar levels of diabetics. Suppose that $n = 10$ for the first investigator (i.e. her sample size was 10). Suppose that for the second investigator, $n = 40$ (i.e. his sample size was 40). The two investigators will estimate $\mu$ by their respective values of $\bar{x}$. Since both are unbiased estimates of $\mu$, they should be reasonably close to each other. Similarly, their respective estimates of $\sigma^2$ should be reasonably close to each other, since both are unbiased estimates of $\sigma^2$.

   On the other hand, the length of the confidence interval for $\mu$ for the second investigator will be about half that of the first investigator, since he will have a $\sqrt{40}$ involved in the denominator in the calculation of the width of his confidence interval, whereas the first investigator has $\sqrt{10}$ in the denominator in the calculation of the width of her confidence interval (see the interval (8.14)). Since $1/\sqrt{40}$ is half of $1/\sqrt{10}$, the conclusion above follows. This leads to the next point.
4. As with the estimation of a binomial parameter $\theta$, when estimating a mean, to be twice as accurate, we need four times the sample size and to be three times as accurate, we need nine times the sample size and so on. This follows from the fact that the length of the confidence interval (8.14) is $3.92s/\sqrt{n}$. The fact that

there is a $\sqrt{n}$ in the denominator and not an $n$ explains this phenomenon. This is why research is often expensive: to get very accurate estimates, one often needs very large sample sizes.

5. One particular case of Eq. (8.13) arises when $n = 1$, that is, we only have one data value $x_1$. In this case, $\bar{x}$ is simply $x_1$ and Eq. (8.13) reduces to 0/0. That ratio is mathematically meaningless and in effect states that it is impossible to estimate a variance given only one data value.

6. How large a sample size do we need before we do our experiment in order to get some desired degree of precision of the estimate of the mean $\mu$? One cannot answer this question in advance, since the precision of the estimate depends on the value of $\sigma^2$, which is unknown. Often, one runs a pilot experiment to estimate $\sigma^2$, and from this, one can get a good idea of what sample size is needed to get the required level of precision, using intervals (8.14) and (8.15).

7. The quantity $s/\sqrt{n}$ is often called "the standard error of the mean". More pedantically, it should be: "the estimated standard deviation of the estimator of the mean", and is used as a shorthand for this more precise statement.

## 8.4 Estimating the Difference Between Two Binomial Parameters $\theta_1 - \theta_2$

We start with an example. We are interested in a possible difference between middle- and high-schoolers in their amount of sleep. We address this question from a statistical point of view as follows.

Let $\theta_1$ be the (unknown) probability that a middle-schooler does not get enough sleep and let $\theta_2$ be the (unknown) probability that a high-schooler does not get enough sleep. We are interested in estimating the difference $\theta_1 - \theta_2$ and in obtaining an approximate 95% confidence interval for $\theta_1 - \theta_2$. We will do this by taking a sample of $n$ middle-schoolers and $m$ high-schoolers and find out for each person whether he or she gets enough sleep.

### 8.4.1 The Estimate of $\theta_1 - \theta_2$

Suppose that $x$ middle-schoolers in the sample of the $n$ middle-schoolers do not get enough sleep and $y$ high-schoolers in the sample of $m$ high-schoolers do not get enough sleep. We would estimate $\theta_1$ by $p_1 = x/n$ and would estimate $\theta_2$ by $p_2 = y/m$. It would be natural to estimate $\theta_1 - \theta_2$ by the difference $d = p_1 - p_2$. What are the properties of this estimate?

Before we take the sample, the number $X$ of middle-schoolers in the sample who will not get enough sleep is a random variable, and similarly, the number $Y$ of high-schoolers in the sample who will not get enough sleep is a random variable. Therefore, before we take our sample, $P_1 = X/n$, the proportion of middle-schoolers who will not get enough sleep and $P_2 = Y/m$, the proportion of high-schoolers who will not get enough sleep, are both random variables. The properties of the *estimate* $d = p_1 - p_2$ depend on the properties of the random variable *estimator* $D = P_1 - P_2$. What are these?

$P_1 - P_2$ is the difference between two proportions, so we have to use the probability theory discussed in Sect. 5.6. This shows that the mean of $P_1 - P_2$ is $\theta_1 - \theta_2$. Thus $P_1 - P_2$ is an unbiased estimator of $\theta_1 - \theta_2$ and correspondingly $p_1 - p_2$ is an unbiased estimate of $\theta_1 - \theta_2$. This is why we use $p_1 - p_2$ to estimate $\theta_1 - \theta_2$. Explicitly,

$$\text{the estimate of } \theta_1 - \theta_2 \text{ is } p_1 - p_2. \tag{8.19}$$

How precise is this estimate? We address this question in the next section.

### 8.4.2   The Precision of the Estimate of $\theta_1 - \theta_2$

The precision of the estimate $p_1 - p_2$ depends on the variance of the estimator $P_1 - P_2$, which is given by the second equation in (5.10). Using Eq. (6.26) applied to the random variable $P_1 - P_2$, we obtain

$$\text{Prob}(\theta_1 - \theta_2 - 1.96\sqrt{\theta_1(1-\theta_1)/n + \theta_2(1-\theta_2)/m} < P_1 - P_2$$
$$< \theta_1 - \theta_2 + 1.96\sqrt{\theta_1(1-\theta_1)/n + \theta_2(1-\theta_2)/m}) \approx 0.95. \tag{8.20}$$

Using the same sort of argument that led to Eq. (8.2), we could then say

$$\text{Prob}(P_1 - P_2 - 1.96\sqrt{\theta_1(1-\theta_1)/n + \theta_2(1-\theta_2)/m} < \theta_1 - \theta_2$$
$$< P_1 - P_2 + 1.96\sqrt{\theta_1(1-\theta_1)/n + \theta_2(1-\theta_2)/m}) \approx 0.95. \tag{8.21}$$

Once we have our data and calculate $p_1$ and $p_2$, we plug them in to Eq. (8.21) to form the following approximate 95% confidence interval for $\theta_1 - \theta_2$:

$$p_1 - p_2 - 1.96\sqrt{\theta_1(1-\theta_1)/n + \theta_2(1-\theta_2)/m} \quad \text{to}$$
$$p_1 - p_2 + 1.96\sqrt{\theta_1(1-\theta_1)/n + \theta_2(1-\theta_2)/m}.$$

This is of no immediate value since we do not know the values of $\theta_1$ and $\theta_2$, but we can replace them with their estimates $p_1$ and $p_2$ in the expression

$1.96\sqrt{\theta_1(1-\theta_1)/n + \theta_2(1-\theta_2)/m}$. This leads to the following (approximate) 95% confidence interval for $\theta_1 - \theta_2$:

$$p_1 - p_2 - 1.96\sqrt{p_1(1-p_1)/n + p_2(1-p_2)/m} \quad \text{to}$$

$$p_1 - p_2 + 1.96\sqrt{p_1(1-p_1)/n + p_2(1-p_2)/m}. \tag{8.22}$$

This formula is rather clumsy, so if $0.3 \leq p_1, p_2 \leq 0.7$, we can use the same approximation that we did when estimating a single binomial parameter (see the discussion leading to the interval (8.6)), and approximate both $p_1(1-p_1)$ and $p_2(1-p_2)$ by $\frac{1}{4}$. We also approximate 1.96 by 2. Since $\sqrt{1/4} = 1/2$, we arrive at the following approximate confidence interval for $\theta_1 - \theta_2$ if $0.3 \leq p_1, p_2 \leq 0.7$:

$$p_1 - p_2 - \sqrt{\frac{1}{n} + \frac{1}{m}} \quad \text{to} \quad p_1 - p_2 + \sqrt{\frac{1}{n} + \frac{1}{m}}. \tag{8.23}$$

This approximate confidence interval is easy to remember and can be used instead of the more clumsy formula (8.22) if $p_1$ and $p_2$ are both between 0.3 and 0.7. The interval (8.23) is conservative because it is wider than the interval (8.22).

*Example* Suppose that we interview $n = 300$ middle-schoolers and $m = 200$ high-schoolers about their sleep durations. We find that 173 of the middle-schoolers do not get enough sleep and 135 of the high-schoolers do not get enough sleep. We therefore estimate $\theta_1$ by $p_1 = 173/300 \approx 0.577$ and estimate $\theta_2$ by $p_2 = 135/200 = 0.675$. From this, we estimate $\theta_1 - \theta_2$ by $0.577 - 0.675 = -0.098$. Since both $p_1$ and $p_2$ are between 0.3 and 0.7, we can use interval (8.23) to say that we are approximately 95% certain that the difference of the two probabilities $\theta_1$ and $\theta_2$ is between

$$-0.098 - \sqrt{\frac{1}{300} + \frac{1}{200}} = -0.098 - 0.091 = -0.189$$

and

$$-0.098 + \sqrt{\frac{1}{300} + \frac{1}{200}} = -0.098 + 0.091 = -0.007.$$

The value 0.091 given in this calculation is sometimes called the "margin of error".

A 99% confidence interval for $\theta_1 - \theta_2$ parallel to the confidence interval for a single binomial parameter is

$$p_1 - p_2 - 2.576\sqrt{p_1(1-p_1)/n + p_2(1-p_2)/m} \quad \text{to}$$

$$p_1 - p_2 + 2.576\sqrt{p_1(1-p_1)/n + p_2(1-p_2)/m}, \tag{8.24}$$

which can be approximated by

$$p_1 - p_2 - 1.288\sqrt{\frac{1}{n} + \frac{1}{m}} \quad \text{to} \quad p_1 - p_2 + 1.288\sqrt{\frac{1}{n} + \frac{1}{m}}. \tag{8.25}$$

if $0.3 < p_1, p_2 < 0.7$.

*Notes on the Estimation of $\theta_1 - \theta_2$*

1. Most of the notes concerning the estimation of a single binomial parameter continue to apply for estimating the difference between two binomial parameters. For example, we have already used the procedure leading to interval (8.6) by replacing interval (8.22) by interval (8.23) when appropriate.

2. The width of the confidence interval prescribed by (8.23), namely $2\sqrt{\frac{1}{n} + \frac{1}{m}}$, introduces an important point concerning the two sample sizes $n$ and $m$. Suppose, for example, that $n = 1000$ and that $m = 10$. Then the width of the confidence interval (8.23) is about 0.69. Given this, we have essentially no good estimate of the difference $\theta_1 - \theta_2$. Even if $n = 1,000,000$ and $m = 10$, the width of the confidence interval is still about 0.69. What makes the most impact is the size of the smaller sample. Good practice is to make $n$ and $m$ as close to each other as possible. Making them equal to each other minimizes the width of the confidence interval for a given total number of people in the sample.

## 8.5   Estimating the Difference Between Two Means $\mu_1 - \mu_2$

As in the previous section, we start with an example. We define the mean blood pressure of women to be $\mu_1$ and the mean blood pressure of men to be $\mu_2$. Our aim is to estimate $\mu_1 - \mu_2$ and to find an approximate 95% confidence interval for $\mu_1 - \mu_2$.

To do this, we plan to measure the blood pressures of a sample of $n$ women and measure the blood pressures of a sample of $m$ men. Before the experiment, the blood pressures of the $n$ women are random variables $X_{11}, X_{12} \ldots X_{1n}$, which we assume to be $iid$, each with mean $\mu_1$ and variance $\sigma_1^2$. Similarly, the blood pressures of the $m$ men are random variables $X_{21}, X_{22} \ldots X_{2m}$, which we assume to be $iid$, each with mean $\mu_2$ and variance $\sigma_2^2$. (The first suffix 1 on the $X$'s indicates "woman" and the second suffix indicates which woman. Similarly, the first suffix 2 on the $X$'s indicates "man" and the second suffix indicates which man.)

### 8.5.1 The Estimate of $\mu_1 - \mu_2$

We now do the experiment. Suppose that the blood pressures of the $n$ women in the sample are $x_{11}, x_{12} \ldots x_{1n}$ and that the blood pressures of the $m$ men in the sample are $x_{21}, x_{22} \ldots x_{2m}$.

As expected, we estimate the mean blood pressure for women by $\bar{x}_1 = \frac{1}{n}(x_{11} + x_{12} + \cdots + x_{1n})$, the average of the blood pressures of the $n$ women in the sample, and similarly, we estimate the mean blood pressure for men by $\bar{x}_2 = \frac{1}{m}(x_{21} + x_{22} + \cdots + x_{2m})$, the average of the blood pressures of the $m$ men in the sample. We would then naturally estimate $\mu_1 - \mu_2$ by $\bar{x}_1 - \bar{x}_2$. Explicitly,

$$\text{the estimate of } \mu_1 - \mu_2 \text{ is } \bar{x}_1 - \bar{x}_2. \tag{8.26}$$

How precise is this estimate? This is discussed in the next section.

### 8.5.2 The Precision of the Estimate of $\mu_1 - \mu_2$

The properties of this estimate (8.26) depend on the properties of the corresponding estimator $\bar{X}_1 - \bar{X}_2$, where $\bar{X}_1 = \frac{1}{n}(X_{11} + X_{12} + \cdots + X_{1n})$ and $\bar{X}_2 = \frac{1}{m}(X_{21} + X_{22} + \cdots + X_{2m})$. The precision of the estimate (8.26) depends on the variance of the random variable $\bar{X}_1 - \bar{X}_2$. This is given in Eq. (5.7). Using Eq. (6.26) as applied to the random variable $\bar{X}_1 - \bar{X}_2$, we get

$$\text{Prob}\left(\mu_1 - \mu_2 - 1.96\sqrt{\sigma_1^2/n + \sigma_2^2/m} \leq \bar{X}_1 - \bar{X}_2 \leq \mu_1 - \mu_2\right.$$

$$\left. + 1.96\sqrt{\sigma_1^2/n + \sigma_2^2/m}\right) \approx 0.95. \tag{8.27}$$

Using the same argument that led from Eq. (8.10) to interval (8.11), we get

$$\text{Prob}\left(\bar{X}_1 - \bar{X}_2 - 1.96\sqrt{\sigma_1^2/n + \sigma_2^2/m} \leq \mu_1 - \mu_2 \leq \bar{X}_1 - \bar{X}_2\right.$$

$$\left. + 1.96\sqrt{\sigma_1^2/n + \sigma_2^2/m}\right) \approx 0.95. \tag{8.28}$$

If we knew the values of $\sigma_1^2$ and $\sigma_2^2$, then once we collected our data, we would have an approximate 95% confidence interval for $\mu_1 - \mu_2$ as

$$\bar{x}_1 - \bar{x}_2 - 1.96\sqrt{\frac{\sigma_1^2}{n} + \frac{\sigma_2^2}{m}} \quad \text{to} \quad \bar{x}_1 - \bar{x}_2 + 1.96\sqrt{\frac{\sigma_1^2}{n} + \frac{\sigma_2^2}{m}}. \tag{8.29}$$

This is of no immediate value since in practice it is very unlikely that we would know the values of $\sigma_1^2$ or $\sigma_2^2$, so we will have to estimate them from the data. From Eq. (8.13), we estimate $\sigma_1^2$ by

$$s_1^2 = \frac{x_{11}^2 + x_{12}^2 + \cdots + x_{1n}^2 - n(\bar{x}_1)^2}{n - 1} \tag{8.30}$$

and estimate $\sigma_2^2$ by

$$s_2^2 = \frac{x_{21}^2 + x_{22}^2 + \cdots + x_{2m}^2 - m(\bar{x}_2)^2}{m - 1}. \tag{8.31}$$

Thus we estimate $\frac{\sigma_1^2}{n} + \frac{\sigma_2^2}{m}$ by $\frac{s_1^2}{n} + \frac{s_2^2}{m}$. This leads, after we do our experiment and get our data, to the following approximate 95% confidence interval for $\mu_1 - \mu_2$ deriving from Eq. (8.28):

$$\bar{x}_1 - \bar{x}_2 - 1.96\sqrt{\frac{s_1^2}{n} + \frac{s_2^2}{m}} \quad \text{to} \quad \bar{x}_1 - \bar{x}_2 + 1.96\sqrt{\frac{s_1^2}{n} + \frac{s_2^2}{m}}. \tag{8.32}$$

A simple convenient rule of thumb approximation to the confidence interval in (8.32) is

$$\bar{x}_1 - \bar{x}_2 - 2\sqrt{\frac{s_1^2}{n} + \frac{s_2^2}{m}} \quad \text{to} \quad \bar{x}_1 - \bar{x}_2 + 2\sqrt{\frac{s_1^2}{n} + \frac{s_2^2}{m}}. \tag{8.33}$$

The approximate 99% confidence interval for $\mu_1 - \mu_2$ is:

$$\bar{x}_1 - \bar{x}_2 - 2.576\sqrt{\frac{s_1^2}{n} + \frac{s_2^2}{m}} \quad \text{to} \quad \bar{x}_1 - \bar{x}_2 + 2.576\sqrt{\frac{s_1^2}{n} + \frac{s_2^2}{m}}. \tag{8.34}$$

Both confidence intervals (8.32) and (8.34) are inexact since they take no account of the fact that they were obtained by replacing unknown variances $\sigma_1^2$ and $\sigma_2^2$ by the estimates $s_1^2$ and $s_2^2$. This matter will be addressed in Sect. 13.6, where more precise confidence intervals are derived.

*Example* This example refers to the data in Table (1.1). The "full sun" assumptions and data were discussed in Sect. 8.3.2. Changing the notation from that in Sect. 8.3.2, we define $\mu_1$ as the mean biomass in containers exposed to full sun and denote the average of the biomass data values in containers exposed to full sun by $\bar{x}_1$ and the estimate of $\sigma^2$ in those containers by $s_1^2$.

In parallel with the assumptions made for the full sun data, we view the "50% shade" data values as the realized values of 11 *iid* random variables each having mean $\mu_2$ and variance $\sigma_2^2$. We denote the average of the biomass data values in containers exposed to 50% shade by $\bar{x}_2$ and the estimate of $\sigma^2$ in those containers by $s_2^2$.

The full sun estimate $\bar{x}_1$ of $\mu_1$ given in (8.16) is 1877.64 and the full sun estimate $s_1^2$ of $\sigma^2$ given in (8.17) is 26,623.05. The average $\bar{x}_2$ of the 50% shade data values is 1765.27 and the 50% shade estimate $s_2^2$ of $\sigma^2$ is 21,284.42.

From these values, the estimate of $\mu_1 - \mu_2$ is 112.37 and the approximate 95% confidence interval for $\mu_1 - \mu_2$ derived from (8.32) is

$$112.37 - 1.96\sqrt{\frac{26,623.05}{11} + \frac{21,284.42}{11}} \quad \text{to}$$

$$112.37 + 1.96\sqrt{\frac{26,623.05}{11} + \frac{21,284.42}{11}}, \tag{8.35}$$

that is, from $-16.98$ to $241.72$.

As stated below Eq. (8.34), any confidence interval deriving from Eq. (8.32) is inexact. Therefore, the confidence interval below (8.35) is inexact. A more exact confidence interval is given in Sect. 13.6.

*Note on Estimating the Difference Between Two Means* Most of the notes concerning the estimation of one mean in Sect. 8.3 continue to apply for the case of estimating the difference between two means. However, a more nuanced note than Note 3 is needed, and this is similar to Note 2 in Sect. 8.4. The width of the confidence intervals (8.32) and (8.34) depends on both $m$ and $n$. If $m = 10$ and $n = 1000$, the width is almost the same as that when $m = 10$ and $n = 10,000$. In other words, it is not wise to have a large imbalance of the two sample sizes, and equal or approximately equal sample sizes are desirable.

A flow-chart of the "estimation and confidence intervals" part of this book is given on the following page to show the various topics covered in perspective.

# Flowchart: Estimation and Confidence Intervals

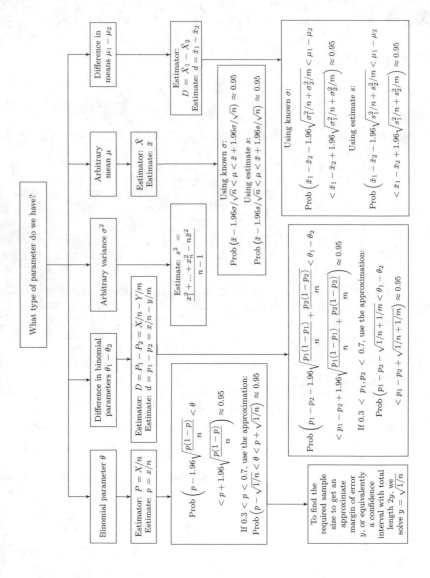

## 8.6 Regression

How does one thing depend on another? How does the gross national product of a country depend on the number of people in full-time employment? How does the reaction time of a person to some stimulus depend on the amount of sleep deprivation administered to that person? How does the growth height of a plant in a greenhouse depend on the amount of water that we give the plant during the growing period? Many practical questions are of the "how does this depend on that?" type. We will use the plant and water example to demonstrate the statistical approach to this sort of question.

These questions are answered by the technique of regression. Regression problems can be quite complicated, so we consider here only one case of regression: How does some random non-controllable quantity $Y$ depend on some non-random controllable quantity $x$? In the plant growth height/water example, the growth height of any plant is a random variable: we do not know, before the experiment, what value it will take. On the other hand, the amount of water that we give any plant is non-random, since it is decided in advance by us.

Notice two things about the notation. The first derives from the fact that we will later plot the data values in the standard $x$–$y$ plane. By convention, the random quantity is plotted on the $y$ axis and the non-random quantity on the $x$ axis. This is why we switched the notation for the random variable from $X$ to $Y$ in the regression context, since in this context $Y$ is the random variable.

Second, we denote the random quantity (the growth height of any plant) in upper case: see $Y$ above. This is in accordance with the notational convention of denoting random variables in upper case. There are many factors that we do not know about, such as the fertility of the soil surrounding each plant, the amount of sunlight that each plant will get, and so on, which imply that $Y$ is a random variable. Second, we denote the controllable non-random quantity (the amount of water) in lower case: see $x$ above. This is in accordance with the notational convention of denoting a non-random quantity in lower case.

We first think of the situation *before* the experiment, and consider some plant to which we plan to give $x$ units of water. At this stage, the eventual growth height $Y$ of this plant is a random variable. We make the assumption that the mean of $Y$ depends on $x$ according to the formula

$$\text{mean of } Y = \alpha + \beta x, \tag{8.36}$$

where $\alpha$ and $\beta$ (the Greek letters "alpha" and "beta") are parameters, that is, quantities whose value we do not know. We also assume that

$$\text{variance of } Y = \sigma^2, \tag{8.37}$$

where $\sigma^2$ is another parameter whose value we do not know. The fact that $Y$ has a variance derives from the fact that it is a random variable.

Equations (8.36) and (8.37) embody the assumptions that we make in the regression procedure described in this book. They are quite strong assumptions and in a given practical situation, they might not be reasonable. There are objective procedures addressing this point which are not discussed in this book; a reasonable subjective procedure will be discussed below.

Before discussing regression further, we review some basic algebra and geometry. Equation (8.36) is similar to the algebraic equation $y = a + bx$ that defines a geometric line in the $x$-$y$ plane, and the regression procedure deriving from Eq. (8.36) is called linear regression. The interpretation of $a$ in the equation $y = a + bx$ is that it is the intercept of this line on the $y$ axis. The interpretation of $b$ in the equation $y = a + bx$ is that it is the slope of the line. If $b = 0$, the line is horizontal and the values of $y$ for all points on the line are all the same, whatever the value of $x$.

Returning to regression, once the experiment is finished, we wish to estimate the numerical values of the three parameters $\alpha$, $\beta$ and $\sigma^2$. Of these three parameters, the most important is $\beta$. This is because Eq. (8.36) implies that if $\beta \neq 0$, the mean growth height of a plant depends on $x$, the amount of water given to it, and thus it is important to estimate $\beta$ and to get some idea of the precision of the estimate.

Now to the details of the experiment. We plan to use some pre-determined number $n$ of plants in our greenhouse experiment, and will give the plants respectively $x_1, x_2, \ldots, x_n$ units of water. These $x$ values are chosen in advance by us: they are therefore not random variables and this is why $x_1, x_2, \ldots, x_n$ are written in lower case. The $x$ values do not have to all be different from each other, but it is essential that they are not all equal. Indeed, there is a strategy question about how we choose the values of $x_1, x_2, \ldots, x_n$ which is discussed later.

Before we conduct the experiment, we conceptualize about the growth heights $Y_1, Y_2, \ldots, Y_n$ of the $n$ plants. $Y_1$ corresponds to the plant getting $x_1$ units of water, $Y_2$ corresponds to the plant getting $x_2$ units of water, and so on. These are all random variables: we do not know in advance of doing the experiment what values they will take. Then from Eq. (8.36), the mean of $Y_1$ is $\alpha + \beta x_1$, the mean of $Y_2$ is $\alpha + \beta x_2$, and so on. From Eq. (8.37), the variance of $Y_1$ is $\sigma^2$, the variance of $Y_2$ is also $\sigma^2$, and so on. We assume that the various $Y_i$ values are independent, a perhaps debatable assumption. However, the various $Y_i$ values are clearly not assumed to be identically distributed, since if, for example, $x_i \neq x_j$, that is, the amount of water to be given to plant $i$ differs from that to be given to plant $j$, the means of $Y_i$ and $Y_j$ are different if $\beta \neq 0$.

The fact that the mean of $Y$ is assumed to be a linear function of $x$ implies that once we have our data, they should, under this assumption, approximately lie on a straight line in the $x$-$y$ plane. We do not expect them to lie exactly on a straight line, since we can expect random deviations from a straight line because each $Y_i$ is a random variable. The fact that deviations of the data values from a straight line are to be expected is captured by the concept of the variance $\sigma^2$. The larger this variance is, the larger these deviations from a straight line would tend to be, even if the assumption in (8.36) is correct. The fact that the variance of $Y$ is assumed to be $\sigma^2$ for all $x$ implies that the amount of scatter around the straight line should not materially change as $x$ changes.

The discussion so far refers to the situation before we conduct our experiment. We now do the experiment and obtain observed growth heights $y_1, y_2, \ldots, y_n$, where the plant getting $x_i$ units of water had growth height $y_i$. The collection of pairs $(x_1, y_1), \ldots, (x_n, y_n)$ form our data. We first plot these data values on a graph in the $x$-$y$ plane. If the data points are more or less on a straight line with consistent scatter, we can go ahead with the analysis, since then the assumption embodied in Eq. (8.36) appears to be reasonable. If they are clearly not close to being on a straight line, then we should not proceed with the analysis described below, since in that case, the assumption embodied in Eq. (8.36) appears to be incorrect. This is the reasonable subjective procedure mentioned above, and it relies only on judgment and common sense. There are objective procedures for assessing whether these data are more or less reasonably close to being on a straight line and for dealing with data that are not reasonably close to being on a straight line, but they are not considered in this book. So from now on, we assume that our common sense subjective procedure leads to the view that the data are reasonably close to being on a straight line.

Our first aim is to use the data to estimate $\alpha$, $\beta$ and $\sigma^2$. To do this, we first have to calculate five auxiliary quantities. These are

$$\bar{x} = \frac{x_1 + x_2 + \ldots + x_n}{n}, \qquad \bar{y} = \frac{y_1 + y_2 + \ldots + y_n}{n}, \tag{8.38}$$

$$S_{xx} = (x_1 - \bar{x})^2 + (x_2 - \bar{x})^2 + \ldots + (x_n - \bar{x})^2, \tag{8.39}$$

$$S_{yy} = (y_1 - \bar{y})^2 + (y_2 - \bar{y})^2 + \ldots + (y_n - \bar{y})^2, \tag{8.40}$$

$$S_{xy} = (x_1 - \bar{x})(y_1 - \bar{y}) + (x_2 - \bar{x})(y_2 - \bar{y}) + \ldots + (x_n - \bar{x})(y_n - \bar{y}). \tag{8.41}$$

The latter equations are written more concisely as

$$S_{xx} = \sum_{i=1}^{n} (x_i - \bar{x})^2, \tag{8.42}$$

$$S_{yy} = \sum_{i=1}^{n} (y_i - \bar{y})^2, \tag{8.43}$$

$$S_{xy} = \sum_{i=1}^{n} (x_i - \bar{x})(y_i - \bar{y}). \tag{8.44}$$

Equations (8.39), (8.40) and (8.41) are often written respectively as the equivalent formulas

$$s_{xx} = x_1^2 + x_2^2 + \ldots + x_n^2 - n\bar{x}^2,$$                                  (8.45)

$$s_{yy} = y_1^2 + y_2^2 + \ldots + y_n^2 - n\bar{y}^2,$$                                  (8.46)

$$s_{xy} = x_1 y_1 + x_2 y_2 + \ldots + x_n y_n - n\bar{x}\,\bar{y}.$$                     (8.47)

The derivation of the unbiased estimates of $\beta$, $\alpha$ and $\sigma^2$ found from these auxiliary quantities is complicated, so only the formulas for the estimates are given, namely: The estimate of $\beta$ is $b$, defined by

$$b = s_{xy}/s_{xx}.$$                                                                    (8.48)

The estimate of $\alpha$ is $a$, defined by

$$a = \bar{y} - b\bar{x}.$$                                                               (8.49)

The estimate of $\sigma^2$ is $s_r^2$, defined by

$$s_r^2 = (s_{yy} - b^2 s_{xx})/(n-2).$$                                                  (8.50)

The suffix "$r$" on $s_r^2$ stands for "regression": the formula (8.50) for $s_r^2$ differs from the formula (8.13) for $s^2$.

Although $b$ is an unbiased estimate of $\beta$, it is still necessary to ask how precise it is. Again, the theory is complicated and the eventual conclusion is that the approximate 95% confidence interval for $\beta$ is

$$b - \frac{1.96 s_r}{\sqrt{s_{xx}}} \quad \text{to} \quad b + \frac{1.96 s_r}{\sqrt{s_{xx}}}.$$   (8.51)

Clearly, the factor 1.96 comes from the normal distribution chart. The factor $s_r/\sqrt{s_{xx}}$ derives from theory that is not given here.

Similarly, the approximate 99% confidence interval for $\beta$ is

$$b - \frac{2.576 s_r}{\sqrt{s_{xx}}} \quad \text{to} \quad b + \frac{2.576 s_r}{\sqrt{s_{xx}}}.$$   (8.52)

Both confidence intervals (8.51) and (8.52) are inexact since they take no account of the fact that they were obtained by replacing an unknown standard deviation $\sigma$ by the estimate $s_r$. This matter will be addressed in Sect. 13.6, where more precise confidence intervals are derived.

An approximate rule of thumb 95% confidence interval is found by replacing (8.51) by

$$b - \frac{2s_r}{\sqrt{s_{xx}}} \quad \text{to} \quad b + \frac{2s_r}{\sqrt{s_{xx}}}. \tag{8.53}$$

In Sect. 13.6, it will be shown that the confidence interval (8.53) is often more precise than is the confidence interval (8.51).

*Example* We have $n = 12$ plants to which we gave varying amounts of water (in coded units). After the experiment, we obtained the following data:

| Plant number | 1 | 2 | 3 | 4 | 5 | 6 | 7 | 8 | 9 | 10 | 11 | 12 |
|---|---|---|---|---|---|---|---|---|---|---|---|---|
| Amount of water | 16 | 16 | 16 | 18 | 18 | 20 | 22 | 24 | 24 | 26 | 26 | 26 |
| Growth height | 76.2 | 77.1 | 75.7 | 78.1 | 77.8 | 79.2 | 80.2 | 82.5 | 80.7 | 83.1 | 82.2 | 83.6 |

In Fig. 8.1, we see that the points fall more or less along a straight line with essentially the same amount of scatter for varying values of $x$, implying that the linearity and constant variance assumptions are valid.

From the data we compute $\bar{x} = 21$ and $\bar{y} = 79.7$. From the definitions of $s_{xx}$, $s_{xy}$ and $s_{yy}$, we find that $s_{xx} = 188$, $s_{yy} = 83.54$ and $s_{xy} = 122.4$.

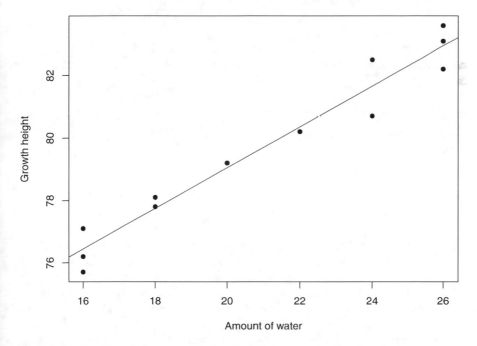

**Fig. 8.1** The data from the plant growth example with the regression line plotted

The estimate $b$ of $\beta$ is $s_{xy}/s_{xx} = 122.4/188 = 0.6511$. This is given to 4 decimal place accuracy so as to not accumulate too much rounding error in subsequent calculations. As the growth heights are given to three significant figures, we are only justified in presenting our estimates to two significant figures. In the final presentation of the results, we would thus write $b = 0.65$.

Next, the estimate $a$ of $\alpha$ is $\bar{y} - b\bar{x} = 79.7 - (0.6511 \times 21) = 66.0277$, given as $a = 66$ in a final presentation.

To find these estimates in R, one option is to use the `lm()` function in R, specifying that our regression is of y on x with the $\tilde{}$ symbol. Printing the object returned by this function will show the estimates of the coefficients for both $\alpha$ and $\beta$.

```
x <- c(16, 16, 16, 18, 18, 20, 22, 24, 24, 26, 26, 26)
y <- c(76.2, 77.1, 75.7, 78.1, 77.8, 79.2, 80.2, 82.5, 80.7, 83.1, 82.2,
83.6)
plot(y ~ x, xlab = "Amount of water", ylab = "Growth height", pch = 16)
model <- lm(y ~ x)
abline(model)   # Add the regression line to the plot
model
model$coefficients["x"] # One way of extracting the value of b
model$coefficients["(Intercept)"] # One way of extracting the value of a
```

The estimate $s_r^2$ of $\sigma^2$ is $\frac{83.54-(0.6511)^2(188)}{10} = 0.3850$. This value, together with (8.51), shows that the approximate 95% confidence interval for $\beta$ is

$$0.65 - \frac{1.96\sqrt{0.3850}}{\sqrt{188}} \quad \text{to} \quad 0.65 + \frac{1.96\sqrt{0.3850}}{\sqrt{188}}, \tag{8.54}$$

that is, 0.56–0.74 (to the appropriate level of accuracy).

In R, we can get this confidence interval with:

```
modelsummary <- summary(model)
model$coefficients["x"] - 1.96 * modelsummary$coefficients["x", "Std. Error"]
model$coefficients["x"] + 1.96 * modelsummary$coefficients["x", "Std. Error"]
```

Alternatively,     we     can     get     this     interval     in     R     with `confint.default(model, parm = "x")`.

*Notes on Regression*

1. The suffix "$r$" in the estimate $s_r^2$ in (8.50) indicates that this is the regression estimate of $\sigma^2$. This variance estimate formula is applicable only in the regression context.

2. The approximate 95% confidence interval for $\beta$ just given introduces a strategy concept into our choice of the values $x_1, x_2, \ldots, x_n$, the amounts of water that we plan to put on the various plants. The values given in interval (8.51) show that the width of this confidence interval is proportional to $1/\sqrt{s_{xx}}$. Thus the larger we make $\sqrt{s_{xx}}$, the shorter the length of this confidence interval will be and the more precise we can expect $b$ to be as an estimate of $\beta$. We can make $\sqrt{s_{xx}}$ large by spreading the $x$ values as far away from their average as we reasonably can (see Eq. (8.39)). There will normally be a range of $x$ values which is of interest

to us, and given this range, we could make $\sqrt{s_{xx}}$ as large as possible by putting half the $x$ values at the lower end of this range and the other half at the upper end of this range.

However, another consideration now comes into play. If we did this, we would have no idea what the growth heights tend to be around the middle of the range of $x$ values. It is important to get an idea of what these growth heights tend to be to so that we can be sure that the linearity assumption implicit in Eq. (8.36) holds for these values. So in practice, we tend to put quite a few $x$ values near the extremes of the interesting range of $x$ values but also put a few $x$ values along the intermediate part of the interesting range. This is illustrated in the choice of numerical values of the $x$'s in the example above. We gave three plants the lowest amount of water (16) and three plants the highest amount of water (26). We also chose a collection of $x$ values between these extremes.

3. A second result goes in the other direction. Suppose that the amounts of water $x_1, x_2, \ldots, x_n$ put on the various plants were close to each other. Then these values would be close to their average, and Eq. (8.39) then shows that $s_{xx}$ would be small. This means in turn that $2s_r/\sqrt{s_{xx}}$ would be large and the confidence interval (8.51) would be wide. We then have little confidence in our estimate of $\beta$.

An even more extreme case arises if all plants are given the same amount of water. In this case, $s_{xx} = 0$ and $s_{xy} = 0$ and the right-hand side in (8.48) becomes $0/0$, which is mathematically meaningless. The expression $0/0$ indicates that it is not possible to estimate $\beta$ in this case. An associated point is that if all plants are given the same amount of water, the confidence interval given by (8.51) would formally extend from minus infinity to plus infinity, so that it is not possible to have any idea what value $\beta$ takes.

4. In the plant growth height example, we would write the estimated regression line as $y = 66.03 + 0.65x$ to the level of accuracy justified by the data. We could use this equation to say that we estimate the mean growth height for a plant given 21 units of water to be $66.03 + 0.65 \times 21 = 79.68$.

5. Never extrapolate outside the $x$ values in the experiment. For example, it is not appropriate to say that we estimate the mean growth height for a plant given 1000 units of water to be $66.03 + 0.65 \times 1000 = 716.03$. We would probably kill the plant if we gave it this much water.

6. Later, we will consider testing the hypothesis that the growth height of the plant does not depend on the amount of water given to it. This is equivalent to testing the hypothesis $\beta = 0$.

7. The confidence intervals (8.51) and (8.52) are not exact, since they use a standard deviation estimate ($s_r$) instead of a known standard deviation. This matter will be discussed in Sect. 13.6.

8. *Assumptions.* We mentioned earlier that linear regression assumes linearity, which we subjectively assess by plotting the data in a scatterplot, as shown in Fig. 8.1.

We also assumed that the variance of $Y$ was $\sigma^2$, regardless of the $x$ value. This "constant variance" notion is known as *homoscedasticity*. One way to subjectively assess this is to look at the same scatterplot of the data and see whether there is a relatively consistent level of spread around the regression line as $x$ changes. In Fig. 8.1, this appears to be a reasonable assumption.

A flow-chart of the "regression" part of this book is given below to show the various topics covered in perspective.

## Flowchart: Linear Regression

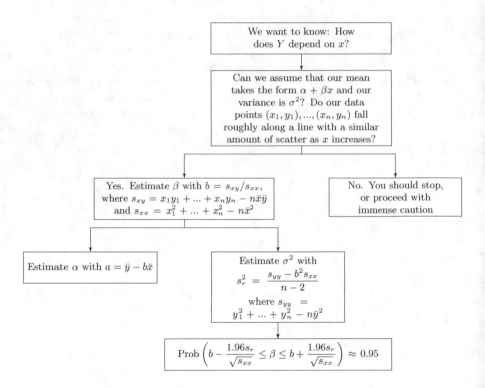

## 8.7   Problems

**8.1** A Gallup pollster wishes to estimate the probability ($\theta$) that a person taken at random will vote for Bauer in an election in 2 weeks' time. (Bauer's opponent is Lee.) She takes a sample of 10,000 people and, of these, 5265 say they will vote for Bauer. Estimate $\theta$ and use Eq. (8.6) to calculate an approximate 95% confidence interval for $\theta$.

**8.2**

(a) A TV station announces, 2 weeks before an election, that they estimate the proportion of people who will vote for candidate Bauer to be 0.53 "with a margin of error of 0.05". Assuming that the margin of error is $1/\sqrt{n}$ as derived from Eq. (8.6), what sample size did they use in arriving at the "margin of error of 0.05"?

(b) If the TV station wanted the "margin of error" to be 0.02, what sample size would they need?

(c) The length of the confidence interval is twice the margin of error. If the TV station wanted the length of the confidence interval to be 0.01, what sample size would they need?

**8.3** There are two expressions for an (approximate) 95% confidence interval for a binomial parameter $\theta$, the probability of "success" on each trial, namely intervals (8.4) and (8.6). Interval (8.4) is more accurate than (8.6) but (8.6) is easier to remember than is (8.4). Also, interval (8.6) is more conservative than interval (8.4) in the sense that it is wider than interval (8.4).

Suppose that in $n = 2500$ binomial trials, we see 1300 successes. Calculate the (approximate) 95% confidence intervals (8.4) and also (8.6) to assess (i) how close they are to each other, and (ii) to check that the confidence interval given by (8.6) is slightly wider than the confidence interval given by (8.4).

**8.4** We wish to estimate the mean weight gain $\mu$ (in pounds) of children between the age of 1 year and 3 years. A sample of 20 children gave the following weight gains:

$$25, 18, 33, 42, 5, 12, 21, 18, 17, 23, 38, 15, 19, 22, 18, 17, 33, 29, 31, 9$$

(a) Estimate $\mu$.

(b) Find two numbers between which we are approximately 95% certain that $\mu$ lies.

Hint: With these data, $\bar{x} = 22.25$ and $s^2 = 92.19737$, so that $s = 9.6019$.

**8.5** We are interested in investigating the mean blood sugar level of diabetics ($\mu$). To do this, we take a sample of six diabetics and find the following blood sugar levels: 127, 144, 140, 136, 118, 138.

Estimate $\mu$ and find two numbers between which we are approximately 95% certain that $\mu$ lies.

**8.6** Different people remember a series of instructions for different lengths of time. A group of 10 people was given special training in remembering these instructions. The times that they remembered them were, respectively, 6.49, 6.75, 6.60, 6.43, 6.63, 7.05, 6.51, 6.71, 6.55, 6.43 h. Use these data to estimate $\mu$, the mean time that people given the special training remember the instructions and also find an approximate 95% confidence interval for $\mu$. (Hint: $\bar{x} = 6.615$, $s = 0.1875$, $s/\sqrt{10} = 0.0593$.)

**8.7**

(a) A medical researcher interested in the genetic basis of chronic bronchitis collects data from 1000 single-child families where at least one parent suffers from this illness. She finds that 375 of the children also suffer from the illness. She also collected data from 1000 single-child families where neither parent suffers from this illness. She finds that 345 of these children suffer from the illness.

Let $\theta_1$ be the probability that a child in single child family suffers from chronic bronchitis for the case where at least one parent suffers from chronic bronchitis and $\theta_2$ be the probability that a child in single child family suffers from chronic bronchitis for the case where neither parent suffers from chronic bronchitis. From the data given, find an unbiased estimate of the difference $\theta_1 - \theta_2$ and calculate a conservative approximate 95% confidence interval for $\theta_1 - \theta_2$.

(b) Suppose the data are changed, so that the researcher collects data from 10,000 single-child families where at least one parent suffers from chronic bronchitis and finds that 3700 of the children also suffer from this illness. The researcher also collects data from 10,000 single-child families where neither parent suffers from chronic bronchitis and finds that 3350 of the children suffer from this illness.

From these new data, find an unbiased estimate of the difference $\theta_1 - \theta_2$ and calculate a conservative approximate 95% confidence interval for $\theta_1 - \theta_2$ .

(c) Comment on the similarities and differences between your answers to parts (a) and (b), basing your comment around the formula for the mean, and also the formula for the variance, of the difference between two proportions.

**8.8** We have two drugs, drug A and drug B, both aimed at curing a certain illness. We wish to compare the two drugs. Define $\theta_1$ as the probability that a person with this illness will be cured if they take drug A and $\theta_2$ as the probability that a person with this illness will be cured if they take drug B. We give drug A to 1000 people and it cures 640 of them. We give drug B to 1200 people and it cures 670 of them. Find two numbers between which you are about 95% certain that $\theta_1 - \theta_2$ lies.

**8.9** Let $\theta_1$ be the probability that a woman is left-handed and $\theta_2$ be the probability that a man is left-handed. We are interested in the question of whether men and women differ in their tendency to be left-handed. Thus we are interested in the difference $\theta_1 - \theta_2$. We took a sample of 2000 women and found that 348 of them are left-handed. We also took a sample of 1500 men and found that 294 of them are left-handed.

(a) Does it make sense to compare the numbers 348 and 294? Why (or why not)?
(b) Estimate the difference $\theta_1 - \theta_2$ from the data given.
(c) Find two numbers between which we are about 95% certain that $\theta_1 - \theta_2$ lies.

**8.10**  We are interested in investigating any potential difference between the mean blood sugar level of diabetics ($\mu_1$) and that of non-diabetics ($\mu_2$). To do this, we took a sample of ten diabetics and found the following blood sugar levels: 127, 144, 140, 136, 119, 138, 145, 122, 132, 129. We also took a sample of eight non-diabetics and found the following blood sugar levels: 125, 128, 133, 141, 109, 125, 126, 122.

*Hint:* To help you with this question, the estimate of the mean blood sugar level among diabetics is $\bar{x}_1 = 133.200$ and the estimate of the variance of blood sugar levels among diabetics is $s_1^2 = 79.7333$. The estimate of the mean blood sugar level among non-diabetics is $\bar{x}_2 = 126.125$ and the estimate of the variance of blood sugar levels among non-diabetics is $s_2^2 = 83.5536$. You may use these values in answering this question.

(a)  Find an unbiased estimate of the difference $\mu_1 - \mu_2$.

(b)  Find two numbers between which we are about 95% certain that $\mu_1 - \mu_2$ lies.

**8.11**  Suppose that in Problem 8.10, there had been 160 diabetics in the sample and 128 non-diabetics, but that (somehow amazingly!) the values of $\bar{x}_1$ (= 133.200), $\bar{x}_2$ (= 126.125), $s_1^2$ (= 79.7333) and $s_2^2$ (= 83.5536) remain unchanged.

(a)  Find an unbiased estimate of the difference $\mu_1 - \mu_2$.

(b)  Find two numbers between which we are about 95% certain that $\mu_1 - \mu_2$ lies.

(c)  Comment on the similarities and differences between your answers to this question and to Problem 8.10.

**8.12**  We wish to estimate the way in which weight ($y$) (in kg) of infant girls between the ages of 12 and 36 months depends on their age ($x$) (in months). A sample of 10 infant girls gave the following data:

| Infant | 1 | 2 | 3 | 4 | 5 | 6 | 7 | 8 | 9 | 10 |
|---|---|---|---|---|---|---|---|---|---|---|
| Age | 33 | 32 | 14 | 20 | 15 | 16 | 30 | 17 | 21 | 23 |
| Weight | 12.9 | 13.8 | 8.2 | 12.2 | 8.5 | 12.9 | 13.7 | 11.2 | 11.9 | 10.4 |

(a)  Calculate the values of $b$ and $a$. [Hint: $\bar{x} = 22.1$, $\bar{y} = 11.57$, $s_{xx} = 464.9$, $s_{xy} = 93.53$, $s_{yy} = 35.841$]

(b)  Plot the data on a graph. Plot your regression line $y = a + bx$ on your data graph. Does it more or less "skewer" through your data points?

(c)  Find two limits between which you are approximately 95% certain that $\beta$ lies.

**8.13**  This question is related to the "plant growth" example. The data are reproduced here for convenience:

| Plant number | 1 | 2 | 3 | 4 | 5 | 6 | 7 | 8 | 9 | 10 | 11 | 12 |
|---|---|---|---|---|---|---|---|---|---|---|---|---|
| Amount of water | 16 | 16 | 16 | 18 | 18 | 20 | 22 | 24 | 24 | 26 | 26 | 26 |
| Growth height | 76.2 | 77.1 | 75.7 | 78.1 | 77.8 | 79.2 | 80.2 | 82.5 | 80.7 | 83.1 | 82.2 | 83.6 |

(a) Plot the data on a graph. Plot your regression line $y = a + bx$ on your data graph using the values $a = 66.03$ and $b = 0.65$. Does the line "skewer" through your data points?

(b) Find the 99% confidence interval for $\beta$.

**8.14** Suppose that the data in the "plant growth" example are as follows:

| Plant number | 1 | 2 | 3 | 4 | 5 | 6 | 7 | 8 |
|---|---|---|---|---|---|---|---|---|
| Amount of water | 5 | 10 | 20 | 8 | 4 | 6 | 12 | 15 |
| Growth height | 27 | 47 | 73 | 40 | 30 | 28 | 46 | 59 |

(a) Estimate the mean growth height of a plant given $x$ units of water, given that $\bar{x} = 10$, $\bar{y} = 43.75$, $s_{xx} = 210$, $s_{yy} = 1835.5$, $s_{xy} = 610$.

(b) Find two limits between which you are approximately 95% certain that $\beta$ lies.

# Chapter 9
# Testing Hypotheses About the Value of a Parameter

As discussed in Sect. 1.2, Statistics is an *inductive* operation and consists of making inductions, or inferences. It uses two things: first, the data from some experiment, and second, the relevant probability calculation associated with those data. In this chapter, the probability calculation starts with the word "if". More precisely, the deductive statement in hypothesis testing procedures will start with: "if such and such a hypothesis is true, then the probability that ...". We now give an example.

*Example* Suppose that we wish to assess whether a newborn is equally likely to be a boy as a girl. To make an assessment about this, we take an unbiased well-conducted representative sample of 2000 newborns and observe, say, 1072 boys. The number 1072 is our single data value. The relevant probability statement is "if a newborn is equally likely to be a boy as a girl, the probability of seeing 1072 or more boys in a sample of 2000 newborns is 0.0006". (We will see later how a more refined approach to this question is made.) Putting this probability statement together with the data, we would say that having actually seen 1072 boys in the sample of 2000 newborns, and taking into account the very small probability 0.0006 of obtaining 1072 or more boys *if a newborn is equally likely to be a boy as a girl*, we make the reasonable inference that we have evidence that a newborn is not equally likely to be a boy as a girl.

The logical structure of this induction is as follows. The experiment gave us a data value, namely 1072 boys. It would be very unlikely to get this value, or one even larger, if a newborn is equally likely to be a boy as a girl. We therefore prefer to believe that a newborn is *not* equally likely to be a boy as a girl. In doing this, we follow the procedures of modern science. We trust our data and we do not accept hypotheses that do not reasonably explain our data.

In the context of hypothesis testing, the relation between probability theory and Statistics is a zig-zag one. This will be illustrated later in a diagram when the procedures of hypothesis testing have been described in more detail.

© The Author(s), under exclusive license to Springer Nature Switzerland AG 2023    115
W. J. Ewens, K. Brumberg, *Introductory Statistics for Data Analysis*,
https://doi.org/10.1007/978-3-031-28189-1_9

## 9.1   Introduction to Hypothesis Testing

In hypothesis testing, we attempt to get information about the answers to various questions. The following are some simple examples that relate to the estimation procedures considered previously.

Is this coin fair? Is the probability of not getting enough sleep the same for middle- and high-schoolers? Is the mean blood pressure for men the same as the mean blood pressure for women? Is there any effect of the amount of water given to a plant on its growth height?

We always rephrase these questions in terms of questions about parameters. The reason for this is that we know how to estimate parameters and to get some idea of the precision of the estimates. So rephrasing these questions in terms of questions about parameters allows us to use that estimation information and thus helps us to answer the hypothesis testing questions. The rephrased questions are as follows.

If the probability of a head is $\theta$, is $\theta = 1/2$? If the probability that a middle-schooler does not get enough sleep is $\theta_1$, and the probability that a high-schooler does not get enough sleep is $\theta_2$, is $\theta_1 = \theta_2$? If the mean blood pressure for a woman is $\mu_1$, and the mean blood pressure for a man is $\mu_2$, is $\mu_1 = \mu_2$? In the plant growth example, is $\beta = 0$? It is because we frame our hypothesis testing procedures as tests about the numerical values of parameters that the concept of a parameter is so important.

## 9.2   Two Approaches to Hypothesis Testing

In this book, we consider two equivalent approaches to hypothesis testing. The first approach pre-dates the availability of statistical packages, while the second approach is to some extent motivated by the availability of these packages. Both approaches may be found in research papers and that is why both approaches are discussed in this book. Both approaches always lead to the same conclusion, so it is only a matter of style, or of preference, or perhaps the availability of a suitable computer package, which determines which approach is used in any specific case. Both approaches involve five steps. The first three steps are the same in both approaches, and we consider these three steps first. We illustrate all five steps, and both approaches, by considering two problems involving the binomial distribution.

### 9.2.1   Both Approaches, Step 1

Statistical hypothesis testing involves the test of a *null hypothesis,* which we write in shorthand as $H_0$, against an *alternative hypothesis*, which we write in shorthand as $H_1$. The first step in a hypothesis testing procedure is to declare the relevant null hypothesis $H_0$ and the relevant alternative hypothesis $H_1$. The choice of null and alternative hypotheses must be made before our experiment is carried out and the data are seen. To base a hypothesis on the data that have already been seen introduces a bias into the procedure and invalidates any conclusion that might be drawn from it.

The null hypothesis, as the name suggests, often states that two parameters have the same numerical value or that one parameter takes some specified numerical value. This will be seen in more detail later through various examples.

The alternative hypothesis will be either "one-sided up", "one-sided down", or "two-sided". These concepts will be discussed in more detail later, using examples. The context of the situation will always make it clear which is the appropriate form of the alternative hypothesis. As stated above, the nature of the alternative hypothesis must be decided upon before the experiment is conducted and the data are seen.

Our eventual aim is to reject or fail to reject the null hypothesis as the result of an objective statistical procedure, using the data and the relevant probability theory in making this decision. In doing this, it is important to clarify the meaning of the expression "we fail to reject the null hypothesis." This expression means that there is no statistically significant evidence for rejecting the null hypothesis in favor of the alternative hypothesis. It is slightly misleading to say "we accept $H_0$", although this statement is often made. It is a shorthand for saying that we have not found enough significant evidence to reject $H_0$.

These abstract concepts are now illustrated by two examples, both involving the binomial distribution.

*Example 9.2.1*  This is an over-simplified example intended to illustrate the procedures involved. We wish to test whether a certain coin is fair. If it is unfair, we have no prior view as to the direction of the bias. If the probability of getting "head" on any flip of the coin is denoted $\theta$, the null hypothesis $H_0$ is that $\theta = 0.5$. From the fact that if the coin is unfair, we have no prior view as to the direction of the bias, the alternative hypothesis $H_1$ is the two-sided alternative $\theta \neq 0.5$.

*Example 9.2.2*  This example comes from the field of medical research. Suppose that we have been using some medicine for some illness for many years (the "current" medicine), and from much experience we are prepared to assume that the probability of a cure with the current medicine is 0.84. A new medicine is proposed and we wish to assess whether it is better than the current medicine. Here, the only interesting possibility is that the new medicine has a higher cure probability than the current medicine. If it is equally effective as the current medicine, or, even worse, less effective than the current medicine, we would not want to introduce it.

Let $\theta$ be the unknown probability of a cure with the new medicine. Here, the null hypothesis is $\theta = 0.84$. If this null hypothesis is true, the new medicine is equally effective as the current one. The natural alternative is that the new medicine is better than the current one, that is, that $\theta > 0.84$. This is the only case of interest to us, so this is a one-sided up alternative hypothesis. As in the coin example, the alternative hypothesis is determined by the context and is decided before the clinical trial begins.


## 9.2.2   Both Approaches, Step 2

Since the decision between rejecting $H_0$ and failing to reject $H_0$ will be made on the basis of data derived from some random sampling process, it is possible that an incorrect decision will be made. More explicitly, it is possible that we reject $H_0$ when it is true (a *Type I error* or a "false positive"), and it is also possible that we fail to reject $H_0$ when it is false (a *Type II error* or a "false negative"). This is illustrated in the table below.

|                  | We fail to reject $H_0$ | We reject $H_0$ |
| ---------------- | ----------------------- | --------------- |
| $H_0$ is true    | OK                      | Type I error    |
| $H_0$ is false   | Type II error           | OK              |

When testing a null hypothesis against an alternative hypothesis, it is often not possible to ensure that the probability of making the Type I error and also the probability of making the Type II error are both small, say less than 0.01, since to make them both small might require a very large number of data values, which might not be possible to obtain.

This dilemma is resolved in practice by observing that there is often an asymmetry in the implications of making a Type I error and a Type II error. In the two examples given above, there might be more concern about making a false positive claim, that is making a Type I error, and less concern about making the false negative claim, that is, making a Type II error. In the medicine example, we are anxious not to claim that the new medicine is better than the current one if it is not better. If we make this claim and it turns out to be untrue, then apart from the disappointed hopes of those hoping to use the new medicine, a lot of wasted time and effort, and perhaps millions of dollars, will possibly have been spent in pointlessly manufacturing it.

For this reason, a frequently adopted procedure in science is to focus on the Type I error, and to fix the numerical value of the probability of making this error at some acceptably low level (usually 1% or 5%), and not to attempt to control the numerical value of the Type II error. The numerical value chosen is often denoted by $\alpha$, and is so denoted in this book. This is the second occasion in this book where a Greek letter denotes something different from a parameter. We use the $\alpha$ notation since it is standard in hypothesis testing procedures.

The choices of the values of 0.01 and of 0.05 for $\alpha$ are both reasonable and are made often, but both are also arbitrary. The choice 0.01 is a more conservative one than the choice 0.05 and is often made in a medical context, since in that context we are very concerned about the possibility of making a false positive claim.

Step 2 of the hypothesis testing procedure is straightforward and simply consists of choosing the numerical value for the Type I error, that is, in choosing the numerical value of $\alpha$. This choice is entirely at our discretion. For purposes of illustration, in the examples discussed above, in accordance with the comment in the previous paragraph, we will choose 0.01 for the medicine example and 0.05 for the coin example.

Since the Type I error is the probability of rejecting the null hypothesis when it is true, all the calculations that we make to ensure that the numerical value of the Type I error is the chosen value $\alpha$ assume that the null hypothesis is indeed true.

### 9.2.3  Both Approaches, Step 3

The third step in the hypothesis testing procedure is to determine the appropriate *test statistic*. This is the quantity calculated from the data whose numerical value leads to acceptance or rejection of the null hypothesis. In the coin example, a reasonable test statistic is the number $x$ of heads that we will get after we have flipped the coin in our testing procedure. In the medicine case, a reasonable test statistic is the number $x$ of people cured with the new medicine in the clinical trial. In more complicated hypothesis testing procedures, the determination of the test statistic is far less straightforward.

In the coin example, it is equally reasonable to use as a test statistic the proportion of flips that come up heads instead of the number of heads. It is equally reasonable to use the proportion of people cured by the new medicine in the clinical trial rather than the number cured. In more complicated testing procedures considered later, we can *only* proceed by considering proportions rather than numbers, and that is why properties of proportions were discussed in Sect. 5.6. The procedure using proportions is discussed later.

### 9.2.4  Steps 4 and 5

As stated above, there are two (equivalent) approaches to hypothesis testing. Steps 4 and 5 differ under the two approaches, so we now consider them separately. Which approach we use is to some extent a matter of preference. However, other considerations are also involved, including the availability of charts for the first approach and the availability of computer packages for the calculations sometimes needed for the second approach. We consider Approach 1 first and Approach 2 later.

## 9.2.5  Approach 1, Step 4, the Medicine Example

Under Approach 1, Step 4 in the procedure consists of determining which observed values of the test statistic lead to rejection of $H_0$. This choice is made so as to ensure that the test has the numerical value $\alpha$ for the Type I error chosen in Step 2.

Suppose that in the medicine example, we plan to give the proposed new medicine to 5000 people and choose $\alpha = 0.01$. We choose the test statistic to be the number $x$ of patients who, after the experiment, were cured with the new medicine. The null hypothesis claims that $\theta = 0.84$ and the natural alternative hypothesis for this example claims that $\theta > 0.84$, so that the test is one-sided up. Because of this, we will reject the null hypothesis if $x$ is large enough. How large does $x$ have to be before we will reject the null hypothesis? This is where we need a probability calculation.

We will reject the null hypothesis if $x \geq a$, where $a$ is chosen so that the Type I error takes the desired value of 0.01. We now do a probability theory calculation and go back to the time before the clinical trial is conducted, when the random variable $X$, the number of people who will be cured with the new medicine, is a random variable. Since we will reject the null hypothesis if $x \geq a$, we have to choose $a$ so that $\text{Prob}(X \geq a$ when $\theta = 0.84) = 0.01$. Choosing $a$ in this way ensures that the numerical value of the Type I error is indeed the required value 0.01.

We calculate the value of $a$ using the Central Limit Theorem as applied to the binomial distribution, a standardization procedure, and the $Z$ chart or a computer package. If the null hypothesis is true, binomial distribution theory shows that the mean of $X$ is $(5000)(0.84) = 4200$ and the variance of $X$ is $(5000)(0.84)(0.16) = 672$. Next, to a very close approximation, $X$ can be taken as having a normal distribution with this mean and this variance when the null hypothesis is true. So to this level of approximation, $a$ has to be chosen so that

$$\text{Prob}\,(X \geq a) = 0.01, \tag{9.1}$$

where X has a normal distribution with mean 4200 and variance 672. The standardization procedure then gives

$$\text{Prob}\left(\frac{X - 4200}{\sqrt{672}} \geq \frac{a - 4200}{\sqrt{672}}\right) = 0.01. \tag{9.2}$$

If the null hypothesis is true, $(X - 4200)/\sqrt{672}$ is a $Z$, so that Eq. (9.2) can be written as

$$\text{Prob}\left(Z \geq \frac{a - 4200}{\sqrt{672}}\right) = 0.01. \tag{9.3}$$

Equation (6.20) shows that

$$\text{Prob}\,(Z \geq 2.326) = 0.01. \tag{9.4}$$

Therefore, $(a - 4200)/\sqrt{672} = 2.326$. Solving this equation for $a$, we find that $a = 4260.30$. To be conservative, we round up and use the value 4261.

In R, we can also find this with the qnorm() function:
```
qnorm(p = 0.01, mean = 4200, sd = sqrt(672),
lower.tail = FALSE).
```

To summarize, if $x$ is the observed number of patients cured with the new drug once the clinical trial has been conducted, we will reject the null hypothesis if $x \geq 4261$ and claim that we have significant evidence that the new medicine is superior to the current one. If $x \leq 4260$, we do not have enough evidence to reject the null hypothesis. The value 4261 is called the "critical point" (or "critical value"). In general, when the alternative hypothesis is one-sided up, as in this case, we reject the null hypothesis if the observed value of the test statistic is equal to or larger than the relevant critical point.

### 9.2.6   Approach 1, Step 5, the Medicine Example

All steps so far are taken before we even do the experiment (field survey, etc.) and get the data. Under Approach 1, the final step in the testing procedure is straightforward. With the information found in Steps 3 and 4 in hand, we now do the clinical trial and count the number $x$ of people cured with the new medicine. If this number is 4261 or larger, we reject the null hypothesis and claim that the new medicine is superior to the current one. If this number is less than 4261, we say that we do not have significant evidence that the new medicine is better than the current one.

Once Steps 1–4 have been completed, Step 5, the only statistical step, involves no theory. In effect, Step 5 simply consists of carrying out the experiment as designed in Steps 1–4.

*Notes on the Medicine Example*

1. In the medicine example, the interval of values "4261 or more" is called the *critical region*. The value 4261 is called the *critical point*, (often called the *critical value*). This terminology is used in all testing procedures carried out under Approach 1.
2. All the hard work arises in Step 4. This is a probability theory step. Once this step is done, the statistical Step 5 is straightforward.
3. It is interesting that under Approach 1, we start with a probability deriving from the chosen Type I error, and then find a number or numbers in the $Z$ chart corresponding to that probability, eventually finding a critical point. By contrast, under Approach 2, discussed later, we start with a $z$ value and then use the $Z$

chart to find the probability corresponding to that number. In other words, under Approach 1 we use the $Z$ chart in a reverse direction, and under Approach 2, we use it in a forward direction.

4. It was stated above that the same test would have been performed if the test statistic had been the proportion of people cured with the new medicine rather than the number cured. We now outline how the testing procedure would proceed using the proportion of people cured as test statistic.

As before, the null hypothesis is $\theta = 0.84$. If this null hypothesis is true, then before the experiment, the mean of the proportion $P$ of people who will be cured is 0.84 and the variance of $P$ is $(0.84 \times 0.16)/5000 = 0.00002688$. (These calculations use Eq. (5.9)). Then, if the null hypothesis is true, to a close approximation

$$\frac{P - 0.84}{\sqrt{0.00002688}}$$

is a $Z$. Therefore, once we have done the clinical trial and have in hand the observed proportion $p$ of patients cured, we would reject the null hypothesis if

$$\frac{p - 0.84}{\sqrt{0.00002688}} \geq 2.326, \tag{9.5}$$

where again the number 2.326 is found either from the $Z$ chart or from Eq. (6.20).

This implies that we would reject the null hypothesis if $p \geq 0.84 + 2.326 \times \sqrt{0.00002688}$, that is, if $p \geq 0.852059$.

In R, we can also find this as we have previously learned with the qnorm() function:

```
qnorm(p = 0.01, mean = 0.84, sd = sqrt(0.84 * 0.16 / 5000),
lower.tail = FALSE).
```

This is equivalent to the approach using the number cured, since if $p$ exceeds 0.852059 (the critical point for $p$), then $x$ (which is $5000p$) exceeds $5000 \times 0.852059 = 4260.30$, and this value was found in deriving the critical point calculated above for $x$.

Another way of seeing the equivalence of the approaches using the number cured and the proportion cured is to note that if both top and bottom lines on the left-hand side in (9.5) are multiplied by 5000, we obtain

$$\frac{(x - 4200)}{\sqrt{672}} \geq 2.326$$

and this leads to our rejecting the null hypothesis if $x \geq 4260.30$. This is exactly the procedure that we arrived at using the number of people cured as the test statistic.

### 9.2.7  Approach 1, Step 4, the Coin Example

In this section, we consider the coin example (Example 9.2.1 of Sect. 9.2.1). We plan to flip the coin 10,000 times to test the null hypothesis ($\theta = \frac{1}{2}$) against the alternative hypothesis ($\theta \neq \frac{1}{2}$). We choose a numerical value for $\alpha$ of 0.05, and use $x$, the number of heads that we will get after we have flipped the coin (say) 10,000 times, as the test statistic.

Step 4. Because the nature of the alternative hypothesis is two-sided, we will reject the null hypothesis if $x$ is either too large or too small. How large or how small? We will reject the null hypothesis if $x \leq a$ or if $x \geq b$, where $a$ and $b$ have to be chosen so that $\alpha = 0.05$. We now use probability theory and consider the random variable $X$, the random number of times we will get heads before the experiment is done. In order to ensure that the Type I error is indeed 0.05, we have to choose $a$ and $b$ so that when the null hypothesis is true,

$$\text{Prob } (X \leq a) + \text{Prob } (X \geq b) = 0.05.$$

We usually adopt the symmetric requirement that when the null hypothesis is true,

$$\text{Prob } (X \leq a) = \text{Prob } (X \geq b) = 0.025.$$

Since we plan to flip the coin 10,000 times, $X$ has a binomial distribution with mean 5000 and variance 2500 when the null hypothesis is true. The standard deviation of $X$ is thus $\sqrt{2500} = 50$. To a sufficiently close approximation, when the null hypothesis is true, $X$ has a normal distribution with this mean and this standard deviation. Thus when the null hypothesis is true, $(X - 5000)/50$ is a $Z$ to a good approximation.

We first calculate $b$. Carrying out a standardizing procedure, we have to choose $b$ such that if the null hypothesis is true,

$$\text{Prob } \left( \frac{X - 5000}{50} \geq \frac{b - 5000}{50} \right) = 0.025.$$

Since $\frac{X-5000}{50}$ is approximately a $Z$ when the null hypothesis is true, this can be written as

$$\text{Prob } \left( Z \geq \frac{b - 5000}{50} \right) = 0.025. \tag{9.6}$$

Equation (6.17) shows that

$$\text{Prob } (Z \geq 1.96) = 0.025. \tag{9.7}$$

A comparison of Eqs. (9.6) and (9.7) shows that $\frac{b-5000}{50} = 1.96$. Solving this equation for $b$, we get $b = 5098$. Carrying out a similar operation for $a$, we find $a = 4902$.

In R, we have qnorm(p = 0.025, mean = 5000, sd = 50, lower.tail = FALSE) and

qnorm(p = 0.025, mean = 5000, sd = 50, lower.tail = TRUE).

### 9.2.8  Approach 1, Step 5, the Coin Example

We now flip the coin 10,000 times. If the number of heads is 4902 or fewer, or 5098 or more, we reject the null hypothesis and claim that we have significant evidence that the coin is biased. If the number of heads is between 4903 and 5097 inclusive, we say that we do not have significant evidence to reject the null hypothesis. That is, we do not have significant evidence to claim that the coin is unfair. For example, suppose that we flipped the coin 10,000 times and saw 5088 heads. Since this is between 4902 and 5098, we do not have enough evidence to reject the null hypothesis that the coin is fair.

*Notes on the Coin Example*

1. Using the same terminology as for the medicine example, the values 4902 and 5098 are the critical points, and the union of the two intervals "$x \leq 4902$" and "$x \geq 5098$" is the critical region.
2. As in the medicine example, all the hard work arises in Step 4. This is entirely a probability theory step. Once this step is done, the statistical Step 5 is straightforward.
3. As in the medicine example, we can use the proportion of flips coming up heads rather than the number of flips coming up heads as the test statistic. Using the proportion of flips coming up heads in effect leads to the same testing procedure as that when the number of flips coming up heads is used as the test statistic. We do not give the details.

### 9.2.9  Approach 2 to Hypothesis Testing

As stated above, Steps 1, 2 and 3 are the same under Approach 2 as they are under Approach 1. We now consider Steps 4 and 5 under Approach 2. We do this by using the medicine and the coin examples discussed above.

## 9.2.10   Approach 2, Step 4, the Medicine and the Coin Examples

Under Approach 2, Step 4 consists of doing our experiment and noting the observed value of the test statistic. Thus in the medicine example, we do the clinical trial and observe the number $x$ of people cured under the new medicine. In the coin example, we flip the coin and observe the number $x$ of heads that turned up. If we used proportions rather than numbers as the test statistic, we would calculate the corresponding proportions.

## 9.2.11   Approach 2, Step 5, the Medicine Example

The first part of Step 5 involves the calculation of a so-called $P$-value. A $P$-value is a central concept in Statistics and is an essential feature of Approach 2 to hypothesis testing, so we now give the formal definition:

**The $P$-value is the probability, if the null hypothesis is true, of getting the observed value of the test statistic or one more extreme than the observed value in the direction that is indicated by the alternative hypothesis.**

Once the data are obtained, we calculate the $P$-value. We then draw a conclusion from the $P$-value. This is that if the $P$-value is less than or equal to the chosen value $\alpha$ for the numerical value of the Type I error, the null hypothesis is rejected. If the $P$-value exceeds $\alpha$, we do not have enough evidence to reject the null hypothesis. This procedure always leads to a conclusion identical to that found under Approach 1.

*Example 9.2.1* Suppose that in the medicine example considered above, the number of people cured under the new medicine was 4272. Using the normal distribution approximation to the binomial, the $P$-value is the probability that a random variable $X$ takes a value 4272 or more, given that under the null hypothesis, $X$ has a normal distribution with mean 4200 and variance 672. This is a probability theory operation, carried out using a standardization procedure and either the normal distribution chart or a computer package. Under these assumptions the $P$-value is

$$P\text{-value} = \text{Prob}(X \geq 4272|H_0 \text{ true}) = \text{Prob}\left(\frac{X - 4200}{\sqrt{672}} \geq \frac{4272 - 4200}{\sqrt{672}}\right).$$

Since $(X - 4200)/\sqrt{672}$ is approximately a $Z$ when the null hypothesis is true, and since $(4272 - 4200)/\sqrt{672} = 2.78$, we get

$$P\text{-value} = \text{Prob}(Z \geq 2.78),$$

and the $Z$ chart then shows that the $P$-value is about 0.0027. This is less than the chosen value $\alpha$ of the Type I error, so we reject the null hypothesis. This is the same conclusion that we would have reached using Approach 1, since the observed value 4272 exceeds the critical point 4261 found under Approach 1.

In R, we can find all this information either with the pnorm() function we have learned previously (pnorm(q = 4272, mean = 4200, sd = sqrt(672), lower.tail = FALSE)) or with the built in prop.test() function: prop.test (x = 4272, n = 5000, p = 0.84, alternative = "greater", conf.level = 0.99, correct = FALSE).

*Example 9.2.2* Suppose that the number of people cured with the new medicine was 4250. We calculate the $P$ value as

$$P\text{-value} = \text{Prob}(X \geq 4250 \mid H_0 \text{ true})$$

$$= \text{Prob}\left( \frac{X - 4200}{\sqrt{672}} \geq \frac{4250 - 4200}{\sqrt{672}} \mid H_0 \text{ true} \right).$$

Since $(X - 4200)/\sqrt{672}$ is a "$Z$" when the null hypothesis is true, and since $(4250 - 4200)/\sqrt{672} = 1.93$, we get

$$P\text{-value} = \text{Prob}(Z \geq 1.93).$$

From the $Z$ chart, the $P$-value is about 0.0268. This is more than the Type I error of 0.01, so we do not have enough evidence to reject the null hypothesis. This conclusion agrees with the one that we would have found under Approach 1, since the observed value 4250 falls short of the critical point 4261 found under Approach 1.

In R, we can use pnorm(q = 4250, mean = 4200, sd = sqrt(672), lower.tail = FALSE) or
prop.test(x = 4250, n = 5000, p = 0.84, alternative = "greater", conf.level = 0.99, correct = FALSE).

In this example, we were able to compute the $P$-value ourselves. In some more complicated examples considered later with different forms of test statistics, it is only possible to find the $P$-value by using a computer package.

### 9.2.12   Approach 2, Step 5, the Coin Example

As in the medicine example, this step involves the calculation of a $P$-value. However, this calculation for a two-sided alternative hypothesis such as that in the coin case is more complicated than in the medicine example.

Suppose, for example, that we obtained 5088 heads from the 10,000 flips. This is 88 more than the null hypothesis mean of 5000. The $P$-value is then the probability of obtaining 5088 or more heads **plus the probability of getting 4912 or fewer heads** if the coin is fair, that is, if the null hypothesis is true. We need the probability of getting 4912 or fewer heads calculation since 4912 is 88 fewer than the null hypothesis mean of 5000. That is, for a two-sided alternative, getting 4912 or fewer heads is as extreme as, or more extreme than, getting the observed value 5088. For example, 4906 is more extreme than 5088 in that it differs from the null hypothesis mean (5000) by 94, whereas 5088 differs from the null hypothesis mean by 88.

Using a normal distribution approximation, the $P$-value is the probability that a random variable having a normal distribution with mean 5000 and standard deviation 50 takes a value 5088 or more, **plus** the probability that this random variable takes a value 4912 or fewer. A standardization procedure shows that this is $0.0392 + 0.0392 = 0.0784$. This exceeds the chosen numerical value chosen for $\alpha$, so we do not have enough evidence to reject the null hypothesis. This agrees with the conclusion that we reached using Approach 1 for the example.

In R, we can find all this information most simply with pnorm(q = 5088, mean = 5000, sd = 50, lower.tail = FALSE) + pnorm(q = 4912, mean = 5000, sd = 50, lower.tail = TRUE) or
prop.test(x = 5088, n = 10000, p = 0.5, alternative = "two.sided", conf.level = 0.95, correct = FALSE).

*Notes on Approach 2*

1. The coin $P$-value calculation is typical of all $P$-value calculations for two-sided tests in that it is the sum of two terms, one on the up side and one on the down side. This is because "more extreme" means more extreme up **or** more extreme down.
2. Under Approach 2, we start with a number (4272 in the first medical example above) and from this calculate a $P$-value. In doing this, we use the $Z$ chart in a forward way. Under Approach 1, we start with a probability (the chosen Type I error) and from this, we find a number or numbers (the critical point or points). In doing this, we use the $Z$ chart in a reverse way.
3. All the calculations in the two examples above involve a normal approximation to the binomial. When the number of trials $n$ is small, say less than 50, the normal approximation is not very accurate and either exact binomial probabilities or an approximating calculation using a continuity correction are needed.

## 9.3   The Hypothesis Testing Procedure and the Concepts of Deduction and Induction

We recall the material in Sect. 1.2 concerning probability calculations, which are deductions, or implications, and statistical operations, which are inductions, or inferences. In both the coin and the medicine examples, we started with a probability theory deduction, or implication. Such a deduction, or implication, starts with the word "if". In the examples considered above, and in all hypothesis testing procedures that follow, this is "if the null hypothesis is true, then...". The calculation that followed was a probability theory "zig". It was later followed by a statistical "zag".

Under Approach 1 for hypothesis testing, which uses critical points, the format of Sect. 1.2 leads to the diagrams below.

Probability theory (deduction, implication)  → → → → → →

| If the null hypothesis is true | Under this assumption we calculate the critical point (points) |

← ← ← ← ← ←  Statistics (induction, inference)

| We accept or reject the null hypothesis | We compare the observed value of the test statistic with the critical point (points) |

Following this general format, the medicine example is formatted as follows:

Probability theory (deduction, implication)  → → → → → →

| If the cure rate of the new medicine is 0.84 | Under this assumption the probability of 4,261 or more cures is 0.01 |

← ← ← ← ← ←  Statistics (induction, inference)

| We reject the null hypothesis and claim that we have good evidence that the new medicine is better than the current one | 4,272 people were cured with the new medicine |

Under Approach 2, carried out via $P$-values, the format of Sect. 1.2 leads to the following general diagram:

Probability theory (deduction, implication)  → → → → → →

| If the null hypothesis is true | We get the data and calculate the $P$-value |

$\leftarrow\leftarrow\leftarrow\leftarrow\leftarrow\leftarrow$ Statistics (induction, inference)

| We reject the null hypothesis | If, for example, the $P$-value is less than the chosen numerical value of the Type I error |

The medicine example formatted in this way is as follows:

Probability theory (deduction, implication) $\rightarrow\rightarrow\rightarrow\rightarrow\rightarrow\rightarrow$

| If the new medicine has the same cure rate as the current one | 4,272 people were cured and under the same cure rate assumption, the $P$-value is 0.0027 |

$\leftarrow\leftarrow\leftarrow\leftarrow\leftarrow\leftarrow$ Statistics (induction, inference)

| We reject the null hypothesis and claim that we have good evidence that the new medicine is better than the current one | We did see 4,272 cured so the $P$-value is less than the numerical value of the Type I error |

## 9.4 Power

So far, we have focused on calculations that assume that the null hypothesis is true. For example, the calculation of the critical point 4261 in the medicine example above, and the calculation of a $P$-value 0.0027 in the same example, all assume that the null hypothesis is true. In this section, we consider calculations which assume various possibilities for the alternative hypothesis.

The numerical value of the Type II error is the probability of failing to reject the null hypothesis when the alternative hypothesis is true. By contrast, the *power* of a test is the probability of successfully rejecting the null hypothesis when the alternative hypothesis is true. This implies that power $= 1-$ the numerical value of the Type II error. It also implies that if the null hypothesis is true, the power is $\alpha$.

In many cases there is no specific alternative hypothesis, so there is no specific value for the power of a given test. Instead, there are a set of power values, each value corresponding to some possible numerical value of the parameter involved in the test. We illustrate this with the medicine example considered in Sect. 9.2.5.

In this example, we planned to give the proposed new medicine to 5000 people and, choosing $\alpha = 0.01$, to reject the null hypothesis ($\theta = 0.84$) if the number of people cured by the proposed new medicine is 4261 or more. Suppose that $\theta = 0.85$. Then if the random number of people who will be cured is denoted by $X$,

$$\text{power of test} = \text{Prob}(X \geq 4261 | \theta = 0.85). \tag{9.8}$$

This probability can be calculated to a sufficient degree of accuracy using a normal distribution approximation to the distribution of $X$. If $\theta = 0.85$, the mean of $X$ is 4250 and the variance of $X$ is 637.5. Thus upon using a normal distribution approximation to the binomial and standardizing,

$$\text{power} = \text{Prob}\left(\frac{X - 4250}{\sqrt{637.5}} \geq \frac{4261 - 4250}{\sqrt{637.5}}\right) \approx \text{Prob}(Z \geq 0.44) \approx 0.3300. \tag{9.9}$$

Similarly, if $\theta = 0.86$, the mean of $X$ is 4300 and the variance is 602 and thus

$$\text{power} = \text{Prob}\left(\frac{X - 4300}{\sqrt{602}} \geq \frac{4261 - 4300}{\sqrt{602}}\right) \approx \text{Prob}(Z \geq -1.59) \approx 0.9441. \tag{9.10}$$

If $\theta = 0.87$, the mean of $X$ is 4350 and the variance is 565.5 and thus

$$\text{power} = \text{Prob}\left(\frac{X - 4350}{\sqrt{565.5}} \geq \frac{4261 - 4350}{\sqrt{565.5}}\right) \approx \text{Prob}(Z \geq -3.74) \approx 1. \tag{9.11}$$

Thus if $\theta = 0.87$, it is almost certain that the null hypothesis will be rejected and the proposed new medicine will correctly be claimed to be significantly superior to the current one.

There is a curve of the power of the test as a function of $\theta$, and this is called the *power curve*. The power curve deriving from calculations such as those in Eqs. (9.8)–(9.11) for the above example is shown in Fig. 9.1. The $S$-shaped nature of the power curve is evident.

For a two-sided test, the power curve is $U$-shaped. We illustrate this with the coin example considered in Sect. 9.2.7. In that example, we planned to flip the coin 10,000 times to test the null hypothesis that the coin is fair ($\theta = 0.5$) against the two-sided alternative hypothesis $\theta \neq 0.5$. The value chosen for $\alpha$ was 0.05, and we found that we would reject the null hypothesis with this value of $\alpha$ if the number of heads that eventually appeared was 4902 or fewer or 5098 or more. This information is sufficient for us to carry our power calculations.

**Fig. 9.1** The power curve for the medicine example

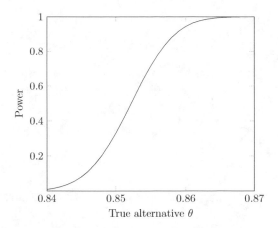

If before the experiment, $X$ is the random number of heads that will appear and if $\theta = 0.505$, the power of the test is $\text{Prob}(X \leq 4902 | \theta = 0.505) + \text{Prob}(X \geq 5098 | \theta = 0.505)$. If $\theta = 0.505$, the mean of $X$ is 5050 and the variance of $X$ is very close to 2500 (standard deviation 50). Thus upon using a normal distribution approximation to the binomial and standardizing,

$$\text{power} = \text{Prob}\left(\frac{X - 5050}{50} \leq \frac{4902 - 5050}{50}\right)$$
$$+ \text{Prob}\left(\frac{X - 5050}{50} \geq \frac{5098 - 5050}{50}\right). \tag{9.12}$$

This is $\text{Prob}(Z \leq -2.96) + \text{Prob}(Z \geq 0.96) = 0.1700$.

If $\theta = 0.495$, the parallel power calculation again yields a value of 0.1700. In this example the power curve is symmetrical around the value $\theta = 0.5$, deriving from the fact that the binomial distribution is symmetrical around the value 5000 when $\theta = 0.5$. It is therefore only necessary to compute probabilities for the case $\theta > 0.5$ and then find probabilities for the case $\theta < 0.5$ by symmetry.

Similar calculations shows that if $\theta = 0.51$, the power of the test is 0.4840, if $\theta = 0.515$, the power of the test is 0.8508, and if $\theta = 0.52$, the power of the test is 0.9793. Values such as these, together with the fact that the power curve is symmetric around $\theta = 0.5$, allow us to draw the power curve, which is shown in Fig. 9.2. The symmetric U-shaped nature of the power curve is evident from this figure.

The flowchart on the following page summarizes the hypothesis testing and power calculation procedures described in this chapter.

**Fig. 9.2** The power curve for
the coin example

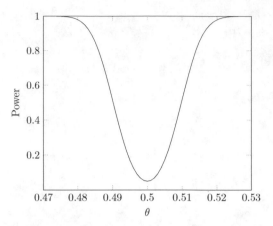

## Flowchart: Hypothesis Testing and Power Calculations

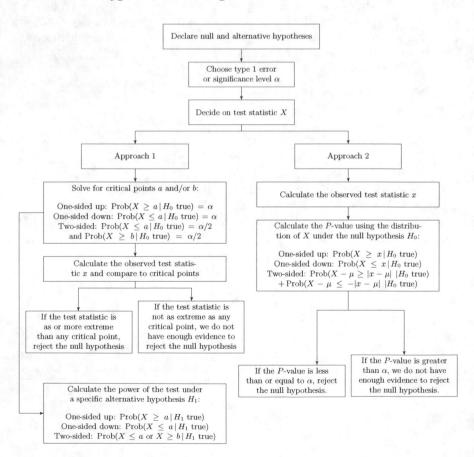

## 9.5 Problems

**9.1** You flip a coin 40 times and you get 22 heads. Typical statistical questions would be: Would you say that there is significant evidence that the coin is biased? What if you got 55 heads from 100 flips? What if you got 110 heads from 200 flips?

(a) Calculate the proportion of heads if you got (i) 22 heads from 40 flips of a fair coin, (ii) 55 heads from 100 flips of a fair coin, or (iii) 110 heads from 200 flips of a fair coin.
(b) Make a start on the probability theory concerning the question of whether the coin is fair by approximating, assuming that the coin is fair, the probability of getting (i) 22 or more heads from 40 flips of a fair coin, (ii) 55 or more heads from 100 flips of a fair coin, (iii) 110 or more heads from 200 flips of a fair coin.
   Note: Use a normal distribution approximation and the $Z$ chart (Charts 2 and 3) in approximating these probabilities.
(c) What do your calculations imply about the usefulness of giving the proportion of heads obtained in any experiment involving coin flipping without also giving the number of flips?

**9.2** We are interested in whether a certain coin is fair. To test the claim (or hypothesis) that it is fair, we plan to flip it 50,000 times and count the number of heads that will turn up. We decide in advance that we will reject the hypothesis that it is fair if the **number of heads** turns out to be less than or equal to some number $c_1$ or greater than or equal to some number $c_2$, where $c_1$ and $c_2$ are chosen so that

Prob(number of heads is less than or equal to $c_1$ if the coin is fair) $= 0.025$

Prob(number of heads is greater than or equal to $c_2$ if the coin is fair) $= 0.025$.

(a) Find the values of $c_1$ and $c_2$ using the $Z$ chart (or R).
(b) What would $c_1$ and $c_2$ be if we replaced both of the two probabilities above (i.e. 0.025) by 0.005?

**9.3**

(a) Under the null hypothesis, a random variable $X$ has a normal distribution with mean 200 and variance 100. Under the alternative hypothesis, the mean exceeds 200. We choose $\alpha = 0.05$. Find the critical point.
(b) As in part (a) of this problem, but now we choose $\alpha = 0.01$. Find the critical point.

**9.4** We are currently using a drug for a certain medical complaint which is known to cure a patient with probability 0.8. A new drug is claimed to have a higher cure rate than the drug that we are currently using. To test this claim, we plan to conduct a clinical trial and give the new drug to 2000 patients. Let $\theta$ be the (unknown) probability of a cure with the proposed new drug. The null hypothesis is that the new drug has the same cure probability as the current one (i.e. $\theta = 0.8$) and the alternative hypothesis is that the proposed new drug has a higher cure probability than the current one (i.e. $\theta > 0.8$). Also, since this is a medical situation, we use a Type I error of 0.01. The test statistic is the **number of people** who will be cured in the clinical trial.

(a)  What is the critical point?
(b)  If, after the trial was conducted, 1634 people were cured, do you reject the null hypothesis?
(c)  Find the $P$-value corresponding to the number 1634 cured. Based on your $P$-value, do you accept or reject the null hypothesis? Does your decision agree with the decision you made in part (b), using Approach 1?
(d)  What if, instead, after the trial was conducted, 1648 people were cured, do you reject the null hypothesis based on the critical point (Approach 1)?
(e)  Find the $P$-value corresponding to the number 1648 cured. Based on your $P$-value, do you accept or reject the null hypothesis? Does your decision agree with the decision you made in part (d), using Approach 1?

**9.5**  We now consider the same situation as in Problem 9.4, but using the **proportion** of people cured as the test statistic.

(a)  Using only the theory for proportions, find the critical point if the test statistic is the proportion of people cured, again choosing $\alpha = 0.01$.
(b)  Check that the "proportions" critical point and the "numbers" critical point, although of course numerically different, correspond appropriately with each other.

**9.6**  A coin is to be flipped 1600 times in order to test the null hypothesis that the coin is fair against the (two-sided) alternative hypothesis that it is not fair at the $\alpha = 0.05$ level.

(a)  Find the two relevant critical points if the test statistic is the **proportion** of times the coin comes up heads in the 1600 flips.
(b)  Suppose that when the coin is flipped 1600 times, we see 844 heads. Do you accept or reject the null hypothesis?
(c)  What is the $P$-value corresponding to the observed number 844? Based on the $P$-value, do you accept or reject the null hypothesis? Does your decision agree with the decision you made in part (b), using Approach 1?

**9.7**  You have decided to become a professional gambler specializing in roulette. If the roulette wheel is fair, each number has an equal chance (1/38) of coming up and the bets are structured such that you will lose in the long run. Your strategy is to find roulette wheels that are not properly balanced and produce some numbers more frequently than 1 out of 38 times. You believe that you have found such a wheel and that it produces the number 29 more frequently than expected.

(a) You observe the wheel for 420 spins and note that the number 29 came up 14 times. Carry out a hypothesis test using **Approach 1** with $\alpha = 0.05$ and with the **proportion** of times that 29 came up as a test statistic.

(b) With the same data as in part (a), carry out a hypothesis test using **Approach 2** with $\alpha = 0.05$ and with the **number** of times that 29 came up as a test statistic.

**9.8** Suppose that $X$ has a binomial distribution with parameter $\theta$. The null hypothesis claims that $\theta = 0.7$ and the alternative hypothesis claims that $\theta > 0.7$. The number of trials $n$ is 1600 and $\alpha$ is chosen to be 0.05. Find the power of the test if in fact (a) $\theta = 0.71$, (b) $\theta = 0.72$, (c) $\theta = 0.73$ (d) $\theta = 0.74$, (e) $\theta = 0.75$.

**9.9** As in Problem 9.8, but now with $n = 400$ trials.

**9.10** This problem refers to Problem 9.6.

(a) Let $\theta$ be the probability of heads on each flip. Find the power of the test when
 (i) $\theta = 0.51$, (ii) $\theta = 0.52$, (iii) $\theta = 0.53$, (iv) $\theta = 0.54$, (v) $\theta = 0.55$.
(b) Use your answers to find, without further calculation, the power of the test when
 (i) $\theta = 0.49$, (ii) $\theta = 0.48$, (iii) $\theta = 0.47$, (iv) $\theta = 0.46$, (v) $\theta = 0.45$.

# Chapter 10
# Testing for the Equality of Two Binomial Parameters

## 10.1 Two-by-Two Tables

Suppose we want to test whether there is any difference between middle- and high-schoolers in terms of getting enough sleep. If there is a difference, suppose for concreteness that we have no a priori view as to whether middle-schoolers are more or less likely to get enough sleep as high-schoolers are. Therefore the eventual test will be two-sided. We consider a one-sided example later.

To make progress, we rephrase this question as a test of whether two binomial parameters are equal. We write $\theta_1$ as the probability that a middle-schooler will not get enough sleep and $\theta_2$ as the probability that a high-schooler will not get enough sleep. The null hypothesis, that there is no difference between middle- and high-schoolers in terms of getting enough sleep, is then equivalent to

$$H_0 : \theta_1 = \theta_2 \ (= \theta, \ \text{unspecified}).$$

This null hypothesis only claims that $\theta_1$ and $\theta_2$ are equal: it does not specify what their common numerical value is and as shown above, we denote their common value by an unknown parameter $\theta$.

Since the context is that we have no a priori view as to whether middle-schoolers are more or less likely to not get enough sleep as high-schoolers are, the alternative hypothesis in this example is two-sided: that is, the alternative hypothesis is

$$H_1 : \theta_1 \neq \theta_2.$$

Declaring $H_0$ and $H_1$ completes Step 1 of the hypothesis testing procedure.

As discussed later in Note 7 of Sect. 10.3, a statement equivalent to the null hypothesis is that there is no association between the row mode of classification and the column mode of classification. In this example, the null hypothesis is that there is no association between between school level and the amount of sleep.

© The Author(s), under exclusive license to Springer Nature Switzerland AG 2023

W. J. Ewens, K. Brumberg, *Introductory Statistics for Data Analysis*,

https://doi.org/10.1007/978-3-031-28189-1_10

Step 2. In Step 2, we choose $\alpha$, the numerical value of the Type I error. Suppose that in this example, we choose $\alpha = 0.05$.

Step 3. In this step, we create a test statistic. This is a much more complicated procedure than it was in the "single binomial" medicine and coin examples. We have to think in advance what the data will look like. Suppose that we plan to ask $r_1$ middle-schoolers whether they get enough sleep and that we plan to ask $r_2$ high-schoolers as well. (The reason for choosing the notation $r_1$ and $r_2$ will be seen in Table (10.1) below: $r$ is the first letter in the word "row".) We write $r_1 + r_2 = n$, the total number of people whose sleep habits we will ask about. Of the middle-schoolers, some number $o_{11}$ will say they do not get enough sleep and some number $o_{12}$ will say they get enough sleep. Some number $o_{21}$ of the high-schoolers will say they do not get enough sleep and some number $o_{22}$ will say they get enough sleep. (The reason for the $o_{ij}$ notation will be discussed later: "o" is the first letter of the word "observed", and these are the four observed data values.)

We can think of these data as being arranged in a so-called "two-by-two" table, the general form of which is as shown below.

|        | column 1 | column 2 | total |
|--------|----------|----------|-------|
| row 1  | $o_{11}$ | $o_{12}$ | $r_1$ |
| row 2  | $o_{21}$ | $o_{22}$ | $r_2$ |
| total  | $c_1$    | $c_2$    | $n$   |

$$(10.1)$$

In the example we are considering, middle-schooler data could be in row 1, high-schooler data could be in row 2, data for sleep-deprived individuals could be in column 1 and data for well-rested individuals could be in column 2. $r_1$ is the total number of middle-schoolers in the sample and $r_2$ is the total number of high-schoolers in the sample. $c_1$ and $c_2$ denote column totals, since $c$ is the first letter in the word "column". In this example, $c_1$ is the total number of people in the sample who are sleep-deprived and $c_2$ is the total number of people in the sample who are well-rested. The grand total $n$ is equal to both $r_1 + r_2$ and $c_1 + c_2$.

If $r_1$ is not equal to $r_2$, it does not make sense to compare $o_{11}$ with $o_{21}$. This is not a fair comparison since if, for example, $r_1$ exceeds $r_2$, we would expect $o_{11}$ to tend to exceed $o_{21}$ even if middle- and high-schoolers had the same sleep habits. This implies that in this test, we can *only* proceed by comparing the proportions $o_{11}/r_1$ and $o_{21}/r_2$. This is in contrast to the case of testing for the value of one binomial parameter, where we can use either counts or proportions. This is why we earlier considered the probability theory relating to proportions. A fair comparison is the difference between the proportion $o_{11}/r_1$ of middle-schoolers who are sleep-deprived and the proportion $o_{21}/r_2$ of high-schoolers who are sleep-deprived.

The difference $o_{11}/r_1 - o_{21}/r_2$ on its own is however not enough as the test statistic. We need to have some idea of the potential random variability in this difference, or in other words, we need to calculate a variance. To do this, it is necessary to go back to the time before we took the survey. At this time, the number of middle-schoolers who will say they are sleep-deprived is a random variable, which we write as $O_{11}$. Similarly, the number of high-schoolers who will say they are sleep-deprived is a random variable, which we write as $O_{21}$. The proportion of middle-schoolers who will say they are sleep-deprived is $O_{11}/r_1$, and this is also a random variable. Similarly, the proportion of high-schoolers who will say they are sleep-deprived is $O_{21}/r_2$, and this is also a random variable.

Suppose now that the null hypothesis is true. Then from the first part of Eq. (5.9), the mean of $O_{11}/r_1$ is $\theta$ and the mean of $O_{21}/r_2$ is also $\theta$. From the first part of Eq. (5.11), the mean of $O_{11}/r_1 - O_{21}/r_2$ is $\theta - \theta = 0$ when the null hypothesis is true.

Thus if the null hypothesis is true, once we have done our experiment and have our data as given in the table above, $o_{11}/r_1 - o_{21}/r_2$ should be close to 0. However, as stated above, this on its own is not enough. We also have to find the variance of $O_{11}/r_1 - O_{21}/r_2$ when the null hypothesis is true. From the second part of Eq. (5.9) the variance of $O_{11}/r_1$ is $\theta(1-\theta)/r_1$ and the variance of $O_{21}/r_2$ is $\theta(1-\theta)/r_2$. Then from the second part of Eq. (5.11), the variance of $O_{11}/r_1 - O_{21}/r_2$ is

$$\frac{\theta(1-\theta)}{r_1} + \frac{\theta(1-\theta)}{r_2}$$

when the null hypothesis is true. This shows that when the null hypothesis is true, the quantity

$$\frac{\frac{o_{11}}{r_1} - \frac{o_{21}}{r_2}}{\sqrt{\frac{\theta(1-\theta)}{r_1} + \frac{\theta(1-\theta)}{r_2}}} \tag{10.2}$$

is a "Z": that is, it has approximately a normal distribution with mean 0 and variance 1 when the null hypothesis is true.

The problem now is that we do not know the numerical value of $\theta$. This implies that we will have to estimate it from the data. We are assuming that the null hypothesis is true, and so we estimate $\theta$ (the probability that a student, middle- or high-schooler, is sleep-deprived) by the overall proportion of people in the sample who are sleep-deprived, namely $c_1/n$. Similarly, we estimate $1 - \theta$ (the probability that a student, middle- or high-schooler, is well-rested) by the overall proportion of people in the sample who are well-rested, namely $c_2/n$. We therefore approximate the statistic in (10.2) by a new "Z", namely

$$\frac{\frac{O_{11}}{r_1} - \frac{O_{21}}{r_2}}{\sqrt{\frac{(c_1/n)(c_2/n)}{r_1} + \frac{(c_1/n)(c_2/n)}{r_2}}}. \tag{10.3}$$

Given the observed data $o_{11}, o_{12}, o_{21}, o_{22}$, this leads to the test statistic for this procedure, usually denoted by $z$ (more accurately as "z"):

$$z = \frac{\frac{o_{11}}{r_1} - \frac{o_{21}}{r_2}}{\sqrt{\frac{(c_1/n)(c_2/n)}{r_1} + \frac{(c_1/n)(c_2/n)}{r_2}}}. \tag{10.4}$$

We call this the original $z$ statistic. It is far more complicated than the test statistic $x$ used when testing for the value of one binomial parameter. When the null hypothesis is true, it is approximately the observed value of a $Z$ random variable, and this explains the notation "$z$". The accuracy of this approximation is discussed later.

It is helpful to think of the statistic in (10.4) as a signal-to-noise ratio. The signal in the numerator, namely $\frac{o_{11}}{r_1} - \frac{o_{21}}{r_2}$, is the data estimate of $\theta_1 - \theta_2$. The noise is the denominator, $\sqrt{\frac{(c_1/n)(c_2/n)}{r_1} + \frac{(c_1/n)(c_2/n)}{r_2}}$. The signal is significant only if it is large enough relative to the noise. The signal on its own is not enough.

For the purposes of computation, the expression (10.4) is more conveniently replaced by the equivalent expression

$$z = \frac{(o_{11} \times o_{22} - o_{21} \times o_{12})\sqrt{n}}{\sqrt{r_1 \times r_2 \times c_1 \times c_2}} \tag{10.5}$$

We call this the computationally convenient form of the $z$ statistic.

Both (10.4) and (10.5) are important. (10.5) is important for the simple reason that it is computationally convenient. However, the $z$ statistic in (10.5) does not indicate directly whether the test is one-sided up or one-sided down for a one-sided test. Only the $z$ statistic in (10.4) in conjunction with the alternative hypothesis can indicate that. This is discussed in connection with Example 10.1.2 below.

This concludes Step 3, the determination of a test statistic. It is a far more complicated procedure than that for testing for the numerical value of a single binomial parameter.

The procedure in Steps 4 and 5 depends on whether we use Approach 1 or Approach 2. We first consider Approach 1.

Approach 1, Step 4. In this step, we ask what values of the test statistic lead us to reject the null hypothesis. Since the alternative hypothesis in the sleep example is two-sided, sufficiently large negative or sufficiently large positive values of $z$ will lead us to reject the null hypothesis. How large positive or how large negative? This depends on the value we chose for $\alpha$. In Step 2, we chose $\alpha$ to be 0.05 for this example. Next, the random variable $Z$ in the expression (10.3) has, to a reasonable approximation, a $Z$ distribution when the null hypothesis is true. Equation (6.16) shows that the probability that a $Z$ is either less than $-1.96$ or is greater than $+1.96$ is 0.05. These are then the upper and lower critical points for $z$. This leads to the procedure described below in Step 5.

Approach 1, Step 5. We get our data and compute the numerical value of the $z$ test statistic (10.5). If this value is $-1.96$ or less, or $+1.96$ or more, we will reject the null hypothesis. If the numerical value of the test statistic (10.5) is between $-1.96$ and $+1.96$, we do not have enough significant evidence to reject the null hypothesis. This procedure guarantees that, given that the approximations referred to above are sufficiently accurate, the Type I error of the procedure is the desired 0.05.

The only statistical step is the simple one, Step 5. Essentially all the other steps are related to the probability theory part of the procedure. That is why so much emphasis is placed in on probability theory in this book.

Approach 2. Under Approach 2, Steps 1, 2 and 3 are the same as for Approach 1, so we start by considering Step 4. Step 4 consists of getting the data and calculating the numerical value of the test statistic (10.5).

Step 5 involves the calculation of the $P$-value corresponding to the observed numerical value of the test statistic (10.5). If this $P$-value is less than or equal to the value of $\alpha$ chosen in Step 2, we reject the null hypothesis. If the $P$-value is greater than the value of $\alpha$ that we chose in Step 2 we do not have enough evidence to reject the null hypothesis.

*Example 10.1.1 (Sleep Deprivation)* Suppose that we ask 300 middle-schoolers whether they get enough sleep, and that 173 of them say they are sleep-deprived. Suppose that we also ask 200 high-schoolers whether they get enough sleep, and that 135 of these say they are sleep-deprived. The data table now looks like this:

| | sleep-deprived | well-rested | total |
|---|---|---|---|
| middle-schoolers | 173 | 127 | 300 |
| high-schoolers | 135 | 65 | 200 |
| total | 308 | 192 | 500 |

(10.6)

The numerical value of the $z$ test statistic (10.5) is then

$$\frac{(173 \times 65 - 127 \times 135)\sqrt{500}}{\sqrt{300 \times 200 \times 308 \times 192}} \approx -2.21. \tag{10.7}$$

Step 5, Approach 1. The alternative hypothesis in this example is two-sided and the chosen value of $\alpha$ was 0.05. As discussed above, we would reject the null hypothesis if the numerical value of the $z$ test statistic (10.5) is $-1.96$ or less or $+1.96$ or more. Given the numerical value of about $-2.21$ of the test statistic, using Approach 1, we would say that we do have significant enough evidence to reject the null hypothesis. In more practical language, we have enough evidence to claim that there is a difference between middle- and high-schoolers in terms of whether they get enough sleep.

Steps 4 and 5, Approach 2. Under Approach 2, Step 4 consists of finding the numerical value of the test statistic, given the data. As shown above, this is $-2.21$. Step 5 consists of finding the $P$-value corresponding to this value. Remembering that the alternative hypothesis in this example is two-sided, the $P$-value is the probability that a "$Z$" is $-2.21$ or less, or 2.21 or more. Charts 2 and 3 show that this probability is about $0.0136 + 0.0136 = 0.0272$. This is less than the value 0.05 chosen for $\alpha$, so we draw the same conclusion that we drew using Approach 1: we have significant evidence to claim that there is a difference between middle- and high-schoolers in terms of getting enough sleep, in agreement with the conclusion reached via Approach 1.

In R, we can use the `prop.test()` function to run two-by-two table tests. Note that to find the $z$ statistic, we will need to take the square root of the "X-squared" statistic that R prints out by default.

```
successes <- c(173, 135)
trials <- c(300, 200)
prop.test(successes, trials, alternative = "two.sided",
conf.level = 0.95, correct = FALSE)
```

*Example 10.1.2 (Clinical Trials)* This example illustrates a one-sided test. Testing a new medicine is often done using a comparison of the new medicine with a placebo (i.e. a harmless mixture made out of (say) flour, sugar and water). Suppose that we plan to give the proposed medicine to $r_1$ people and the placebo to $r_2$ people. We write $\theta_1$ as the probability that the new medicine leads to a cure and $\theta_2$ as the probability that the placebo leads to a cure. The null hypothesis is $H_0$: $\theta_1 = \theta_2$ (= $\theta$, unspecified). If the null hypothesis is true, the proposed new medicine is ineffective: its cure probability is the same as that for the placebo.

Since we are only interested in the possibility that the proposed medicine is beneficial, the alternative hypothesis is one-sided up: $H_1$: $\theta_1 > \theta_2$. Declaring $H_0$ and $H_1$ completes Step 1 of the hypothesis testing procedure.

Step 2. In this step, we choose $\alpha$. Since this is a medical example, we choose $\alpha = 0.01$.

Step 3. In this step, we create a test statistic. Suppose that $o_{11}$ of the $r_1$ people given the proposed medicine are cured, and that $o_{21}$ of the $r_2$ people given the placebo are cured. We can form the data in a table just like the one above, as follows:

|                          | cured    | not cured | total |
|--------------------------|----------|-----------|-------|
| given proposed medicine  | $o_{11}$ | $o_{12}$  | $r_1$ |
| given placebo            | $o_{21}$ | $o_{22}$  | $r_2$ |
| total                    | $c_1$    | $c_2$     | $n$   |

With this interpretation of $o_{11}, o_{12}, o_{21}, o_{22}, r_1, r_2, c_1, c_2$ and $n$, the test statistic is as in (10.4), or for purposes of computation as in (10.5).

Step 4, Approach 1. We have to find what values of the test statistic leads us to reject the null hypothesis. To do this, we have to consider the test statistic (10.4). We would reject the null hypothesis if the proportion $o_{11}/r_1$ of people cured with the proposed medicine is sufficiently larger than the proportion $o_{21}/r_2$ of people cured with the placebo. The expression (10.4) shows that we would reject the null hypothesis if the numerical value of expression (10.4) is sufficiently large and positive. That is, it is a "one-sided up" test when this test statistic is used. Since the two test statistics (10.4) and (10.5) are equivalent, this implies that if we use the computationally convenient test statistic (10.5), we would also reject the null hypothesis if the value of this statistic is sufficiently large and positive.

How large positive is sufficient? When the null hypothesis is true, the test statistic (10.5) can be taken as a $z$, and since the Type I error was chosen to be 0.01, the $Z$

chart shows that we will reject the null hypothesis if the value of the test statistic (10.5) is 2.326 or more, and otherwise, we will say that we do not have enough evidence to reject the null hypothesis. Equivalently, the value 2.326 for the critical point can be found directly from Eq. (6.20).

Step 5, Approach 1. This is now straightforward. We get the data, compute the value of the test statistic (10.5), and reject the null hypothesis if this numerical value is equal to, or exceeds, 2.326. If it is less than 2.326, we say that we do not have enough evidence to reject the null hypothesis.

We illustrate the above using the data for the clinical trial of the proposed Moderna vaccine against COVID-19 given in Sect. 1.1. With these data, the numerical value of the test statistic (10.5) is

$$\frac{(15,199 \times 185 - 11 \times 15,025)\sqrt{30,420}}{\sqrt{15,210 \times 15,210 \times 30,224 \times 196}} = 12.47.$$

We start with Approach 1. The null hypothesis is that the vaccine is ineffective: that is, it is no better than the placebo. The alternative hypothesis is that the vaccine is beneficial, that is, that the probability of not developing COVID if one is given the vaccine is higher than if one is given the placebo. The test is therefore one-sided up. Because this is a medical situation, in which we want to guard as much as is reasonable against making a false positive claim, the chosen value of $\alpha$ is 0.01. This means that we would reject the null hypothesis if the value of the test statistic (10.5) is 2.326 or more. Since the observed value is greater than 2.326, we reject the null hypothesis and claim that we have significant evidence that the proposed new vaccine is effective, in the sense that it has a beneficial effect. However, it is not 100% effective, as shown by the fact that 11 people given the proposed vaccine did develop COVID.

In Approach 2, Step 5, we calculate the $P$-value corresponding to the statistic 12.47. This is well beyond the values in Chart 3, so we only know that the $P$-value is less than 0.0002. We reject the null hypothesis since this is less than the $\alpha$ level 0.01.

How effective is the proposed vaccine? In the paper referred to in Sect. 1.1, it is stated that the vaccine is "about 94.1% effective". This value was found from the fact that 185 of the 15,210 people given the placebo developed COVID, so that if the vaccine were ineffective, we would expect about 185 of the 15,210 people given the vaccine would also develop COVID. However, only 11 people given the vaccine did develop COVID, so the vaccine prevented an estimated 174 vaccinated people from getting COVID. This leads to an efficacy of $174/185 \approx 94.1\%$.

It should be noted that the analysis of the COVID data provided in the reference given in Sect. 1.1 is far more detailed and complex than that given here. Here we have used aspects of it to give an example of the analysis of data in a two-by-two table.

## 10.2   Simpson's Paradox and Fisher's Exact Test

In this section, we discuss two important matters relating to two-by-two table tests, namely Simpson's paradox and Fisher's exact test.

*Simpson's Paradox*  Simpson's paradox arises to a variety of situations in Statistics and here we focus on it as it relates to two-by-two tables.

We are interested in comparing two treatments for some medical complaint, Treatment A and Treatment B. The alternative hypothesis is that Treatment A is more successful than Treatment B. Suppose that data are gathered from two clinical trials concerning the success or otherwise of the two treatments. The data from trial 1 are as follows:

|             | successful | unsuccessful | total |
|-------------|------------|--------------|-------|
| Treatment A | 320        | 20           | 340   |
| Treatment B | 960        | 160          | 1120  |
| total       | 1280       | 180          | 1460  |

The data from trial 2 are as follows:

|             | successful | unsuccessful | total |
|-------------|------------|--------------|-------|
| Treatment A | 760        | 280          | 1040  |
| Treatment B | 220        | 100          | 320   |
| total       | 980        | 380          | 1360  |

The combined data from the two trials are as follows:

|             | successful | unsuccessful | total |
|-------------|------------|--------------|-------|
| Treatment A | 1080       | 300          | 1380  |
| Treatment B | 1180       | 260          | 1440  |
| total       | 2260       | 560          | 2820  |

The value of $z$ as calculated from (10.5) in trial 1 is approximately 4.13, strongly suggesting that Treatment A is more successful than Treatment B. The value of $z$ from trial 2 is approximately 1.51, which although not significant, is at least positive and suggests, although not significantly, Treatment A is more successful than Treatment B. It is thus consistent with the data from trial 1. The value of $z$ for the combined data is approximately $-2.45$, significantly suggesting that Treatment B is more successful than Treatment A. Thus the combined data have led to a conclusion which contradicts the conclusions reached when using the data from the two trials separately.

Simpson's paradox can arise when data are accumulated from two distinct groups, or populations, and a spurious association can arise in the accumulation of data from the two groups into a two-by-two table. This is important in the context of using genetic data to locate disease genes. If two alleles (gene types) at two different gene loci show a significantly high association with each other, it is often assumed, for reasons not discussed here, that the loci at which these alleles are close to each other on the same chromosome. If the location of one of these alleles is known and the other is a purported disease allele, the approximate location of the disease allele is then sometimes inferred. But if the data from which this inference is made are derived from, for example, two different geographical regions, this might be a spurious association, with the disease locus being nowhere near the marker locus.

The take-home message is that one must be very careful in using data in a two-by-two table which are derived from two or more distinct groups.

*Fisher's Exact Test*   The reason why the hypergeometric distribution was in Sect. 4.6 is that it leads to another approach for hypothesis testing for the data in a two-by-two table. The data discussed in Sect. 4.6 can be put into a two-by-two table as follows, using now the notation established in (10.1) for two-by-two tables:

|  | drawn out | not drawn out | total |  |
|---|---|---|---|---|
| red marble | $o_{11}$ | $o_{12}$ | $r_1$ |  |
| blue marble | $o_{21}$ | $o_{22}$ | $r_2$ | (10.8) |
| total | $c_1$ | $c_2$ | $n$ |  |

Using this notation, the number $r_1$ of red marbles and the number $r_2$ of blue marbles were fixed in advance, as was the number $c_1$ of marbles to be drawn from the urn.

Suppose that we wish to test whether the marbles were drawn at random from the urn. The null hypothesis is that they were indeed drawn out at random, and if this null hypothesis is true, then before the drawing is made, the probability that $o_{11}$ of the marbles drawn will be red is given by the hypergeometric probability described in Eq. (4.9), reproduced here with the new notation:

$$\text{Prob}(O_{11} = o_{11}) = \frac{\binom{r_1}{o_{11}}\binom{r_2}{o_{21}}}{\binom{n}{c_1}}. \qquad (10.9)$$

This implies that given that the marginal totals in a two-by-two table were fixed in advance, and assuming that the null hypothesis is true, exact probabilities, and hence exact $P$-values, can be found from the hypergeometric distribution formula (10.9). This enables a comparison with an exact $P$-value and the approximate $P$-value found from the $z$ statistic. We illustrate this with the following example, where the alternative hypothesis is that there is a preference for drawing out red marbles.

*Example* Suppose that the data are as follows:

|              | drawn out | not drawn out | total |
|--------------|:---------:|:-------------:|:-----:|
| red marble   | 6         | 2             | 8     |
| blue marble  | 2         | 6             | 8     |
| total        | 8         | 8             | 16    |

(10.10)

The hypergeometric distribution shows that the exact *P*-value, which is the probability that 6 or more red marbles are drawn at random, is

$$\frac{\binom{8}{6}\binom{8}{2}}{\binom{16}{8}} + \frac{\binom{8}{7}\binom{8}{1}}{\binom{16}{8}} + \frac{\binom{8}{8}\binom{8}{0}}{\binom{16}{8}} = \frac{849}{12,870} = 0.0660.$$

In R, we can use the built in function `fisher.test()`:
`fisher.test(x = matrix(c(6, 2, 2, 6), nrow = 2), alternative = "greater")` to find this *P*-value as well as calculating the hypergeometric probabilities directly.

The value of $z$ as calculated from (10.5) is $\frac{(6 \times 6 - 2 \times 2)\sqrt{16}}{\sqrt{8 \times 8 \times 8 \times 8}} = 2$, so using the $z$ procedure, the *P*-value would be calculated as 0.0228. Clearly for a sample of this small size, the $z$ approximation is not accurate. This is referred to again below.

In Sect. 10.3 below, it is pointed out that the test in a two-by-two table is often more conveniently thought of as a test of association between row and column modes of classification. The fact that the marbles are drawn out of the urn at random is equivalent to there being no association between the color of any marble and the event that it is drawn out from the urn. This in turn is equivalent to the independence of the events "marble is red" and "marble drawn out".

Advanced theory shows that if the row totals are fixed in advance, but not the column totals, exactly the same procedure as that just described is appropriate. An example of this is provided by the Moderna clinical trial data given in Sect. 1.1, where the row totals, both 15,210, were clearly fixed in advance. However, with the large numbers in the Moderna data, an exact hypergeometric calculation would be extremely difficult. Fortunately, when the sample sizes are large in a two-by-two table, the $z$ procedure is sufficiently accurate for all practical purposes.

The theoretical position is not so clear when neither the row totals nor the column totals are fixed in advance, and is perhaps controversial. We do not discuss this controversy here. Our view is that the exact procedure using the hypergeometric distribution is always reasonable.

*Continuity Correction in Two-by-Two Tables* A continuity correction can be made when carrying out a two-by-two table test. Application of a continuity correction in effect replaces the data in (10.8) by those in (10.11) below.

|  | drawn | not drawn | total |
|---|---|---|---|
| red marble | $o_{11} - \frac{1}{2}$ | $o_{12} + \frac{1}{2}$ | $r_1$ |
| blue marble | $o_{21} + \frac{1}{2}$ | $o_{22} - \frac{1}{2}$ | $r_2$ |
| total | $c_1$ | $c_2$ | $n$ |

(10.11)

Calculation of $z$ using these "data" leads to a new value of $z$ given by

$$z = \frac{(o_{11} \times o_{22} - o_{21} \times o_{12} - \frac{1}{2}n)\sqrt{n}}{\sqrt{r_1 \times r_2 \times c_1 \times c_2}}.$$

(10.12)

The quantity $\frac{1}{2}n$ in (10.12) is known as Yates' correction.

We illustrate this in the "marbles" example when the alternative hypothesis is that there is a preference for a red marble to be drawn compared to a blue marble. The test is one-sided up and we will therefore reject the null hypothesis if $z$ in (10.12) is sufficiently large and positive. Calculation of this new $z$ for the data in (10.10) leads to a value of 1.5, corresponding to a $P$-value of 0.0668. This is quite close to the exact $P$-value of 0.0660 found from the hypergeometric distribution. Further examples of the value of using a continuity correction are given in the problems.

In R, the argument `correct` of the `prop.test()` function is set to `TRUE` to use the continuity correction: `prop.test(c(6, 2), c(8, 8), alternative = "greater", correct = TRUE)`. R performs the continuity correction by default, which is why we have been careful to set this argument to `FALSE` in earlier examples.

It has been claimed that use of Yates' correction leads to an over-conservative test. On the other hand, failure to use a continuity correction when using $z$ can lead to an anti-conservative test. Since our aim is to guard against making a Type I error, it can be argued that we are willing to run the risk of making an over-conservative test. Our view, as illustrated by the example in the previous paragraph, is that for purposes of a $P$-value calculation, use of a continuity correction is desirable. Fortunately, when sample sizes are not small, the hypergeometric procedure and the $z$ procedure using a continuity correction usually lead to the same conclusion.

## 10.3  Notes on Two-by-Two Tables

1. For obvious reasons, tests of the kind just considered are often called "two-by-two table tests" (two rows of data, two columns of data).
2. It is useful to summarize the various probability theory results that were used in the two-by-two table test procedure. First, a two-by-two table test procedure concerns two binomial parameters. Second, in carrying out the test, we have to use proportions and not raw numbers, implying the need for the formulas for

the mean and the variance of a proportion. Next, the test involves the difference between two proportions, implying the need for the formulas for the mean and the variance of a difference. Then, the procedure uses a normal distribution approximation and a standardization procedure. Finally, it involves the use of the $Z$ chart. There are therefore eight probability theory concepts and results involved in this testing procedure.

3. What are we testing in the sleep example? We are **not** testing whether people are more likely to be sleep deprived than not. We are testing for a **difference** between middle- and high-schoolers in their rates of sleep deprivation.

4. There were various approximations that we used. For example, we did not know the numerical value of $\theta$, so we did not know the numerical value of the null hypothesis variance of $O_{11}/r_1 - O_{21}/r_2$, namely $\theta(1 - \theta)/r_1 + \theta(1 - \theta)/r_2$. We therefore had to estimate this variance by the estimate $(c_1/n)(c_2/n)/r_1 + (c_1/n)(c_2/n)/r_2$. Next, when the null hypothesis is true, the random variable (10.2) does not exactly have a normal distribution with mean 0, variance 1. However, for large sample sizes, its distribution is very close to this $Z$ distribution, so we are happy to use this approximation in that case. On the other hand, no approximations are made in Fisher's exact test in cases where it is appropriate.

5. It is arbitrary, in the data table, which row we use for middle-schoolers (row 1 or row 2), and also arbitrary which column we use for sleep-deprived (column 1 or column 2). We also could have used the columns for middle/high-schoolers and the rows for sleep-deprived/not. Similarly in the medicine example, we could have used column 1 for "not cured" and column 2 for "cured".

   This shows that one has to be careful about noting the labeling of the rows and columns and what this labeling implies about the sidedness of the test. Suppose, for example, in the medicine example, we decided to use column 1 for "not cured" and column 2 for "cured". With this labeling, the fraction $\frac{o_{11}}{r_1}$ would mean the proportion of people given the new medicine who were **not** cured and the fraction $\frac{o_{21}}{r_2}$ would mean the proportion of people given the placebo who were **not** cured. Then we would reject the null hypothesis if this numerical value in the expression (10.4) is significantly large and *negative*.

   There is no contradiction involved here because with this new labeling the value of $z$ would be the exact negative of the original value of $z$. If, for example, the test is one-sided up with the original labeling, it would be one-sided down with the new labeling, and a significantly large positive value of the original value of $z$ would imply a significantly large negative value of the new value of $z$. Therefore, the same conclusion would be reached under both labeling choices.

6. It is *essential* to use the original numbers, and not, for example, percentages, in the data table and the resulting calculations. Consider two data tables where the numbers in the second table are all 100 times the corresponding numbers in the first table. Although the percentages are the same in both tables, the value of $z$ in the second table will be 10 times the value of $z$ in the first table. The reason

for this is that the sample size matters. Suppose, for example, that the data in a two-by-two table are as in (10.13):

|       | column 1 | column 2 | total |
|-------|----------|----------|-------|
| row 1 | 5        | 3        | 8     |
| row 2 | 3        | 5        | 8     |
| total | 8        | 8        | 16    |

$$(10.13)$$

The value of $z$ as calculated from (10.13) is 1, and this is not a significantly large value and we would not reject any null hypothesis. On the other hand, suppose that the data are:

|       | column 1 | column 2 | total |
|-------|----------|----------|-------|
| row 1 | 500      | 300      | 800   |
| row 2 | 300      | 500      | 800   |
| total | 800      | 800      | 1600  |

$$(10.14)$$

Each value in this table is 100 times larger than the corresponding value in (10.13). The value of $z$ as calculated from (10.14) is 10, and this is a significantly large value and we would reject the null hypothesis with any normally chosen Type I error value $\alpha$.

If percentages were used, the same conclusion would be reached with both data sets. But this would not be correct: as shown above, we would not reject the null hypothesis with the first data set but we would reject the null hypothesis with the second data set.

7. A two-by-two table test is sometimes most naturally though of as a test of association. For example, in the vaccine example, the null hypothesis is that there is no association between vaccine status (given vaccine or given placebo) and outcome status (did develop COVID or did not develop COVID). In the red and blue marbles example discussed in connection with Fisher's exact test, to say that the marbles were drawn at random from the urn is the same as saying that there is no association between the color of any marble and its propensity to be drawn from the urn. In general, the null hypothesis in a two-by-two table becomes the claim that there is no association between row and column modes of classification.

8. In both the sleep example and the medicine example, the row totals were assumed to be chosen in advance of getting the data, but not the column totals. In some other cases, both the row totals and the columns totals are chosen in advance of getting the data. In other cases again, neither the row totals nor the column totals are chosen in advance of getting the data. Despite these differences, the procedures described above apply in all three cases.

## 10.4    Two-Sided Two-by-Two Table Tests

In this section about two-by-two table tests, it is assumed that the alternative hypothesis is two-sided. In terms of the association concept, the only alternative hypothesis considered is that there is some association, but of an unspecified type, between row and column modes of classification. This concludes Step 1: only this null hypothesis and this alternative hypothesis are considered.

Step 2. As always in this step, we choose the numerical value of $\alpha$.

Step 3. The test statistic is, at this stage, the $z$ statistic as given in (10.5). However, we now change it to something equivalent but which is more convenient and flexible.

Suppose that we had chosen $\alpha$ to be 0.05, so that we reject the null hypothesis if the $z$ statistic in (10.5) is less than or equal to $-1.96$ or if it is greater than or equal to $+1.96$. This is the same as rejecting the null hypothesis if $z^2$ is greater than or equal to $(1.96)^2 = 3.8415$.

From (10.5), we can calculate $z^2$ as

$$z^2 = \frac{(o_{11} \times o_{22} - o_{21} \times o_{12})^2 \times n}{r_1 \times r_2 \times c_1 \times c_2}, \tag{10.15}$$

so we will reject the null hypothesis if $z^2$ as given in (10.15) is greater than or equal to 3.8415.

$z^2$ is usually called "chi-square" and written as $\chi^2$. (More precisely, it is called "chi-square with one degree of freedom". We will discuss degrees of freedom later.) $\chi$ is a Greek letter and this is the third occasion in this book where we use a Greek letter for something that is not a parameter. We do this because it is standard statistical practice. So from now on, we will use the notation $\chi^2$ instead of $z^2$ for two-by-two tables, and write Eq. (10.15) as

$$\chi^2 = \frac{(o_{11} \times o_{22} - o_{21} \times o_{12})^2 \times n}{r_1 \times r_2 \times c_1 \times c_2}. \tag{10.16}$$

We will later generalize this type of problem to data tables that are bigger than two-by-two. To do this, it is convenient to re-write $\chi^2$ in a different form. We first form a table of so-called "expected numbers" corresponding to the observed data values in the data table (10.1). This table of expected numbers is as shown below.

|        | column 1 | column 2 | total |
|--------|----------|----------|-------|
| row 1  | $e_{11}$ | $e_{12}$ | $r_1$ |
| row 2  | $e_{21}$ | $e_{22}$ | $r_2$ |
| total  | $c_1$    | $c_2$    | $n$   |

(10.17)

The definition of the "expected numbers" $e_{11}, e_{12}, e_{21}$ and $e_{22}$ is that

$$e_{11} = r_1 c_1/n, \quad e_{12} = r_1 c_2/n, \quad e_{21} = r_2 c_1/n, \quad e_{22} = r_2 c_2/n. \tag{10.18}$$

The logic behind these definitions is explained by referring to the sleep data table (10.6). The proportion of middle-schoolers in the sample is $300/500 = 0.6$, or 60%. If there is no difference between middle- and high-schoolers in their sleep habits, we would expect that about 60% of the 308 people who were sleep-deprived would be middle schoolers. 60% of 318 is $(300)(308)/500 = 184.8$. Using the notation of the general data Table (10.1), the numerical value of $r_1 c_1 / n$ is $(300)(308)/500$, and this is then the numerical value of $e_{11}$ as defined in (10.18). Thus "expected" means the number that we would more or less expect to see in the upper left-hand cell if the null hypothesis is true.

More precisely, given the row and column totals and assuming that the null hypothesis is true, the mean of the random number in the upper left-hand cell of a two-by-two table is given by Eq. (4.29), which in the notation of Table (10.17) is $\frac{r_1 c_1}{n}$, which is the definition of $e_{11}$. Similar arguments lead to the calculations and the interpretations of $e_{12}$, $e_{21}$ and $e_{22}$ defined in (10.18).

Calculating $\chi^2$ using these expected numbers leads to an equivalent alternative formula for $\chi^2$ as

$$\chi^2 = \frac{(o_{11} - e_{11})^2}{e_{11}} + \frac{(o_{12} - e_{12})^2}{e_{12}} + \frac{(o_{21} - e_{21})^2}{e_{21}} + \frac{(o_{22} - e_{22})^2}{e_{22}}. \qquad (10.19)$$

Although the calculations for $\chi^2$ using this formula are more cumbersome than those using (10.16), we have introduced this formula here since, unlike (10.16), it leads to a generalization to tables bigger than two-by-two.

This concludes Step 3: $\chi^2$ as given in (10.19) is the test statistic.

Approach 1, Step 4. What values for $\chi^2$ lead us to reject the null hypothesis? The calculations given above show that if we had chosen $\alpha$ to be 0.05, we would reject the null hypothesis if $\chi^2$ is greater than or equal to 3.8415.

Approach 1, Step 5. We get the data, calculate $\chi^2$, and if $\alpha = 0.05$, we accept or reject the null hypothesis as specified in Step 4. The procedure if $\alpha = 0.01$ is discussed in Note 7 below.

*Example* In this example, we re-do the $z$ calculation (10.7) for the sleep example in terms of $\chi^2$. This is allowed since the alternative hypothesis for this example is two-sided. We choose 0.05 for $\alpha$ as in our previous analysis of the sleep data. The data were:

|                  | sleep-deprived | well-rested | total |
|------------------|:--------------:|:-----------:|:-----:|
| middle schoolers |       173      |     127     |  300  |
| high schoolers   |       135      |      65     |  200  |
| total            |       308      |     192     |  500  |

From (10.18), the numerical values of the $e_{ij}$ are

$$e_{11} = 184.4, e_{12} = 115.2, e_{21} = 123.2, e_{22} = 76.8. \qquad (10.20)$$

Equation (10.19) then leads to a calculation of $\chi^2$ as

$$\chi^2 = \frac{(173 - 184.4)^2}{184.4} + \frac{(127 - 115.2)^2}{115.2} + \frac{(135 - 123.2)^2}{123.2} + \frac{(65 - 76.8)^2}{76.8} = 4.9.$$

$$(10.21)$$

Since this value is greater than 3.8415, we have significant evidence to reject the null hypothesis.

As a check on these calculations, the square of the $z$ value $-2.21$ given in (10.7) is 4.9, and this agrees with the $\chi^2$ calculation above. Alternatively, we could calculate $\chi^2$ from (10.16) and arrive at the same numerical value 4.9.

In R, the function prop.test() that we used in Sect. 10.1 prints out the $\chi^2$ value as "X-squared" by default.

*Notes on the Use of $\chi^2$ in Two-by-Two Tables*

1. The formula (10.19) for $\chi^2$ has been introduced because it generalizes to tables that are bigger than two-by-two, as described in the next Chapter. For two-by-two tables, it is computationally more convenient to use the equivalent expression (10.16) for $\chi^2$.
2. A more precise definition of the "expected value" in any cell in the two-by-two table is that it is the mean of the number in this cell, given only the data in the row and column totals of the table, and given that the null hypothesis is true.
3. $\chi^2$ as defined in (10.19) can be thought of as a measure of the "distance" between the set $\{o_{11}, o_{12}, o_{21}, o_{22}\}$ of observed values and the set $\{e_{11}, e_{12}, e_{21}, e_{22}\}$ of null hypothesis mean values. The larger this distance is, the more likely we are to reject the null hypothesis.
4. The $\chi^2$ approach may be used only if the original alternative hypothesis is two-sided.
5. When each $e_{ij}$ is calculated, the value obtained will usually not be a whole number. To be sufficiently accurate, we should try to compute each $e_{ij}$ value with more decimal place accuracy than is needed in the final answer.
6. Only sufficiently large positive values of $\chi^2$ lead to rejection of the null hypothesis.
7. Since in the "sleep" example, $\alpha$ was chosen to be 0.05, we would reject the null hypothesis if $\chi^2 \geq 3.8415$. What would be the critical point of $\chi^2$ if $\alpha$ had been chosen to be 0.01? We calculated 3.8415 as the square of 1.96, where $\text{Prob}(Z \leq -1.96) + \text{Prob}(Z \geq +1.96) = 0.05$. Equation (6.23) shows that $\text{Prob}(Z \leq -2.576) + \text{Prob}(Z \geq +2.576) = 0.01$. Thus the critical point of $\chi^2$ if the numerical value of our Type I error had been chosen to be 0.01 is $(2.576)^2 = 6.6349$. This value will be seen in the $\chi^2$ chart, as discussed in the next note.
8. *Continuation from Note 7.* Chart 5 is the chi-square chart and has the numbers 3.8415 and 6.6349 on it for $\alpha$ values 0.05 and 0.01 respectively and one degree of freedom $(df)$. This leads to the question: what are degrees of freedom and what is one degree of freedom?

Suppose that the four marginal totals $r_1$, $r_2$, $c_1$ and $c_2$ are given. Then we can only freely fill in one number in the four inner cells of the table. The remaining three numbers will then automatically be defined. We only have one degree of freedom in filling out the numbers in the table. This concept becomes important when we consider tables that are bigger than two-by-two in the next chapter.

9. All the analysis of the $\chi^2$ procedure considered so far follows Approach 1. Approach 2 would require us, in Step 4, to get the data and calculate the value of $\chi^2$. Step 5 would require us to find the $P$-value corresponding to the observed value of $\chi^2$. Doing this is possible by considering the original $z$ statistic, but this is roundabout and not straightforward. On the other hand, any reasonable statistical computer package will show this $P$-value for a chi-square test. If this $P$-value is less than or equal to the value of $\alpha$ chosen in Step 2, the null hypothesis is rejected.

10. In the testing procedure described above, the use of the test statistic $z$, together with the use of the $Z$ chart, is an approximate one. The same comment is true for the $\chi^2$ procedure: the procedure is only as accurate as the normal approximation to the binomial is accurate as justified by the Central Limit Theorem. Accepted wisdom is that if the expected numbers calculated from the data values in the table are all sufficiently large, the approximation is reasonably accurate. In practice, "sufficiently large" is often taken as being "5 or more".

11. It is essential when carrying out this and any other $\chi^2$ test that the data used are the original data values and not, for example, percentages.

12. The chi-square test discussed above is, more exactly, the chi-square test of association in a two-by-two contingency table. There are various other chi-square procedures: a generalization of the two-by-two table chi-square is discussed in the next chapter. Other chi-square procedures are discussed later in this book.

## 10.5   Problems

**10.1** In the discussion of two-by-two tables, it is stated that the test of whether or not two binomial probabilities are equal must be carried out using the original raw number counts, and not (for example) percentages. This question is intended to illustrate this point, and to ask you to explain why this is so.

It is claimed that "trained" mice are more likely to make a correct decision in a T-maze than are "untrained" mice. To test this hypothesis, 26 mice (14 of which were trained, 12 of which were untrained) were put in a T-maze. We choose the value of $\alpha$ to be 0.05. The following data were observed (data set 1):

Decision made:

|           | correct | incorrect | total |
|-----------|---------|-----------|-------|
| trained   | 8       | 6         | 14    |
| untrained | 5       | 7         | 12    |
| total     | 13      | 13        | 26    |

(a) State the appropriate null and alternative hypotheses in terms of two parameters $\theta_1$ and $\theta_2$, first defining what you mean by $\theta_1$ and $\theta_2$.
(b) Indicate whether the test is one-sided up, one-sided down, or two-sided, and give the reason for your answer.
(c) Calculate the value of $z$ (defined by Eq. (10.5)), given the data in the above two-by-two table.
(d) Approach 1. Calculate the relevant critical point. Indicate whether you would accept or reject the null hypothesis based on a comparison of the observed value of $z$ and the critical point.
(e) Approach 2. Calculate the $P$-value. Indicate whether you would accept or reject the null hypothesis based on a comparison of the $P$-value and the chosen value of $\alpha$.
(f) Do your conclusions reached via Approaches 1 and 2 agree? If so, why? If not, why not?

**10.2** With reference to the data in Problem 10.1, suppose now the data values had been (data set 2):

|          | correct | incorrect | total |
|----------|---------|-----------|-------|
| trained  | 80      | 60        | 140   |
| untrained| 50      | 70        | 120   |
| total    | 130     | 130       | 260   |

(a) Comment on the relationship between the two data sets from the point of view of percentages.
(b) Calculate the value of $z$ as defined in (10.5), given the data in the new two-by-two table.
(c) Approach 1. Calculate the relevant critical point. Indicate whether you would accept or reject the null hypothesis based on a comparison of the observed value of $z$ and the critical point.
(d) Approach 2. Calculate the $P$-value. Indicate whether you would accept or reject the null hypothesis, based on a comparison of the $P$-value and the chosen value of $\alpha$.
(e) Do your conclusions reached via Approaches 1 and 2 agree? If so, why? If not, why not?
(f) Do you reach the same conclusion for data set 1 as for data set 2? If so, why? If not, why not?

**10.3** A new medicine is used to attempt to cure a certain illness. We know little about the properties of this new medicine and in particular, we know nothing about whether there is a difference in cure rate between adults and children. In other words, if there is an age difference in cure rate, we have no prior idea whether adults or children have the higher cure rate. We choose $\alpha = 0.05$.

In a sample of 300 people, of whom 140 are children and 160 adults, the following results arise:

|          | cured | not cured | total |
|----------|-------|-----------|-------|
| children | 116   | 24        | 140   |
| adults   | 137   | 23        | 160   |
| total    | 253   | 47        | 300   |

(a) State the appropriate null and alternative hypotheses in terms of two parameters $\theta_1$ and $\theta_2$, first defining what you mean by $\theta_1$ and $\theta_2$.

(b) Indicate whether the test is one-sided up, one-sided down, or two-sided, and give the reason for your answer.

(c) Calculate the value of $z$ given the data in the above two-by-two table.

(d) Approach 1. Calculate the relevant critical point(s). Indicate whether you would accept or reject the null hypothesis, based on a comparison of the observed value of $z$ and the critical point(s).

(e) Approach 2. Calculate the $P$-value. Indicate whether you would accept or reject the null hypothesis, based on a comparison of the $P$-value and the chosen value of $\alpha$.

(f) Do your conclusions reached via Approaches 1 and 2 agree? If so, why? If not, why not?

**10.4** The following data arose in a clinical trial testing for a proposed new vaccine:

|               | contracted illness | did not contract illness | total  |
|---------------|--------------------|--------------------------|--------|
| given vaccine | 50                 | 9950                     | 10,000 |
| given placebo | 150                | 9850                     | 10,000 |
| total         | 200                | 19,800                   | 20,000 |

We choose a numerical value 0.01 for $\alpha$.

(a) State the appropriate null and alternative hypotheses in terms of two parameters $\theta_1$ and $\theta_2$, first defining what you mean by $\theta_1$ and $\theta_2$.

(b) Indicate whether the test is one-sided up, one-sided down, or two-sided, and give the reason for your answer.

(c) Calculate the relevant value of $z$.

(d) Approach 1. Calculate the relevant critical point(s). Indicate whether you would accept or reject the null hypothesis based on a comparison of the observed value of $z$ and the critical point(s).

(e) Approach 2. Calculate the $P$-value. Indicate whether you would accept or reject the null hypothesis based on a comparison of the $P$-value and the chosen value of $\alpha$. (Note: If the value of $z$ is "off the chart", the $P$-value will be of the form "less than 0.0002".)

(f)  Do your conclusions reached via Approaches 1 and 2 agree? If so, why? If not, why not?

**10.5**  A new vaccine is tested to cure a certain illness involving a virus. The data for the clinical trial are given below. We choose a numerical value 0.01 for $\alpha$. State the null and alternative hypotheses in terms of two parameters $\theta_1$ and $\theta_2$ where $\theta_1 =$ the probability that the proposed vaccine prevents the development of the virus and $\theta_2$ = the probability that the placebo prevents the development of the virus. Carry out a hypothesis test using the $z$ statistic and the approach of your choice.

|          | did not develop illness | did develop illness | total  |
|----------|-------------------------|---------------------|--------|
| vaccine  | 15,995                  | 5                   | 16,000 |
| placebo  | 15,800                  | 200                 | 16,000 |
| total    | 31,795                  | 205                 | 32,000 |

**10.6**  The data values in an artificially small clinical trial are as follows:

|                | recovered | did not recover | total |
|----------------|-----------|-----------------|-------|
| given medicine | 8         | 2               | 10    |
| given placebo  | 5         | 5               | 10    |
| total          | 13        | 7               | 20    |

Before the trial, it was decided that 10 people would be given the medicine and 10 would be given the placebo. Calculate

(a)  an exact $P$-value using the hypergeometric distribution,
(b)  the $P$-value found by using $z$ as defined in (10.5),
(c)  the $P$-value found by using the "continuity corrected" $z$ as defined in (10.12).
(d)  Comment on your answers.

**10.7**  The data values in another artificially small clinical trial are as follows:

|                | recovered | did not recover | total |
|----------------|-----------|-----------------|-------|
| given medicine | 10        | 4               | 14    |
| given placebo  | 6         | 8               | 14    |
| total          | 16        | 12              | 28    |

Before the trial, it was decided that 14 people would be given the medicine and 14 would be given the placebo. Calculate

(a)  an exact $P$-value using the hypergeometric distribution,
(b)  the $P$-value found by using $z$ as defined in (10.5),
(c)  the $P$-value found by using the "continuity corrected" $z$ as defined in (10.12).
(d)  Comment on your answers.

# Chapter 11
# Chi-Square Tests (i): Tables Bigger Than Two-by-Two

## 11.1 Large Contingency Tables

We developed the alternative form (10.19) of the two-by-two table $\chi^2$ statistic since when $\chi^2$ is written in that form it generalizes easily to the case of tables that have some arbitrary number $r$ of rows and some arbitrary number $c$ of columns. We call this an $r$-by-$c$ table.

As an example, suppose that we have $r = 4$ strains of mice, strains 1, 2, 3 and 4. Suppose also that there are $c = 5$ possible coat colors for any mouse: black, brown, white, yellow and gray. We plan to take a sample of $n$ mice. Each mouse in the sample will be categorized by its strain and its coat color. We will then have a 4-by-5 table of counts. For example, the number in row 1, column 1 in this table is the number of mice in the sample who are of strain 1 and have a black coat color.

Step 1. In any $r$-by-$c$ table bigger that two-by-two, the null hypothesis always is that there is no association between the row mode of categorization and the column mode of categorization. Thus in the "mouse-coat color" example, the null hypothesis claims that there is no association between the strain of a mouse and its coat color. Another way of saying this is that the null hypothesis claims that the probability that the coat of any mouse is, for example, brown, is the same for all the strains of the mice. The alternative hypothesis claims that there is some unspecified association between row and column categorizations, in this example between the strain of a mouse and its coat color. The alternative hypothesis therefore is not very specific and is often described as being diffuse.

Step 2. We choose a value for $\alpha$, the numerical value of the Type I error. In the "mouse-coat color", example the Type I error is claiming that there is an association between the strain of a mouse and the coat color of that mouse when in fact there is no such association.

© The Author(s), under exclusive license to Springer Nature Switzerland AG 2023
W. J. Ewens, K. Brumberg, *Introductory Statistics for Data Analysis*,
https://doi.org/10.1007/978-3-031-28189-1_11

Step 3. To carry out Step 3, we first put the data into an $r$-by-$c$ table. Suppose, for example, that in the "mouse-coat color" example, the data are as in the following table:

|  |  | Black | Brown | White | Yellow | Gray | Total |
|---|---|---|---|---|---|---|---|
|  |  |  |  | Color |  |  |  |
|  | 1 | 34 | 41 | 20 | 23 | 32 | 150 |
| Strain | 2 | 40 | 47 | 27 | 31 | 55 | 200 |
|  | 3 | 71 | 77 | 38 | 51 | 63 | 300 |
|  | 4 | 80 | 81 | 44 | 56 | 89 | 350 |
|  | Total | 225 | 246 | 129 | 161 | 239 | 1000 |

(11.1)

For example, of the 1000 mice in the data set, 34 were of strain 1 and had a black coat color, 41 were of strain 1 and had a brown coat color, and so on, and finally, 89 were of strain 4 and had a gray coat color.

In general, the data can be written algebraically in an $r$-by-$c$ table as in the table below. As in a two-by-two table, the collection of "$o_{ij}$" values are the observed data values in the various cells of the table, for example as in Table (11.1).

|  |  | 1 | 2 | 3 | ... | $c$ | Total |
|---|---|---|---|---|---|---|---|
|  |  |  |  | column |  |  |  |
|  | 1 | $o_{11}$ | $o_{12}$ | $o_{13}$ | ... | $o_{1c}$ | $r_1$ |
| row | 2 | $o_{21}$ | $o_{22}$ | $o_{23}$ | ... | $o_{2c}$ | $r_2$ |
|  | ⋮ | ⋮ | ⋮ | ⋮ | ⋮ | ⋮ | ⋮ |
|  | $r$ | $o_{r1}$ | $o_{r2}$ | $o_{r3}$ | ... | $o_{rc}$ | $r_r$ |
|  | Total | $c_1$ | $c_2$ | $c_3$ | ... | $c_c$ | $n$ |

(11.2)

We next compute the "expected values" corresponding to the observed values. For the cell in row $i$, column $j$, this is $e_{ij}$, defined by $e_{ij} = r_i c_j / n$. This formula applies for all of the $r \times c$ cells in the table and is the generalization to $r$-by-$c$ tables of the values given in (10.18). The test statistic is then

$$\chi^2 = \frac{(o_{11} - e_{11})^2}{e_{11}} + \frac{(o_{12} - e_{12})^2}{e_{12}} + \ldots + \frac{(o_{rc} - e_{rc})^2}{e_{rc}}, \tag{11.3}$$

the sum being over all cells in the table, and thus having $r \times c$ terms in it. This is the immediate generalization of the test statistic (10.19). In terms of "sigma" notation, this statistic is

$$\chi^2 = \sum_{i=1}^{r} \sum_{j=1}^{c} \frac{(o_{ij} - e_{ij})^2}{e_{ij}}. \tag{11.4}$$

As in the two-by-two table case, $\chi^2$ can be regarded as a measure of the "distance" between the collection of observed values $o_{ij}$ and the collection of "expected" values $e_{ij}$. This is the end of Step 3: the quantity in (11.3) is the test statistic.

Approach 1, Step 4. The theory behind Step 4 is very difficult, and we will only describe the procedure. The first question is: "what values of $\chi^2$ will lead us to reject the null hypothesis?" The broad answer is: "sufficiently large positive values". The next question is: "how large?" The answer to this question depends first on the value of $\alpha$ chosen in Step 2, and also on the number of degrees of freedom. For an $r$-by-$c$ table we have $(r-1) \times (c-1)$ degrees of freedom. (Why there are $(r-1) \times (c-1)$ degrees of freedom for an $r$-by-$c$ table test will be discussed later.) Then the null hypothesis will be rejected if $\chi^2 \geq a$, where $a$ is the appropriate critical point for the value of $\alpha$ chosen in Step 2 and the number $(r-1) \times (c-1)$ of degrees of freedom for the test. These critical points are given in the chi-square chart, Chart 5, for various values of $\alpha$ and various values for the degrees of freedom (df).

Approach 1, Step 5. Get the data, calculate $\chi^2$, and reject the null hypothesis if the observed value of $\chi^2$ is greater than or equal to the relevant critical point in the chi-square chart for the value of $\alpha$ chosen in Step 2 and the appropriate number of degrees of freedom.

Suppose that in the "mouse - coat color" example, we choose $\alpha$ to be 0.05 in Step 2. For Step 4, we have to calculate the various $e_{ij}$ values, using the formula $e_{ij} = r_i c_j / n$ given above. For example, the expected value in the upper left-hand cell (strain 1, black coat color) is $(150)(225)/1000 = 33.7500$. Continuing in this way, we get the following table of expected values.

|  |  | Black | Brown | White | Yellow | Gray | Total |
|---|---|---|---|---|---|---|---|
|  |  |  |  | Color |  |  |  |
|  | 1 | 33.7500 | 36.9000 | 19.3500 | 24.1500 | 35.8500 | 150 |
| Strain | 2 | 45.0000 | 49.2000 | 25.8000 | 32.2000 | 47.8000 | 200 |
|  | 3 | 67.5000 | 73.8000 | 38.7000 | 48.3000 | 71.7000 | 300 |
|  | 4 | 78.7500 | 86.1000 | 45.1500 | 56.3500 | 83.6500 | 350 |
|  | Total | 225 | 246 | 129 | 161 | 239 | 1000 |

$$(11.5)$$

With these values, $\chi^2$ is

$$\chi^2 = \frac{(34 - 33.7500)^2}{33.7500} + \ldots + \frac{(89 - 83.6500)^2}{83.6500} \approx 5.02. \qquad (11.6)$$

Step 5 is straightforward. There are 12 degrees of freedom and we chose $\alpha = 0.05$. The chi-square chart shows that the critical point is 21.0261. Since 5.02 is less than 21.0261, we have no reason to reject the null hypothesis.

We can also find this critical point using R: `qchisq(0.05, df = 12, lower.tail = FALSE)`.

All the $r$-by-$c$ table analysis considered so far follows Approach 1. In Approach 2, Step 4, we would calculate the numerical value of $\chi^2$ (in the mouse example, 5.02

as given above). In Step 5, we would then have to find the $P$-value corresponding to this value of $\chi^2$. This is extremely difficult and can only be done by using a computer package. In the mouse example, a computer package shows that the $P$-value is about 0.957. Since this exceeds the chosen value of $\alpha$, namely 0.05, we would not reject the null hypothesis. This conclusion agrees with that found under Approach 1.

In R, we find this $P$-value using: pchisq(5.02, df = 12, lower.tail = FALSE).

The code to run this example using the built in chisq.test() function in R is as follows. When entering a table of data in R, always make sure it looks as expected. If the table is loaded row by row, make sure to set byrow = TRUE in the matrix() function.

```
tab <- matrix(c(34, 41, 20, 23, 32, 40, 47, 27, 31, 55,
                71, 77, 38, 51, 63, 80, 81, 44, 56, 89),
              nrow = 4, ncol = 5, byrow = TRUE,
              dimnames = list(NULL, c("black", "brown",
              "white", "yellow", "gray")))
tab
chisq.test(tab)
```

*Notes on r-by-c Tables*

1. Most of the notes for a two-by-two table continue to hold for general $r$-by-$c$ tables. One exception is that while in a two-by-two table $\chi^2$ is the square of a $z$ statistic, in the case of tables bigger than two-by-two, there is no corresponding $z$ statistic.
2. As a matter of terminology, two-by-two tables, and more generally $r$-by-$c$ tables, are called "contingency tables".
3. *Degrees of freedom.* In an $r$-by-$c$ contingency table analysis, the number of degrees of freedom is $(r-1)(c-1)$. Thus in the mouse example, the number of degrees of freedom is $3 \times 4 = 12$. Why is this?

   In calculating the number of degrees of freedom, we take the row and column totals to be given. Then in the mouse example, we can freely choose four of the five numbers in row 1, but having done this, we cannot freely choose the fifth number: it must be such that the numbers in this row add up to the given total in row 1. Similarly, we can freely choose four of the five numbers in rows 2 and 3, but cannot freely choose the fifth number in those rows. Having done this, we cannot freely choose any numbers in row 4: given the choices that we have already made in rows 1, 2 and 3, the numbers in row 4 must be such as to lead to the given column totals. They therefore cannot be chosen freely. Thus in this case, we have $4 + 4 + 4 = 12$ degrees of freedom. Similar arguments lead to the general value $(r-1) \times (c-1)$ for the number of degrees of freedom in an $r$-by-$c$ contingency table. As a special case, in a two-by-two table we have $(2-1) \times (2-1) = 1$ degree of freedom, as found earlier when considering this table.

4. The use of the test statistic $z$ and deriving critical points from the $Z$ chart when testing procedure for a 2-by-2 table is an approximate one. In effect, the procedure approximates a binomial probability calculation by a normal distribution probability calculation. This is reasonable if the numbers in the table are sufficiently large, as justified by the Central Limit Theorem. In practice, "sufficiently large" is often taken as being enough if the expected numbers are all 5 or more. The same is true in the testing procedure for an $r$-by-$c$ table. In such tables, the use of the $\chi^2$ chart to find critical points as a reasonable approximation to exact critical points is only justified if the expected values are all 5 or more.

5. As was the case for two-by-two tables, it is essential that the data used in the table are the original counts (numbers observed), and not, for example, percentages.

6. Finally, the details of the probability theory deductive/implication parts of the procedure are not obvious, since the math is very difficult for tables bigger than two-by-two. In the mouse example it is, in effect, the following:

   *If there is no association between strain and coat color*, the probability that the eventually computed value of $\chi^2$ will be greater than or equal to 21.0261 is 0.05. (The value 21.0261 is only arrived at in the chi-square chart after a mathematically difficult deductive probability calculation, hidden to us because of the complexities of the math.) The corresponding statistical induction/inference is this. The observed value of $\chi^2$ is 5.02. Based on the value 21.0261 calculated by deductive probability theory methods, we have no significant evidence of an association between the strain of a mouse and its coat color.

## 11.2  Problems

**11.1**  Consider the data values in the following "two-by-two contingency table":

|  | col 1 | col 2 | total |
|---|---|---|---|
| row 1 | $o_{11} = 10$ | $o_{12} = 16$ | $r_1 = 26$ |
| row 2 | $o_{21} = 8$ | $o_{22} = 14$ | $r_2 = 22$ |
| total | $c_1 = 18$ | $c_2 = 30$ | $n = 48$ |

For two-sided tests, there are two equivalent $\chi^2$ test statistics, namely

$$\chi^2 (= z^2) = \frac{(o_{11} \times o_{22} - o_{12} \times o_{21})^2 \times n}{r_1 \times r_2 \times c_1 \times c_2}$$

and

$$\chi^2 = (o_{11} - e_{11})^2 / e_{11} + (o_{12} - e_{12})^2 / e_{12} + (o_{21}e_{21})^2 / e_{21} + (o_{22} - e_{22})^2 / e_{22},$$

where in the second test statistic, $e_{11}$, $e_{12}$, $e_{21}$ and $e_{22}$ are respectively defined by (10.18). Check that the two formulas give the same numerical value for the two test statistics, given the above data.

**11.2**  Suppose that the value of chi-square ($\chi^2$) in a 5 × 7 table is 38.33.

(a)  How many degrees of freedom are there?
(b)  If $\alpha = 0.05$, would you accept or reject the null hypothesis?
(c)  If you wanted to use Approach 2, can you find the $P$-value exactly from the chi-square chart? If not, can you find it exactly some other way?

**11.3**  Suppose that the value of chi-square ($\chi^2$) in a 4 × 6 table is 28.68.

(a)  How many degrees of freedom are there?
(b)  If $\alpha = 0.01$, would you accept or reject the null hypothesis?
(c)  If you wanted to use Approach 2, can you find the $P$-value exactly from the chi-square chart? If not, can you find it exactly some other way?

**11.4**  We wish to test for an association between ABO blood type and the severity of a certain disorder. We obtain the following data:

|                     | blood type | | | | |
| severity of disorder | O | A | B | AB | total |
| --- | --- | --- | --- | --- | --- |
| absent | 529 | 220 | 95 | 476 | 1320 |
| mild | 58 | 13 | 8 | 26 | 105 |
| severe | 28 | 9 | 7 | 31 | 75 |
| total | 615 | 242 | 110 | 533 | 1500 |

Carry out a chi-square test of whether there is a significant association between blood type and severity of the disorder, choosing the value of $\alpha = 0.05$.

**11.5**  A manager wishes to determine whether or not there is a relationship between the proportion of defective products and the machine used. Carry out a chi-square test of association with $\alpha = 0.05$.

|               | machine A | machine B | machine C | total |
| --- | --- | --- | --- | --- |
| defective | 8 | 6 | 12 | 26 |
| non-defective | 54 | 62 | 58 | 174 |
| total | 62 | 68 | 70 | 200 |

# Chapter 12
# Chi-Square Tests (ii): Testing for a Specified Probability Distribution

## 12.1 Introduction

Chi-square procedures can be used for several different purposes. In this section, we consider a new form of the chi-square statistic that is different from the form used in contingency tables. It is important not to confuse the form of chi-square discussed in this chapter with the form used in contingency tables.

We start with an example. Is this die fair? Asking this question is the same as asking the question "If $X$ is the random number to turn up on a future roll of the die, is the probability distribution of $X$ given by the following table?"

$$\begin{array}{c|cccccc} \text{Possible values of } X & 1 & 2 & 3 & 4 & 5 & 6 \\ \hline \text{Probability} & 1/6 & 1/6 & 1/6 & 1/6 & 1/6 & 1/6 \end{array} \qquad (12.1)$$

The hypothesis testing procedure is as follows.

Step 1. The null hypothesis in this die example is that the die is fair. Equivalently, the null hypothesis is that (12.1) is the probability distribution of $X$. The alternative hypothesis that we consider is that the die is unfair, but in an unspecified way. Other more structured choices for the alternative hypothesis are possible, for example, $\text{Prob}(X = 1) < \text{Prob}(X = 2) < \ldots < \text{Prob}(X = 6)$, but we do not consider them in this book.

Step 2. As usual, in this step, we choose the numerical value of $\alpha$. In this example, this is the probability that we will claim the die is unfair when it is, in fact, fair.

Step 3. The choice of test statistic is not so obvious. Suppose that we plan to roll the die $n$ times and record the number that turns up on each roll. One possibility for the test statistic is the average of the numbers that will turn up on these $n$ rolls. Before we roll the die, this average is a random variable. We know the mean of this average if the null hypothesis is true (3.5) and we also know the variance of

© The Author(s), under exclusive license to Springer Nature Switzerland AG 2023
W. J. Ewens, K. Brumberg, *Introductory Statistics for Data Analysis*,
https://doi.org/10.1007/978-3-031-28189-1_12

this average if the null hypothesis is true ($\frac{35}{12n}$), and thus we could easily form a $z$ statistic from the eventual data which would allow us to test the null hypothesis.

However, this is not a good test statistic, as the following example shows. Suppose that we roll the die 10,000 times, and that a "1" turns up 5000 times and a "6" turns up 5000 times. No other number turns up. Clearly this is almost certainly a biased die. Yet the average of the numbers that turned up is 3.5, which is the mean of the (random variable) average to turn up when the null hypothesis is true. The value of the $z$ statistic would then be zero and we would not reject the null hypothesis. This is obviously unreasonable. So we need a better test statistic.

This observation shows that the choice of a test statistic is not a straightforward matter. Some test statistics are "better" than others. There is a deep mathematical theory which leads to the choice of a test statistic that should be used in any given testing procedure. We do not consider this theory in this book. Instead, we go straight to what this theory shows is a good test statistic in the rolling a die example, namely a chi-square statistic.

First, the chi-square statistic for the situation discussed in this section is similar to that in a contingency table in that it considers a test statistic of the form "sum over all possibilities of (observed − expected)$^2$/expected." However, apart from this similarity, the details of the procedure, in particular the details about how we calculate the expected numbers and the form of the eventual $\chi^2$ statistic, differ from those in a contingency table. We illustrate this with the die example.

Suppose that we plan to roll the die $n$ times. Then by the expected number of times that 1 turns up, we mean the mean number of times that 1 turns up if the null hypothesis is true (that there is a 1/6th probability of each number turning up). Similarly for the numbers $2, 3, \ldots, 6$. If we consider a 1 turning up as a success and any other number as a failure, then the binomial distribution applies. The short formula for the mean of the number of 1s to show up is then exactly $n/6$. The same holds for all six numbers, 1 through 6. Thus in the die example, all six expected numbers are $n/6$.

Suppose now that we have rolled the die $n$ times and that a 1 turned up $n_1$ times, a 2 turned up $n_2$ times, $\ldots$, a 6 turned up $n_6$ times. Then the appropriate test statistic is of the form "sum over all possibilities of (observed - expected)$^2$/expected", which is

$$\chi^2 = \frac{(n_1 - \frac{n}{6})^2}{\frac{n}{6}} + \frac{(n_2 - \frac{n}{6})^2}{\frac{n}{6}} + \cdots + \frac{(n_6 - \frac{n}{6})^2}{\frac{n}{6}}. \tag{12.2}$$

This concludes Step 3 for the die example. The appropriate test statistic in more general cases will be discussed later.

Step 4, Approach 1. What values of the test statistic (12.2) lead us to reject the null hypothesis that the die is fair? First, only sufficiently large positive values lead us to reject the null hypothesis. How large? This depends on two things: first, the value of $\alpha$ chosen in Step 2 and second, the number of degrees of freedom that we have. To find the number of degrees of freedom, we have to ask how many of the numbers $n_1, n_2, \ldots, n_6$ can be chosen freely, given that the number of rolls $(n)$ is fixed in advance. The answer is five. For example, once $n_1, n_2, \ldots, n_5$ are given, $n_6$ is automatically determined as $n - n_1 - n_2 - n_3 - n_4 - n_5$, so there are five degrees of freedom. While the concept of degrees of freedom is similar here as in contingency tables, the calculation differs from that in contingency tables.

Suppose that in Step 2, we had chosen $\alpha = 0.05$. This implies that we will reject the null hypothesis if $\chi^2 \geq a$, where $a$ is chosen so that the probability of eventually getting a value of $\chi^2$ greater than or equal to $a$ is 0.05 when the null hypothesis is true. The calculation of $a$ is quite complicated, and the relevant value is given in the chi-square chart, Chart 5. Since $\alpha = 0.05$ and we have five degrees of freedom, the chart shows that $a = 11.0705$.

Step 5, Approach 1. As always, this step is easy. We compute the value of $\chi^2$ as defined in (12.2) and reject the null hypothesis if this value is 11.0705 or larger. This concludes the procedure under Approach 1.

We next consider Steps 4 and 5 under Approach 2. In Step 4, we compute the value of $\chi^2$. In Step 5, we find the $P$-value associated with the calculated value of $\chi^2$. This can only be done via a statistical computer package. The null hypothesis is rejected if the $P$-value given by the computer package is less than or equal to the chosen value of $\alpha$.

*Example (The "Die" Case)* Suppose that in Step 2, we choose $\alpha = 0.05$. As shown above, we will reject the null hypothesis if, once we get the data and calculate $\chi^2$, we find that $\chi^2 \geq 11.0705$.

Suppose that we now roll the die $n = 5000$ times and get the following data:

| Number turning up: | 1 | 2 | 3 | 4 | 5 | 6 |
|---|---|---|---|---|---|---|
| Number of times seen: | 861 | 812 | 820 | 865 | 821 | 821 |

$$(12.3)$$

Each expected number is $5000/6 = 833.3333$ (to four decimal place accuracy). The value of $\chi^2$ is thus

$$\frac{(861 - 833.3333)^2}{833.3333} + \frac{(812 - 833.3333)^2}{833.3333} + \frac{(820 - 833.3333)^2}{833.3333} +$$

$$+ \frac{(865 - 833.3333)^2}{833.3333} + \frac{(821 - 833.3333)^2}{833.3333} + \frac{(821 - 833.3333)^2}{833.3333} \approx 3.25.$$

$$(12.4)$$

Since this is less than the critical point 11.0705 when $\alpha = 0.05$, we do not have enough evidence to reject the null hypothesis that the die is fair. The same conclusion would be reached under Approach 2.

In R, we can conduct this test as follows:

```
chisq.test(x = c(861, 812, 820, 865, 821, 821), p = rep(1/6, 6)).
```

Without carrying out a statistical procedure, it is not obvious that the numbers in Table (12.9) do not suggest that the die is unfair. Only the formal statistical procedure just described can help us with this question.

*Notes on the Die Example*

1. The expected numbers ($n/6$) for the die example are all the same. This is not usually the case in other situations, as will be seen later.
2. As shown by the die example, the expected numbers are not necessarily whole numbers. They should be calculated to four decimal place accuracy, and the value of $\chi^2$ presented to two decimal place accuracy.
3. Although the statistic (12.2) is different from that in a contingency table, it does share the same characteristic of the contingency table chi-square statistic in that it can be thought of as a measure of the difference between, or distance between, the various observed numbers and the various numbers expected if the null hypothesis is true. The larger these differences are, the larger $\chi^2$ is, and if these differences are large enough, $\chi^2$ will be large enough for us to reject the null hypothesis.

## 12.2   Generalization

In the die example, the null hypothesis specified equal probabilities for all categories. We now generalize to a broader null hypothesis.

Suppose that in general, we have $k$ categories, which we call categories $1, 2, \ldots, k$. The null hypothesis states that the probability that any of these observations will fall in category 1 is $P_0(1)$, the probability that an observation is in category 2 is $P_0(2)$, ..., the probability that an observation is in category $k$ is $P_0(k)$. (The suffix "0" denotes "under the null hypothesis".) These probabilities are assumed to be specific numerical values appropriate to the case in hand, for example 1/6, 1/6, 1/6, 1/6, 1/6, 1/6 in the die example. That is, the probabilities $P_0(1), P_0(2), \ldots, P_0(k)$ do not involve unknown parameters.

Step 2. In this step, we choose the value of $\alpha$, in this case, the probability that we will claim that the null hypothesis probabilities are not correct when in fact they are correct.

Step 3. The test statistic is the general form of that used in the die example. To describe this explicitly, suppose that we have done our experiment and that $n_1$ observations fell in category 1, $n_2$ fell in category 2, ..., $n_k$ fell in category $k$, with $n_1 + \cdots + n_k = n$. The test statistic $\chi^2$ is now defined by

$$\chi^2 = \frac{(n_1 - n P_0(1))^2}{n P_0(1)} + \ldots + \frac{(n_k - n P_0(k))^2}{n P_0(k)}. \tag{12.5}$$

Step 4, Approach 1. The values of $\chi^2$ that lead to rejection of the null hypothesis are sufficiently large (positive) values. How large? This depends on the value of $\alpha$ chosen in Step 2, and the number of degrees of freedom. Generalizing from the "die" example, the number of degrees of freedom is $k - 1$.

Step 5, Approach 1. Get the data, calculate $\chi^2$, and if the value found is greater than or equal to the appropriate $\chi^2$ chart value, reject the null hypothesis. If the value found is less than the appropriate chart value, we do not have enough evidence to reject the null hypothesis.

Step 4, Approach 2. Get the data and calculate $\chi^2$.

Step 5, Approach 2. Find the $P$-value associated with the observed value of $\chi^2$. This can only be done by a computer statistical package.

Examples of this procedure are given in the problems.

## Notes on the "Testing for a Specified Probability Distribution" $\chi^2$ Procedure

1. Although, as emphasized above, the "testing for a specified probability distribution" chi-square procedure described above is different from the chi-square procedure used in $r \times c$ tables, many of the notes for $r \times c$ tables also apply for this form of chi-square procedure. In particular, we have to use the actual counts and not percentages.
2. It is important to be clear about the meanings of, and distinction between, $k$ and $n$. $k$ is the number of categories, for example 6 in the die case. $n$ is the number of observations, 5000 in the die example. The value of $n$ can be chosen by the investigator and depends on the amount of time and money at his/her disposal. The value of $k$ often cannot be chosen by the investigator: for example, for a die, $k$ must be 6. This is an important distinction since the number of degrees of freedom is $k - 1$, not $n - 1$.
3. In many cases, the categories are descriptive. In the die example, we would say that category 1 is "a 1 turns up", that category 2 is "a 2 turns up", etc.
4. Generalizing binomial testing. The $\chi^2$ procedure discussed above can be viewed as a generalization of testing in the binomial distribution case. This is shown by the following example.

    Suppose that we plan to conduct 1000 binomial trials. The probability of success on each trial is $\theta$. The null hypothesis claims that $\theta = 0.3$. The alternative hypothesis is two-sided ($\theta \neq 0.3$). We observe 321 successes in the 1000 trials. Our aim is to compare three ways of testing the null hypothesis against the alternative hypothesis.

    (a) Focus on the number of successes. Calculate a $z$ statistic, using the observed number of successes and the null hypothesis mean and variance of the number of successes in 1000 trials. From $z$, calculate $z^2$.
    (b) Focus on the proportion of trials giving success. Calculate a $z$ statistic, using the observed value of this proportion of successes and the null hypothesis mean and variance of this proportion in 1000 trials. From $z$, calculate $z^2$.
    (c) Calculate a $\chi^2$ statistic using Eq. (12.5). (This will be the sum of two terms, one relating to successes, one relating to failures).

In order to compare these three procedures, we will use exact fractions, not decimals, and thus calculate $z^2$ exactly for all three cases.

Under method (a), $z = \dfrac{(321 - 300)}{\sqrt{(1000(0.3)(0.7)}} = \dfrac{21}{\sqrt{210}}$, so that $z^2 = \dfrac{441}{210} = 2.1$ (exactly).

Under method (b), $z = \dfrac{(0.321 - 0.3)}{\sqrt{(0.3)(0.7)/1000}} = \dfrac{0.021}{\sqrt{0.00021}}$, so that $z^2 = \dfrac{0.000441}{0.00021} = 2.1$ (exactly).

Under method (c), $\chi^2 = \dfrac{(321 - 300)^2}{300} + \dfrac{(679 - 700)^2}{700} = \dfrac{441}{300} + \dfrac{441}{700} = 1.47 + 0.63 = 2.1$ (exactly).

Thus all three methods give the same answer. The first two rely on binomial calculations, which are possible here since there are only two categories (success and failure). The $\chi^2$ method works for two categories, as just shown, but also extends to any number of categories, for example, six categories as in the die example.

## 12.3　A More Complicated Situation

In the examples considered so far, the probabilities for the $k$ categories as given by the null hypothesis were all explicit specific numbers, for example $1/6, 1/6, \ldots, 1/6$ in the die example. In some more complex cases, the probabilities are given in terms of an unknown parameter or several unknown parameters. The procedure in such cases is as follows.

(i) Estimate the parameters from the data. There is advanced statistical theory, generally not considered in this book, that shows how this is done. In the example below, the required procedure is simply indicated.

(ii) Calculate $\chi^2$ in the normal way, but with the parameter(s) replaced by the parameter estimate(s).

(iii) One further degree of freedom in the chi-square is lost for every parameter that is estimated. So if there are $k$ categories and $m$ parameters are estimated, the number of degrees of freedom is $k - m - 1$.

*Example from Genetics*　Under the null hypothesis, individuals in a certain population are either of genetic type $aa$ with probability $(1 - \theta)^2$, of genetic type $Aa$ with probability $2\theta(1 - \theta)$, or of genetic type $AA$ with probability $\theta^2$. Here $\theta$ is a parameter whose numerical value is not known. The alternative hypothesis is that the null hypothesis is not true, but the alternative hypothesis is diffuse and does not specify in what way the null hypothesis not is true.

Steps 3 and 4 are the complicated steps. What is our test statistic and what values of the test statistic will lead us to reject the null hypothesis?

Suppose first that the numerical value of $\theta$ is known. In the data, there are $n_1$ individuals of type $aa$, $n_2$ individuals of type $Aa$, and $n_3$ individuals of type $AA$, with $n_1 + n_2 + n_3 = n$. Plugging these data and the probabilities above into expression (12.5), we have the chi-square statistic

$$\chi^2 = \frac{(n_1 - n(1-\theta)^2)^2}{n(1-\theta)^2} + \frac{(n_2 - 2n\theta(1-\theta))^2}{2n\theta(1-\theta)} + \frac{(n_3 - n\theta^2)^2}{n\theta^2}. \tag{12.6}$$

We would then use this to test the null hypothesis using the chi-square chart with two degrees of freedom.

However, as stated above, the numerical value of $\theta$ is not known, and will have to be estimated from the data. This is best done by focusing on the number of genes and not on the number of individuals, thus looking at $2n$ genes. The null hypothesis assumption implies that any gene is of type $a$ with probability $1 - \theta$ and of type $A$ with probability $\theta$ (taking the genes to be independent, these probabilities agree with those above for people of type $aa$, $Aa$, and $AA$). Following binomial distribution procedures, we then estimate $\theta$ by the proportion of the $2n$ genes in the sample which are of type $A$, namely $p = \dfrac{n_2 + 2n_3}{2n}$. Then by analogy with (12.6), we form the appropriate $\chi^2$ statistic by replacing $\theta$ wherever we see it in the expression (12.6) by $p$. This gives the test statistic

$$\chi^2 = \frac{(n_1 - n(1-p)^2)^2}{n(1-p)^2} + \frac{(n_2 - 2np(1-p))^2}{2np(1-p)} + \frac{(n_3 - np^2)^2}{np^2}. \tag{12.7}$$

We refer the value so calculated to chi-square charts with $3 - 1 - 1 = 1$ degree of freedom, since we always lose one degree of freedom, and we lose a further degree of freedom here because we estimated one parameter.

*Example* Suppose that $n_1 = 466$, $n_2 = 444$ and $n_3 = 90$, so that $n = 1000$. Then $p = (444 + 180)/2000 = 0.312$. Then $\chi^2$ is calculated as

$$\chi^2 = \frac{(466 - 1000(0.688)^2)^2}{1000(0.688)^2} + \frac{(444 - 2000(0.312)(0.688))^2}{2000(0.312)(0.688)}$$

$$+ \frac{(90 - 1000(0.312)^2)^2}{1000(0.312)^2} \approx 1.17. \tag{12.8}$$

If we choose $\alpha = 0.05$ in Step 2, the relevant critical point from the chi-square chart is 3.8415. Since 1.17 is less than this, we do not have enough evidence to reject the null hypothesis.

## 12.4   Problems

**12.1** In order to test if a given die is fair, we now roll it $n = 6000$ times and get the following data:

$$
\begin{array}{l|cccccc}
\text{Number turning up:} & 1 & 2 & 3 & 4 & 5 & 6 \\
\hline
\text{Number of times seen:} & 1009 & 984 & 1038 & 988 & 1002 & 979
\end{array}
\tag{12.9}
$$

Test whether we have significant evidence that the die is unfair, using a Type I error $\alpha$ of 0.05.

**12.2** A genetic theory claims that the probability that an individual is of genetic type A, genetic type B or genetic type C are as follows:

$$
\begin{array}{l|ccc}
\text{Genetic type} & A & B & C \\
\hline
\text{Respective probabilities} & \frac{1}{4} & \frac{1}{2} & \frac{1}{4}
\end{array}
\tag{12.10}
$$

This claim becomes the null hypothesis.

In a well-conducted representative sample of 1000 individuals, the following numbers were found in these categories:

$$
\begin{array}{l|ccc}
\text{Genetic type} & A & B & C \\
\hline
\text{number seen} & 210 & 484 & 306
\end{array}
\tag{12.11}
$$

Test the null hypothesis using a Type I error $\alpha$ of 0.05.

**12.3** A genetic theory claims that the probability that an individual is of genetic type A, genetic type B or genetic type C are as follows:

$$
\begin{array}{l|ccc}
\text{Genetic type} & A & B & C \\
\hline
\text{Respective probabilities} & (1 - \theta)^2 & 2\theta(1 - \theta) & \theta^2
\end{array}
\tag{12.12}
$$

Here $\theta$ is an unknown parameter. The observed data are as in Problem 12.2. The appropriate estimate of $\theta$ in this case is $p = (n_B + 2n_C)/2n$, where $n_B$ is the number of individuals in the sample of genetic type $B$ and $n_C$ is the number of individuals in the sample of genetic type $C$. Test the null hypothesis using a Type I error $\alpha$ of 0.05.

**12.4** A genetic theory claims that the probability that an individual is of genetic type A, genetic type B, genetic type C or genetic type D are as follows:

$$
\begin{array}{l|cccc}
\text{Genetic type} & A & B & C & D \\
\hline
\text{Respective probabilities} & \frac{1}{8} & \frac{3}{8} & \frac{3}{8} & \frac{1}{8}
\end{array}
\tag{12.13}
$$

This claim becomes the null hypothesis.

In a well-conducted representative sample of 2000 individuals, the following numbers were found in these categories:

$$\begin{array}{c|cccc} \text{Genetic type} & A & B & C & D \\ \hline \text{number seen} & 244 & 782 & 742 & 232 \end{array} \qquad (12.14)$$

Test the null hypothesis using a Type I error $\alpha$ of 0.01.

# Chapter 13
# Tests on Means

Perhaps the most frequently used tests in Statistics concern tests on means. In this book, tests on means are carried out using $t$ tests. We shall discuss four different $t$ tests in this book, the first three of which are tests about means. Other tests on means for data more complicated than that which we consider use Analysis of Variance (ANOVA) procedures, which are not considered in this book.

## 13.1 The One-Sample $t$ Test

We start with an example. Different people have different natural body temperatures, due to differences in physiology, age, and so on. That is, the temperature of a person taken at random cannot be known in advance and is therefore a (continuous) random variable. So there is a probability distribution of temperatures. From considerable past experience, suppose that we know that the mean of this distribution is 98.6 degrees Fahrenheit for normal healthy individuals.

We are concerned that the mean temperature for people 24 hours after an operation exceeds 98.6. To investigate this, we plan to take the temperatures of $n$ people 24 hours after they have had this operation. At this stage, these temperatures are random variables: we do not know what values they will take, since we are still in the planning phase. Because these temperatures at this stage are random variables, we denote them in upper case: $X_1$ for the first person's temperature, ..., $X_n$ for the $n$th person's temperature. We assume that these random variables have a normal distribution. This assumption is discussed below in Notes 9 and 10. We also assume that $X_1, X_2, \ldots, X_n$ are identically and independently distributed ($iid$). This assumption is discussed below in Note 10. One has to be careful in practice that these two assumptions are reasonable and the judgment on these assumptions is largely a matter of experience and common sense. These practical considerations

© The Author(s), under exclusive license to Springer Nature Switzerland AG 2023
W. J. Ewens, K. Brumberg, *Introductory Statistics for Data Analysis*,
https://doi.org/10.1007/978-3-031-28189-1_13

are of great importance and are not discussed as much as they should be in this book, since the focus in this book is on theory.

We denote the unknown mean temperature of people 24 hours after the operation by $\mu$. This mean is a parameter, that is, it is an unknown number, and this is why we use the Greek notation $\mu$ for it. The null hypothesis claims that the mean body temperature of people 24 hours after the operation is the same as that for normal healthy people. In terms of parameters, the null hypothesis claims that $\mu = 98.6$. From the context of the situation, the natural alternative hypothesis is one-sided up, that is, the alternative hypothesis claims that $\mu$ is greater than 98.6. This concludes Step 1 in the hypothesis testing procedure: we have declared our null and alternative hypotheses. They both relate to the parameter $\mu$.

As always, Step 2 consists of choosing a value of $\alpha$. In this example, it is the probability that we are prepared to accept the claim that $\mu$ is greater than 98.6 when it is in fact equal to 98.6. Since this is a medical situation, we choose $\alpha$ to be 0.01.

Step 3 consists of choosing the test statistic. Looking ahead to the time after we have conducted our survey, the data that we will have will be the actual temperatures $x_1, x_2, \ldots, x_n$ that we observed for the $n$ people after the operation. A key component in the test statistic will be a comparison of the average $\bar{x}$ of these data values with the null hypothesis mean 98.6. That is, a key component in the test statistic will be the difference $\bar{x} - 98.6$.

This difference is the comparison of an average with a mean. This is why it has been emphasized so frequently in this book that an average and a mean are two entirely different concepts. Using these two words as meaning the same thing makes it almost impossible to understand $t$ tests.

The difference $\bar{x} - 98.6$ on its own is not enough. To see why this is so, we consider first the unrealistic case where we know the variance $\sigma^2$ of the distribution of the $X$'s. We consider the realistic case, where we do not know this variance, later.

We first do a probability theory calculation. Before the data were obtained, the average $\bar{X}$ of $X_1, X_2, \ldots, X_n$ is a random variable. If the null hypothesis is true, $\bar{X}$ has mean 98.6 (from the first part of Eq. (5.4)) and variance $\sigma^2/n$ (from the second part of Eq. (5.4)). Since we also assume that the $X$'s have a normal distribution,

$$\frac{\bar{X} - 98.6}{\sigma/\sqrt{n}}$$

has a normal distribution with mean 0 and variance 1 if the null hypothesis is true. That is, it is a $Z$. So once we have our data, we can compute

$$\frac{(\bar{x} - 98.6)}{\sigma/\sqrt{n}} \tag{13.1}$$

and reject the null hypothesis if the value of this is 2.326 or more. The value 2.326 is found from Eq. (6.20) given that $\alpha = 0.01$, or can be found by interpolation in the normal distribution chart.

Although our interest is in testing a hypothesis about a mean, the numerator $(\bar{x} - 98.6)$ in the test statistic (13.1) is not enough. The standard deviation $\sigma/\sqrt{n}$ of $\bar{X}$ in the denominator is a crucial ingredient in the test statistic. Using the normal distribution chart is possible only because we created a $Z$ when the null hypothesis is true, and to do this, we had to use the known standard deviation $\sigma/\sqrt{n}$ of $\bar{X}$ as part of the test statistic.

The above procedure suggests what to do in the more realistic case where we do not know the variance $\sigma^2$ of the $X$'s. Equation (8.13) shows how $\sigma^2$ is estimated, so it makes sense to replace $\sigma$ in the test statistic (13.1) by $s$ as defined from Eq. (8.13). Doing this results in a new statistic called $t$, defined as

$$t = \frac{(\bar{x} - 98.6)}{s/\sqrt{n}}. \tag{13.2}$$

This is the test statistic for the temperatures example. This concludes Step 3 of the testing procedure in the temperatures example: the test statistic is $t$, as defined in (13.2).

More generally, if the null hypothesis claims that the mean of whatever quantity we are interested in is $\mu_0$, the test statistic is

$$t = \frac{(\bar{x} - \mu_0)}{s/\sqrt{n}}. \tag{13.3}$$

Step 4, Approach 1. What values of $t$ will lead us to reject the null hypothesis? In the "temperatures" example, the alternative hypothesis is that the mean temperature exceeds 98.6 after the operation. If this alternative hypothesis is true, the value of $\bar{x}$ should tend to exceed 98.6. The form of the $t$ statistic (13.2) shows that if the alternative hypothesis is true, $t$ should tend to be positive. Thus this is a one-sided up example: sufficiently large positive values of $t$ will lead us to reject the null hypothesis.

How large? To answer this question, we go back to the situation before we do our experiment. In the general situation, we assume that the random variables $X_1, \ldots, X_n$ are $iid$ with a normal distribution with mean $\mu$. The random variable analogue of $t$ is the random variable $T$, defined in parallel with the right-hand side in Eq. (13.3):

$$T = \frac{(\bar{X} - \mu)}{S/\sqrt{n}}, \tag{13.4}$$

where

$$S^2 = \frac{X_1^2 + X_2^2 + \ldots + X_n^2 - n(\bar{X})^2}{n-1}.$$

So the random variable $T$ is similar to the random variable $Z$. The only difference is that $T$ has the estimator of a standard deviation in the denominator instead of a known standard deviation. Because of this difference, $T$ does not have a normal distribution. Instead, it has the so-called $t$ distribution with $n-1$ degrees of freedom. The reason why there are $n-1$ degrees of freedom in the procedure will be discussed later. If the null hypothesis is true, the probability density function $f_T(t)$ of $T$ is found by a mathematical procedure not given here, and is given in (13.5):

$$f_T(t) = C \left( 1 + \frac{t^2}{\nu} \right)^{-(\nu+1)/2}, \qquad -\infty < t < +\infty. \qquad (13.5)$$

In this expression, the suffix "$T$" indicated that the random variable is $T$, $C$ is a mathematical function depending on $n$ which we do not write down but which ensures that $\int_{-\infty}^{+\infty} f_T(f)dt = 1$, and $\nu$ (the Greek letter "nu") is the number of degrees of freedom, $n - 1$ in the one-sample $t$ test considered in this section, but different from $n - 1$ for the $t$ tests considered in later sections. The distribution (13.5) is well-studied and, like the normal distribution, is of central importance in Statistics.

The form of the distribution (13.5) is used to indicate how large $t$ has to be for us to reject the null hypothesis. For example, if $n = 10$, so that $\nu = 9$, Eq. (13.5) shows (after some difficult mathematics) that if the null hypothesis is true, $\text{Prob}(T \geq 2.821) = 0.01$. The critical point 2.821 in the $t$ chart (Chart 4) derives from this fact. Therefore, in the temperatures example, where $n = 10$ and $\alpha = 0.01$, we will reject the null hypothesis if $t \geq 2.821$. The logic of this is as follows. Equation (13.5) shows that if the null hypothesis is true, it is very unlikely (probability 0.01) that we will obtain a value of $t$ exceeding 2.821 when $\nu = 9$. If we do obtain a value of $t$ exceeding 2.821, we have sufficient evidence to reject the null hypothesis.

In R, we can find this critical point with qt(p = 0.01, df = 9, lower.tail = FALSE).

The above comments relate to a one-sided up test, the form of test for which the $t$ chart is designed. How the $t$ chart is used for one-sided down and two-sided tests will be discussed later.

Approach 1, Step 5. Get the data, compute $t$, compare the value with the relevant critical point in Chart 4, and accept or reject the null hypothesis accordingly.

*Example  (The Temperatures Case)* Suppose that we get the temperatures of $n = 10$ people 24 hours after they have the operation. These values are 98.9, 98.6, 99.3, 98.7, 98.7, 98.4, 99.0, 98.5, 98.8, 98.8. The average ($\bar{x}$) of these is 98.77. The value of $s^2$ is found, from Eq. (8.13), to be 0.066778. From this, $s = 0.258414$. Thus the value of $t$ is

$$t = \frac{(98.77 - 98.6)}{0.258414/\sqrt{10}} = \frac{0.17}{0.0817177} = 2.0803.$$

Since there are 9 degrees of freedom and we chose $\alpha = 0.01$, the critical point is 2.821, as given above. The observed value $t$ is less than this, so we do not have enough evidence to reject the null hypothesis. In other words, we do not have enough evidence to claim that there is a significant increase in temperature 24 hours after the operation.

Step 4, Approach 2. Get the data and calculate the value of the test statistic $t$. As shown above, we get $t = 2.0803$.

Step 5, Approach 2. Find the $P$-value corresponding to the observed value of the test statistic. In the temperatures example, this is the $P$-value corresponding to the observed value 2.0803 of $t$. This can only be done with a statistical computer package.

If you use R or another statistical program, you can calculate such $P$-values. In R: `pt(q = 2.0803, df = 9, lower.tail = FALSE)`.

This yields a $P$-value of 0.0336. Since this is not less than or equal to the chosen value 0.01 of $\alpha$, we draw the same conclusion as we did under Approach 1: we do not have enough evidence to claim that there is a significant increase in temperature 24 hours after the operation.

We can use the built-in R `t.test()` function to calculate the observed $t$ statistic in addition to the $P$-value by entering the data, the hypotheses, and the significance level as follows. This approach will generally lead to the least amount of calculation errors and is the most practical for large data sets.

```
t.test(x = c(98.9, 98.6, 99.3, 98.7, 98.7, 98.4, 99.0, 98.5,
         98.8, 98.8), alternative = "greater", mu = 98.6, conf.level = 0.99)
```

*Notes on the One-Sample t Test*

1. The general form of a one-sample $t$ statistic given in (13.3) is often written more conveniently as $t = \dfrac{(\bar{x} - \mu_0)\sqrt{n}}{s}$.

2. *Degrees of freedom.* The formula for the number of degrees of freedom in a $t$ test differs from that in a two-by-two table test and in $\chi^2$ tests. The logic for deriving the number of degrees of freedom differs in the two different situations. In the one-sample $t$ test case, there are $n - 1$ degrees of freedom since once the value of $\bar{x}$ is given, only $n - 1$ of the values $x_1, x_2, \ldots, x_n$ can be freely chosen. In other $t$ tests, there will be other values for the number of degrees of freedom.

3. The numerator $\bar{x} - \mu_0$ in the $t$ statistic emphasizes the importance of distinguishing between the concepts of an average $\bar{x}$ and a mean $\mu_0$. Without distinguishing between these two concepts, the numerator in the $t$ statistic would not make sense: using the word "mean" for $\bar{x}$ implies that the numerator in $t$ would be called "the mean minus the mean".

4. It is helpful to think of $t$ as a signal-to-noise ratio. The signal is the numerator quantity $(\bar{x} - \mu_0)$ in (13.3), the difference between the average of the data values and the null hypothesis mean. The noise is $s/\sqrt{n}$, the denominator in the $t$ statistic (13.3). Both the signal and the noise are important. An example will be given later illustrating the importance of the noise.

5. The only difference between a one-sample $t$ statistic and a $z$ statistic is that $t$ has a standard deviation estimate in the denominator ($s$) and $z$ has a known standard deviation ($\sigma$) in the denominator. Explicitly,

$$t = \frac{(\bar{x} - \mu_0)}{s/\sqrt{n}}, \quad z = \frac{(\bar{x} - \mu_0)}{\sigma/\sqrt{n}}.$$

6. *Continuation from Note 5.* If, in the "temperatures" example, we knew the variance $\sigma^2$ of the temperatures of people 24 hours after the operation, and if we chose $\alpha = 0.01$, we would use the $z$ chart to show that we reject the null hypothesis if $z \geq 2.326$. How many degrees of freedom does the number 2.326 correspond to in a $t$ test? The $t$ chart shows that if $\alpha = 0.01$, the critical point 2.326 for $t$ corresponds to infinitely many degrees of freedom. So we can think of knowing a variance as having infinitely many degrees of freedom.

7. Although the $t$ chart is designed for one-sided up tests, it can still be used for one-sided down and two-sided tests. This is now illustrated in the temperatures example.

   If the alternative hypothesis had been that $\mu$, the mean temperature for people 24 hours after the operation, is less than 98.6, then the test is one-sided down, and with $n = 10$ and $\alpha = 0.01$ we would reject the null hypothesis if $t \leq -2.821$. In general, for a one-sided down test, we reject the null hypothesis if the observed value of $t$ is less than or equal to the negative of the value shown in the $t$ chart.

   If the alternative hypothesis had been $\mu \neq 98.6$, then with $n = 10$ and $\alpha = 0.01$, we would reject the null hypothesis if $t \leq -3.250$ or if $t \geq +3.250$. The value 3.250 comes from the $t$ chart and corresponds to the column for $\alpha = 0.005$. For a two-sided test, we put half of the $\alpha$ probability 0.01 on the "down" side and half on the "up" side, thus explaining the numerical value 0.005 (half of 0.01). Despite this, the total value of $\alpha$ for this two-sided test is still 0.01.

8. The various critical points in a $t$ chart are calculated under the assumption that the random variables $X_1, X_2, \ldots, X_n$ have a *normal* distribution and were calculated by advanced mathematics under this normal distribution assumption. If you do a $t$ test and use the $t$ chart to assess significance, you are implicitly assuming that the random variables $X_1, X_2, \ldots, X_n$ have a normal distribution. If you are not prepared to assume that $X_1, X_2, \ldots, X_n$ have a normal distribution, you can use a non-parametric (= distribution-free) test. One of these is considered in Chap. 14 as an alternative to the one-sample $t$ test.

9. *Continuation from Note 8. Robustness.* What level of error is made in using a $t$ test if $X_1, X_2, \ldots, X_n$ do *not* have a normal distribution? The answer is "not much". The $t$ test is said to be *robust* against the assumption of a normal distribution for $X_1, X_2, \ldots, X_n$. The critical points in the $t$ chart are often quite accurate even if $X_1, X_2, \ldots, X_n$ do not have a normal distribution. In part, this happens because of the Central Limit Theorem: a crucial component of the $t$ statistic is $\bar{x}$, and from the Central Limit Theorem, one can reasonably assume

that $\bar{X}$ has close to a normal distribution whatever the probability distribution of $X_1, X_2, \ldots, X_n$ might be, at least if $n$ is about 30 or more.

10. It is assumed in the $t$ test procedure that $X_1, X_2, \ldots, X_n$ are $iid$ random variables. This might not be a reasonable assumption in practice. For example, the probability distribution of the temperature for older people might differ from that for younger people. The probability distribution of the temperature for men might differ from that for women. Practical questions such as these are important and decisions concerning them might rely on experience and judgment. If the $iid$ assumption is not thought to be reasonable, more complicated procedures are available. However, these are not discussed in this book.

11. The $t$ statistic is scale-free. If one person measures temperature in degrees Fahrenheit and uses a null hypothesis mean of 98.6, and another person measures the same temperatures in degrees Celsius and uses the equivalent null hypothesis Celsius mean of 37.0, they would get the same numerical value for $t$. The $t$ test would be useless if this did not happen.

12. Approach 2 relies on the calculation of a $P$-value. This calculation is very difficult and is only possible via a computer package.

*Example 2* This example (a) gives an example of a one-sided down test, and (b) shows the importance of the noise $s/\sqrt{n}$ in the denominator of the one-sample $t$ statistic.

The 12 $iid$ random variables $X_1, X_2, \ldots, X_{12}$ each have a normal distribution with unknown mean $\mu$ and unknown variance $\sigma^2$. The null hypothesis is that $\mu = 5$ and the alternative hypothesis is $\mu < 5$. We choose a Type I error value $\alpha = 0.05$.

Step 3. Since we do not know the value of $\sigma^2$, the test statistic will be the $t$ statistic (13.3) with $\mu_0 = 5$.

Step 4. Because of the nature of the alternative hypothesis and the fact that $n = 12$, so that there are 11 degrees of freedom, the $t$ chart shows that we will reject the null hypothesis if our eventual value of $t$ is -1.796 or less.

*Case 1* Suppose that, having carried out the experiment, the observed data values are

$$4.96, 5.04, 4.93, 5.06, 4.92, 4.96, 5.03, 4.91, 4.98, 5.01, 5.00, 4.96.$$

From these values, we find $\bar{x} = 4.98$ and $s^2 = 0.00236$. From this,

$$t = \frac{(4.98 - 5.00)}{\sqrt{0.00236}/\sqrt{12}} = -1.4251.$$

Because this is not less than $-1.796$, we do not have enough evidence to reject the null hypothesis.

*Case 2* As above, but suppose that the observed data values are

$$4.98, 4.97, 4.99, 4.99, 5.01, 4.97, 4.98, 4.96, 4.99, 4.96, 4.97, 4.99.$$

From these values, we find $\bar{x} = 4.98$, the same as in Case 1, but now $s^2 = 0.0002182$, which is much less than the value in Case 1. From this,

$$t = \frac{(4.98 - 5.00)}{\sqrt{0.0002182}/\sqrt{12}} = -4.6904.$$

Because this is less than $-1.796$, we have enough evidence to reject the null hypothesis. This is despite the fact that the averages are the same in Cases 1 and 2.

Note 4 stated that it is useful to think of a $t$ statistic as a signal-to-noise ratio. The two examples above illustrate the importance of the denominator, or the noise, in the $t$ statistic. The numerator, that is, the signal, is the same in both Case 1 and Case 2, but the $t$ statistic is only significant in the second case, where the signal stands out loud and clear relative to the noise in the denominator. This happens because in the second example $s$ is much smaller than it is in the first example, and this occurs because, in the second example, the data values do not vary much one from another, suggesting a smaller value of $\sigma^2$.

Approach 2, Steps 4 and 5 combined. This approach is only possible using R or another statistical program.

*Case 1* As calculated above, the observed $t$ value is $-1.4251$. The $P$-value is Prob($T \leq -1.4251$), which can be shown to be 0.0909, found in R by running pt(q = -1.4251, df = 11, lower.tail = TRUE). As with Approach 1, we fail to reject the null hypothesis since the $P$-value 0.0909 is greater than the significance level $\alpha = 0.05$.

*Case 2* As calculated above, the observed value of $t$ is $-4.6904$. The $P$-value is Prob($T \leq -4.6904$), which is 0.00033, found in R by running pt(q = -4.6904, df = 11, lower.tail = TRUE). As with Approach 1, we reject the null hypothesis since the $P$-value 0.00033 is less than the significance level $\alpha = 0.05$.

We can also have R calculate the observed $t$ statistic in addition to the $P$-value just by entering the data and hypotheses as follows. This is equivalent to Approach 2, without manually calculating the observed $t$ statistic or the $P$-value. Note that the default confidence level is 0.95, so since we chose $\alpha = 0.05$, we do not need to specify the conf.level argument.

*Case 1*

```
t.test(x = c(4.96, 5.04, 4.93, 5.06, 4.92, 4.96, 5.03, 4.91,
         4.98, 5.01, 5.00, 4.96), alternative = "less", mu = 5)
```

*Case 2*

```
t.test(x = c(4.98, 4.97,  4.99, 4.99, 5.01, 4.97, 4.98, 4.96,
         4.99, 4.96, 4.97, 4.99), alternative = "less", mu = 5)
```

## 13.2   The Two-Sample *t* Test

The two-sample *t* test is used often and is thus important. As the name suggests, with two-sample *t* tests, we have two sets of data. Here is an example.

We suspect that as people get older, their reaction time to a certain stimulus tends to get longer. To test this suspicion, we plan to get a sample of *n* people aged 18–45 ("group 1") and a sample of *m* people aged 60–75 ("group 2"), subject each person to the stimulus, and measure the reaction time of each person. It is not necessary that $n = m$, although it is wise to make these two numbers equal, or at least reasonably close to each other.

We are still in the planning phase. We will get our data tomorrow. So at this stage, the reaction times for each of the *n* people in group 1 are random variables, which we denote by $X_{11}, X_{12}, \ldots, X_{1n}$. Similarly, the reaction times for each of the *m* people in group 2 are random variables, which we denote by $X_{21}, X_{22}, \ldots, X_{2m}$. For each person, the first suffix indicates the group (1 or 2) that each person is in and the second suffix indicates membership number (1, 2, 3, ..., *n* or *m*) in the group each person is in.

We assume that $X_{11}, X_{12}, \ldots, X_{1n}$ are *iid* random variables, each having a normal distribution with unknown mean $\mu_1$ and unknown variance $\sigma^2$. Similarly, we assume that $X_{21}, X_{22}, \ldots, X_{2m}$ are *iid* random variables, each having a normal distribution with unknown mean $\mu_2$ and unknown variance $\sigma^2$. The numerical values of $\mu_1$, $\mu_2$ and $\sigma^2$ are all unspecified. Note that we assume the same variance in both groups. A more complicated procedure, discussed in Note 2 below, applies if we are not willing to make the equal-variance assumption.

Step 1. The null hypothesis in this reaction time example claims that $\mu_1 = \mu_2$. However, the null hypothesis does not specify the identical values it assumes for $\mu_1$ and $\mu_2$, so that the null hypothesis might more precisely be written as $\mu_1 = \mu_2 (= \mu$, unspecified). The value of $\sigma^2$ is also unspecified.

The alternative hypothesis comes from the context. As stated above, we suspect that a person's reaction time tends to increase as that person gets older. This means that the natural alternative hypothesis in this example is $\mu_1 < \mu_2$, namely that the mean reaction time for a younger person is less than the mean reaction time for an older person. So this will be a one-sided test. Whether it will be one-sided up or one-sided down will be discussed later. In other cases, the alternative hypothesis could be two-sided ($\mu_1 \neq \mu_2$), depending on the context.

Step 2. In this step, we decide on the value of $\alpha$. In the reaction time example, it is the probability that we reject the null hypothesis that the mean reaction time is the same for both age groups when it is true. Since this is a medical example, we choose $\alpha = 0.01$.

Step 3. What is the test statistic? Suppose that we now have our data. We will have data values $x_{11}, x_{12}, \ldots, x_{1n}$ from the people in group 1 and data values $x_{21}, x_{22}, \ldots, x_{2m}$ from the people in group 2. The "signal" in the *t* statistic that we are developing will be the difference between the averages $\bar{x}_1$ and $\bar{x}_2$, where

$$\bar{x}_1 = \frac{x_{11} + x_{12} + \cdots + x_{1n}}{n}, \quad \bar{x}_2 = \frac{x_{21} + x_{22} + \cdots + x_{2m}}{m}. \tag{13.6}$$

We could use either the difference $\bar{x}_1 - \bar{x}_2$ or the difference $\bar{x}_2 - \bar{x}_1$ for the "signal": there is no reason why one difference is to be preferred to the other. Some computer packages and people use $\bar{x}_1 - \bar{x}_2$ as the signal and others use $\bar{x}_2 - \bar{x}_1$ as the signal. This matter is discussed further below.

As with the one-sample $t$ test, the signal on its own is not enough. We have to consider the noise. To see what this should be, we pretend for the moment that the variance $\sigma^2$ is known. We now consider the situation before we get our data and do a probability theory calculation. Since we know that our eventual $t$ statistic will have either $\bar{x}_1 - \bar{x}_2$ or $\bar{x}_2 - \bar{x}_1$ in the numerator, we have to think about the random variables $\bar{X}_1 - \bar{X}_2$ and $\bar{X}_2 - \bar{X}_1$.

Equation (5.7) provides the mean and variance of $\bar{X}_1 - \bar{X}_2$, so that if the various assumptions we have made are correct and the null hypothesis is true, the quantity

$$\frac{\bar{X}_1 - \bar{X}_2}{\sqrt{\frac{\sigma^2}{n} + \frac{\sigma^2}{m}}} = \frac{\bar{X}_1 - \bar{X}_2}{\sigma\sqrt{\frac{1}{n} + \frac{1}{m}}} \tag{13.7}$$

is a $Z$, that is, it is a random variable having a normal distribution with mean 0 and variance 1. Similarly, if the various assumptions we have made are correct and if the null hypothesis is true, the quantity

$$\frac{\bar{X}_2 - \bar{X}_1}{\sqrt{\frac{\sigma^2}{n} + \frac{\sigma^2}{m}}} = \frac{\bar{X}_2 - \bar{X}_1}{\sigma\sqrt{\frac{1}{n} + \frac{1}{m}}} \tag{13.8}$$

is also a $Z$.

Given our data values $x_{11}, x_{12}, \ldots, x_{1n}$ from the people in group 1 and data values $x_{21}, x_{22}, \ldots, x_{2m}$ from the people in group 2, we could use (13.7) to calculate

$$\frac{\bar{x}_1 - \bar{x}_2}{\sqrt{\frac{\sigma^2}{n} + \frac{\sigma^2}{m}}} = \frac{\bar{x}_1 - \bar{x}_2}{\sigma\sqrt{\frac{1}{n} + \frac{1}{m}}} \tag{13.9}$$

and refer the value so calculated to the $Z$ chart to test for its significance. Similarly, we could use (13.8) to calculate

$$\frac{\bar{x}_2 - \bar{x}_1}{\sqrt{\frac{\sigma^2}{n} + \frac{\sigma^2}{m}}} = \frac{\bar{x}_2 - \bar{x}_1}{\sigma\sqrt{\frac{1}{n} + \frac{1}{m}}} \tag{13.10}$$

and refer the value so calculated to the $Z$ chart to test for its significance.

However, we do not know the numerical value of $\sigma^2$, so we have to estimate it from the data. This will eventually lead us to a $t$ statistic since, as discussed in the previous section, the only difference between a $z$ statistic and a $t$ statistic is that in a $t$ statistic, we have an estimate of a standard deviation in the denominator, whereas in a $z$ statistic, we have a known standard deviation in the denominator, as in (13.9) and (13.10).

We want to use the data from both groups, combined in some way, to estimate $\sigma^2$, and from this, to estimate $\sigma$. The data $x_{11}, x_{12}, \ldots, x_{1n}$ from group 1, taken on their own, would lead to the estimate

$$s_1^2 = \frac{x_{11}^2 + x_{12}^2 + \cdots + x_{1n}^2 - n(\bar{x}_1)^2}{n - 1}. \tag{13.11}$$

Similarly, the data $x_{21}, x_{22}, \ldots, x_{2m}$ from group 2, taken on their own, would lead to the estimate

$$s_2^2 = \frac{x_{21}^2 + x_{22}^2 + \cdots + x_{2m}^2 - m(\bar{x}_2)^2}{m - 1}. \tag{13.12}$$

The following must be taken on trust. The correct estimate of $\sigma^2$, combining the estimates $s_1^2$ from group 1 and $s_2^2$ from group 2, is $s^2$, defined by

$$s^2 = \frac{(n - 1)s_1^2 + (m - 1)s_2^2}{n + m - 2}. \tag{13.13}$$

This is a weighted average of $s_1^2$ and $s_2^2$, the weights being the respective degrees of freedom in the two groups. The value of $s$ will form part of the denominator in the eventual $t$ statistic. One must be careful to only use the estimate (13.13) in the two-sample $t$ test, and not in other situations, where other estimates for $\sigma^2$ are used instead.

There are two versions of the $t$ statistic in current use. The first of these, $t_1$, is found by replacing $\sigma$ by $s$ in (13.9), so that

$$t_1 = \frac{\bar{x}_1 - \bar{x}_2}{s\sqrt{\frac{1}{n} + \frac{1}{m}}}. \tag{13.14}$$

The second of these, namely $t_2$, is found by replacing $\sigma$ by $s$ in (13.10), so that

$$t_2 = \frac{\bar{x}_2 - \bar{x}_1}{s\sqrt{\frac{1}{n} + \frac{1}{m}}}. \tag{13.15}$$

Clearly $t_2 = -t_1$. Both $t_1$ and $t_2$ are valid test statistics. Some computer packages use $t_1$ as the test statistic while other computer packages use $t_2$. One has to be careful, once one has chosen a computer package and therefore the test statistic that is used, about whether the test is one-sided up or one-sided down. This will be discussed below using a numerical example.

This is the end of Step 3. We have arrived at the test statistic, either (13.14) or (13.15). Both are valid.

Step 4, Approach 1. What values of $t_1$ as defined in (13.14), and what values of $t_2$ as defined in (13.15), will lead us to reject the null hypothesis? We discuss this question using the reaction time example.

In the reaction time example, the alternative hypothesis is $\mu_1 < \mu_2$. We now ask: what value of the test statistic chosen ($t_1$ or $t_2$) would we expect to get if this alternative hypothesis is true? If the alternative hypothesis is true, $\bar{x}_1$ will tend to be less than $\bar{x}_2$ and so $t_1$, as defined in (13.14), will tend to be negative. Thus sufficiently large negative values of $t_1$ as defined in (13.14) will lead us to reject the null hypothesis in this example. On the other hand, the value of $t_2$, as defined in (13.15), will tend to be positive if this alternative hypothesis is true. Thus sufficiently large positive values of $t_2$ as defined in (13.15) will lead us to reject the null hypothesis. There is no contradiction here and one reaches the same conclusion whichever test statistic is used. This is because $t_2$ is the negative of the value of $t_1$. If $t_1$ is sufficiently large positive to reject the null hypothesis, then $t_2$ will be sufficiently large negative to reject the null hypothesis.

If the test were to be two-sided, sufficiently large positive or sufficiently large negative values of $t_1$ and also of $t_2$ will lead us to reject the null hypothesis.

To summarize: the values of $t_1$ and of $t_2$ that lead to rejection of the null hypothesis depend on the nature of the alternative hypothesis and on whether $t_1$ or $t_2$ is chosen as the test statistic. If this is kept in mind, the same conclusion is reached whichever test statistic is used.

How large do $t_1$ and $t_2$ have to be (positive or negative, or both, whichever is relevant) for us to reject the null hypothesis? If the various assumptions we made as described above are correct and if the null hypothesis is true, then both $t_1$ and $t_2$ are the observed values of a random variable having the $t$ distribution with $m + n - 2$ degrees of freedom. The degrees of freedom calculation, the value of $\alpha$, and the $t$ chart together indicate how large positive, or how large negative, or how large positive or negative, $t_1$ and $t_2$ have to be before the null hypothesis is rejected.

*Case 1.* Suppose that $n = 10$ and $m = 13$, so that there are $10 + 13 - 2 = 21$ degrees of freedom. Suppose that we chose $\alpha = 0.01$. Since in the reaction time example, the alternative hypothesis is $\mu_1 < \mu_2$, use of the test statistic $t_1$ as given in (13.14) leads to a one-sided down test and the $t$ chart (Chart 4) shows that we reject the null hypothesis if $t_1$ is less than or equal to $-2.518$. Using the test statistic $t_2$ as given in (13.15), we have a one-sided up test and the $t$ chart shows that we reject the null hypothesis if $t_2$ is greater than or equal to $+2.518$. The two conclusions agree since $t_2$ as defined in (13.15) is the negative of the value of $t_1$ as defined in (13.14).

*Case 2.* Suppose that $n = 12$ and $m = 15$, so that there are $12 + 15 - 2 = 25$ degrees of freedom. Suppose that even though this is a medical example, we chose $\alpha = 0.05$. Then using the test statistic $t_1$ as given in (13.14), we have a one-sided down test and the $t$ chart shows that we reject the null hypothesis if $t_1$ is less than or equal to $-1.708$. Using the test statistic $t_2$ as given in (13.15), we have a one-sided up test and the $t$ chart shows that we reject the null hypothesis if $t_2$ is greater than or equal to $+1.708$. The two conclusions agree since $t_2$ as defined in (13.15) is the negative of the value of $t_1$ as defined in (13.14).

*Case 3.* Suppose that $n = 17$ and $m = 14$, giving $17 + 14 - 2 = 29$ degrees of freedom. If the alternative hypothesis had been $\mu_1 \neq \mu_2$, we have a two-sided test and with $\alpha = 0.01$, we put half the value of $\alpha$, that is, 0.005, on the "up" side and half on the "down" side. As a result, we would reject this null hypothesis if $t_1$ (or $t_2$) is greater than or equal to 2.756 or if $t_1$ (or $t_2$) is less than or equal to $-2.756$. If $\alpha = 0.05$, we again put half the value of $\alpha$, that is, 0.025, on the "up" side and half on the "down" side. As a result, we would reject the null hypothesis if $t_1$ (or $t_2$) is greater than or equal to 2.045 or if $t_1$ (or $t_2$) is less than or equal to $-2.045$. Thus for a two-sided test, the procedure is the same whichever test statistic is used.

Step 5 is straightforward. Get the data, calculate $t_1$ (or, if preferred, $t_2$), refer the value obtained to the appropriate value on the $t$ chart, and accept or reject the null hypothesis depending on this comparison.

Step 4, Approach 2. Get the data and from the data, calculate the value of $t_1$ or, if preferred, $t_2$.

Step 5, Approach 2. Find the $P$-value associated with the value of $t_1$ (or $t_2$) calculated in Step 4. This can only be done via a statistical computer package.

*Example* The background and Steps 1, 2 and 3 for the reaction time example have already been described, so we only consider Steps 4 and 5.

Suppose that the data are as follows. For the $n = 10$ young people, the reaction times were

$$382, \ 446, \ 483, \ 378, \ 414, \ 420, \ 452, \ 391, \ 399, \ 426$$

and for the $m = 8$ older people, the reaction times were

$$423, \ 474, \ 456, \ 432, \ 513, \ 480, \ 498, \ 448.$$

From these values, we compute $\bar{x}_1 = 419.1$ and $\bar{x}_2 = 465.5$. We also compute $s_1^2 = 1135.878$ and $s_2^2 = 988.5714$. Combining these using Eq. (13.13), we get
$$s^2 = \frac{9 \times 1135.878 + 7 \times 988.5714}{16} = 1071.43125, \text{ so that } s = 32.73272445.$$
Thus from formula (13.15),

$$t_2 = \frac{(465.5 - 419.1)}{32.73272445\sqrt{\frac{1}{10} + \frac{1}{8}}} = \frac{46.4}{15.5264949} = 2.98844.$$

We first consider Approach 1. In using $t_2$ as the test statistic, the test is one-sided up, and since the observed value 2.98844 of $t_2$ exceeds the relevant $t$ chart critical point 2.583 for $\alpha = 0.01$ and 16 degrees of freedom, we reject the null hypothesis and claim that we have significant evidence that the mean reaction time for older people exceeds that for younger people. If we had chosen to use the $t_1$ statistic as defined in (13.14), the test would be one-sided down and we would reject the null hypothesis if $t_1$ as defined in (13.14) is less than or equal to $-2.583$. With the definition of $t_1$ as given in (13.14),

$$t_1 = \frac{(419.1 - 465.5)}{32.73272445\sqrt{\frac{1}{10} + \frac{1}{8}}} = -2.98844.$$

Since this value of $t_1$ is less than the critical point $-2.583$, we reject the null hypothesis and claim that we have significant evidence that the mean reaction time for older people exceeds that for younger people. This is the same conclusion as the one we reached using $t_2$ as the test statistic. As stated above, the same conclusion is always reached whether one uses $t_1$ or $t_2$ as the test statistic, provided one is careful about the statistic used for $t$ in the computer package used and the consequent "sidedness" of the test.

Under Approach 2, it is necessary to use a computer package to evaluate the $P$-value corresponding to the observed value of $t_1$ (or $t_2$).

In R, we can calculate the $P$-value with pt(q = -2.98844, df = 16). We can also use R for the whole test. R will use the $t_1$ form of the test statistic and label the two groups x and y:

```
t.test(x = c(382, 446, 483, 378, 414, 420, 452, 391, 399, 426),
       y = c(423, 474, 456, 432, 513, 480, 498, 448),
       alternative = "less", var.equal = TRUE, conf.level = 0.99)
```

This gives a $P$-value of 0.0043 for a one-sided that $\mu_1$ is less than $\mu_2$, and since this is less than the value 0.01 chosen for $\alpha$, we reject the null hypothesis. This agrees with the conclusion reached under Approach 1.

The reaction time example is a one-sided test. Some two-sample $t$ tests are two-sided. For two-sided tests, we do the same as for the one-sample $t$ test and put half the Type I error on the up side and the other half on the down side. For example, suppose that $n = 12$ and $m = 10$, that $\alpha = 0.05$, that the alternative hypothesis is two-sided, and that we decide to use $t_2$ as the test statistic. Then we have 20 degrees of freedom and we will have to consult the $\alpha = 0.025$ column in the $t$ chart. This shows that we will reject the null hypothesis if $t_2 \geq 2.086$ or if $t_2 \leq -2.086$. If we had chosen $t_1$ as the test statistic we will reject the null hypothesis if $t_1 \geq 2.086$ or if $t_1 \leq -2.086$. This means that the procedure using $t_1$ is exactly the same as the procedure using $t_2$ for a two-sided test.

*Generalization* The null hypothesis $\mu_1 = \mu_2$ is equivalent to $\mu_1 - \mu_2 = 0$. Another null hypothesis that is often of interest is $\mu_1 - \mu_2 = d$, where $d$ is some given number. $d$ can be either positive or negative, and the alternative hypothesis is either $\mu_1 - \mu_2 > d$, $\mu_1 - \mu_2 < d$ or $\mu_1 - \mu_2 \neq d$, depending on the context. The two relevant test statistics, parallel to $t_1$ and $t_2$ and with the same notation as that used in the definition of $t_1$ and $t_2$, are

$$t_1^* = \frac{\bar{x}_1 - \bar{x}_2 - d}{s\sqrt{\frac{1}{n} + \frac{1}{m}}} \quad \text{and} \quad t_2^* = \frac{\bar{x}_2 - \bar{x}_1 + d}{s\sqrt{\frac{1}{n} + \frac{1}{m}}}. \tag{13.16}$$

If the alternative hypothesis $\mu_1 - \mu_2 > d$ is true, $t_1^*$ would tend to be positive and $t_2^*$ would be tend to be negative. Therefore, with $t_1^*$ as the test statistic, the test is one-sided up and with $t_2^*$ as the test statistic, the test is one-sided down. There is no contradiction here since $t_2^* = -t_1^*$. If the alternative hypothesis is $\mu_1 - \mu_2 < d$, the test is one-sided down if $t_1^*$ is the test statistic and one-sided up if $t_2^*$ is the test statistic. If the alternative hypothesis is $\mu_1 - \mu_2 \neq d$, the procedure using $t_1^*$ is identical to that using $t_2^*$. In all cases, the test is conducted using the $t$ chart with $n + m - 2$ degrees of freedom.

*Example* This example considers the biomass data in Table (1.1). The background, the assumptions and the data are given in the example in Sect. 8.5. Suppose that the null hypothesis is $\mu_1 - \mu_2 = 50$ and the alternative hypothesis is $\mu_1 - \mu_2 \neq 50$. Since this a two-sided alternative hypothesis, the procedure using $t_1^*$ as test statistic is the same as that using $t_2^*$ as test statistic. We choose $\alpha = 0.05$, so that since there are 20 degrees of freedom, we will reject the null hypothesis if $t_1^* \leq -2.086$ or if $t_1^* \geq +2.086$, or equivalently if $t_2^* \leq -2.086$ or if $t_2^* \geq +2.086$.

The values of $s_1^2$ and $s_2^2$ are reasonably close, so we assume that $\sigma_1^2 = \sigma_2^2$ and use Eq. (13.13) to find the estimate 23,953.735 of their common value. This gives $s = 154.77$. The value of $t_1^*$ is then

$$t_1^* = \frac{1877.64 - 1765.27 - 50}{154.77\sqrt{\frac{1}{11} + \frac{1}{11}}} = 0.945. \tag{13.17}$$

Since this value lies between -2.086 and + 2.086, we do not have enough evidence to reject the null hypothesis.

*Notes on the Two-Sample $t$ Test*

1. A similarity with the one-sample $t$ test is that for both tests, it is assumed that the data are the observed values of random variables having a normal distribution. If we are unwilling to make this assumption, we can use a non–parametric test: an example is given in Sect. 14.3. However, the two-sample $t$ test, as with the one-sample $t$ test, is "robust": it works quite well even if the data are not the observed values of random variables having a normal distribution.

2. A key assumption made in the discussion of two-sample $t$ tests so far is that the variance corresponding to group 1 is the same as that corresponding to group 2. The assumption of equal variances is one that we might, or might not, like to make, depending perhaps on our experience with the sort of data we are involved with, or via a histogram plot of the data at hand. Unfortunately, there is no known exact testing procedure for the "unequal variance" test procedure, and the best

that is available is a very close approximation, usually very accurate when $n$ and $m$ are both larger than 5. This is as follows.

First, compute $\bar{x}_1$ and $\bar{x}_2$ as specified in (13.6) and then compute $s_1^2$ and $s_2^2$ as in (13.11) and (13.12) respectively. Then calculate $t_3$, defined by

$$t_3 = \frac{\bar{x}_1 - \bar{x}_2}{\sqrt{\frac{s_1^2}{n} + \frac{s_2^2}{m}}}. \tag{13.18}$$

Having done this, refer the value of $t_3$ to the critical point in the $t$ chart for the value of $\alpha$ chosen and with

$$\frac{(\frac{s_1^2}{n} + \frac{s_2^2}{m})^2}{\frac{1}{n-1}(\frac{s_1^2}{n})^2 + \frac{1}{m-1}(\frac{s_2^2}{m})^2} \tag{13.19}$$

degrees of freedom. This quantity will usually not be an integer, so in practice, we use the integer immediately less than this as the number of degrees of freedom.

Because of the complicated calculations involved, this procedure is normally carried out by a computer package and not by hand. When using R for a two-sample $t$ test, we can specify whether we want to make the equal variance assumption or not with the var.equal argument. R will compute the value of $t$ and its $P$-value corresponding to whatever choice we make.

3. There is no need, in a two-sample $t$ test, for $m$ and $n$ to be equal. However, in practice it is wise to make them as close to each other as possible in order to minimize the total noise.

4. The main part of the "signal" in a one-sample $t$ test is the difference between an average and the null hypothesis mean, i.e. $\bar{x} - \mu_0$. The main part of the "signal" in a two-sample $t$ test is the difference, either $\bar{x}_1 - \bar{x}_2$ or $\bar{x}_2 - \bar{x}_1$, between two averages.

5. The null hypothesis in any two-sample $t$ test is that two means are equal (in the notation above, that $\mu_1 = \mu_2$). However, no statement is made or required as to what the common value of the mean is under the null hypothesis.

6. Both $t_1$ and $t_2$ defined above have been discussed as test statistics since both are in common use. Similarly, both Approach 1 and Approach 2 have been discussed as testing procedures since both are in common use.

## 13.3    The Paired Two-Sample $t$ Test

This test is carried out when we have data from two samples with the further feature that there is a natural pairing of the data between the two samples. We illustrate the procedure for this test, and show how the pairing is used, by an example which naturally involves pairing.

Suppose that we are interested in whether there is a difference between the mean blood pressure of women and the mean blood pressure of men. The null hypothesis is that the mean blood pressure of women is the same as that of men. To be concrete, suppose that if the means differ, we expect, on physiological grounds, that the mean blood pressure of men exceeds that of women. Suppose we choose a Type I error ($\alpha$) of 0.05, and that we are willing to assume that the probability distribution of blood pressure among both males and females has a normal distribution. This concludes Steps 1 and 2 of the hypothesis testing process.

Step 3. What is the test statistic? Suppose that the data consists of $n$ brother-sister pairs, with blood pressures $x_{11}, x_{12}, \ldots, x_{1n}$ for the $n$ sisters and blood pressures $x_{21}, x_{22}, \ldots, x_{2n}$ for their respective brothers. Thus $x_{11}$ and $x_{21}$ are the respective blood pressures from the sister and the brother in family 1, $x_{12}$ and $x_{22}$ are the respective blood pressures from the sister and the brother in family 2, and so on. The natural pairing is between the sister and the brother in the same family.

We could ignore this pairing and do the two-sample $t$ test described in the previous section. But doing this does not take advantage of this natural within-family pairing. Our aim is to take advantage of this pairing to obtain a procedure that is more efficient than that of the previous section.

To take advantage of the pairing, we calculate, for each family, the brother's blood pressure minus his sister's blood pressure. That is, we calculate the differences $d_1 = x_{21} - x_{11}, \ldots, d_n = x_{2n} - x_{1n}$. Thus $d_1$ is the "brother minus sister" difference in family 1, $d_2$ is this difference in family 2, and so on. From now on, we discard the original $x_{ij}$ data values and use only these differences. This means that we will be doing a $one$-sample $t$ test on the $d_i$ values, even though the original data formed two samples.

Following the standard procedure for a one-sample test, we form a $t$ statistic from the respective differences $d_1, d_2, \ldots, d_n$. The numerator in this statistic is the average $\bar{d}$ of these differences. If the null hypothesis is true, the $d$ values are the observed values of random variables with mean zero, so that $\mu_0$ in the test statistic (13.3) will be zero. Since the alternative hypothesis is that the mean blood pressure for men exceeds that for women, and the various $d$ values were the brother reading minus the sister reading, this implies that the test will be one-sided up: if the alternative hypothesis is true, the average $\bar{d}$ will tend to be positive.

Following the formula (8.13) for estimating $\sigma^2$ in one-sample tests, we calculate $s_d^2$ as

$$s_d^2 = \frac{d_1^2 + d_2^2 + \cdots + d_n^2 - n(\bar{d})^2}{n - 1}. \tag{13.20}$$

The eventual $t$ statistic is then found, following the one-sample formula (13.3), to be

$$t = \frac{\bar{d}}{s_d/\sqrt{n}}. \tag{13.21}$$

This is the end of Step 3: (13.21) is the test statistic.

Steps 4 and 5, Approach 1. If the alternative hypothesis is true, then as noted above, the test is one-sided up, so we refer the calculated value of $t$ as defined in (13.21) to the $t$ chart with $n - 1$ degrees of freedom and reject the null hypothesis if the value of $t$ is equal to or greater than the relevant critical point in the $t$ chart.

The advantage of using the paired $t$ test is that it eliminates the natural family-to-family variation in blood pressure, and this eliminates an unwanted addition to the noise in the denominator of the $t$ statistic, thus increasing the signal-to-noise ratio. This is illustrated by the following example.

*Example* Suppose that we take the blood pressures of $n = 12$ women and their brothers, and get the following blood pressure readings:

| Family | 1 | 2 | 3 | 4 | 5 | 6 | 7 | 8 | 9 | 10 | 11 | 12 |
|---|---|---|---|---|---|---|---|---|---|---|---|---|
| Sister | 107 | 134 | 111 | 141 | 121 | 118 | 145 | 110 | 164 | 126 | 148 | 132 |
| Brother | 110 | 136 | 115 | 140 | 124 | 119 | 148 | 113 | 168 | 129 | 148 | 137 |

We first do a paired two-sample $t$ test. To do this, we calculate the brother-sister differences:

| Family | 1 | 2 | 3 | 4 | 5 | 6 | 7 | 8 | 9 | 10 | 11 | 12 |
|---|---|---|---|---|---|---|---|---|---|---|---|---|
| Difference | 3 | 2 | 4 | −1 | 3 | 1 | 3 | 3 | 4 | 3 | 0 | 5 |

The average $\bar{d}$ of these differences is 2.5. Next, a calculation using Eq. (13.20) shows that $s_d^2 = 3$, so that the numerical value of the paired $t$ statistic (13.21) is

$$t = \frac{2.5}{\sqrt{3}/\sqrt{12}} = 5. \tag{13.22}$$

There are $12 - 1 = 11$ degrees of freedom and with $\alpha = 0.05$, the critical point is 1.796. Therefore, this value of $t$ is significant so that we would now reject the null hypothesis.

In R, we can either use the one sample procedure performed on the differences, or we can use the t.test() function with two samples but set the paired argument to TRUE. Note that R will look at the first group minus the second. Since we have set the sisters as the first group, we have a one sided down test in R.

```
t.test(x = c(107, 134, 111, 141, 121, 118, 145, 110, 164, 126, 148, 132),
       y = c(110, 136, 115, 140, 124, 119, 148, 113, 168, 129, 148, 137),
       alternative = "less", paired = TRUE, var.equal = TRUE, conf.level
       = 0.95)
```

We next see what would happen if we (incorrectly) carried out the unpaired two-sample $t$ test, using the procedures described in the previous section.

The average $(\bar{x}_1)$ of the blood pressures of the sisters is 129.75 and the average $(\bar{x}_2)$ of the blood pressures of the brothers is 132.25. The difference $(\bar{x}_2 - \bar{x}_1)$ between these two averages is 2.50. Further calculation shows that the pooled estimate $s^2$ of variance given by (13.13) is $s^2 = 302.931818$ and from this, $s = 17.4049$. Thus under this approach, the numerical value of the unpaired two-sample $t_2$ statistic (13.15) is

$$t_2 = \frac{2.50}{17.4049\sqrt{\frac{1}{12} + \frac{1}{12}}} = 0.3518, \tag{13.23}$$

and this is nowhere near significant if $\alpha = 0.05$ and there are $12 + 12 - 2 = 22$ degrees of freedom.

The numerators in the unpaired and the paired $t$ statistics, $\bar{x}_2 - \bar{x}_1$ and $\bar{d}$, are mathematically identical as is confirmed by the value 2.50 for each, so that the signal is the same for both tests. The difference between the numerical values of the two $t$ statistics thus derives entirely from the difference between their respective denominators, or in other words, the difference between the respective values of the noise. The noise in the two-sample $t$ statistic includes unwanted family-to-family variation which is not of interest. By taking differences within each family, this component of the noise is eliminated, thus leading to a sharper test.

Examination of the original data supports this claim. In some families (for example, families 2, 4, 7, 9 and 11), both the brother and the sister have high blood pressures, while in other families (for example, families 1, 3, 6, and 8), both the brother and the sister have low blood pressures. This family-to-family variation contributes to the noise in the unpaired two-sample $t$ test, so that the signal is not significant relative to this noise. By taking differences within families, this family-to-family variation is eliminated from the paired $t$ test, diminishing the noise, so that now the signal is significant relative to the noise.

The two take-home messages are: (a) The denominator in a $t$ statistic is just as important as the numerator, and therefore (b) if there is a logical reason to pair, do a paired $t$ test.

Steps 4 and 5, Approach 2. Under Approach 2, in Step 4 we calculate the value of $t$ as given in (13.22) and then, in Step 5, find the $P$-value corresponding to this. This can only be done by a computer package.

In R, the t.test() function used earlier for the paired test will display a $P$-value in the result. However, we can also calculate it directly from the calculated statistic with pt(5, df = 11, lower.tail = FALSE). The $P$-value is 0.0002, leading to rejection of the null hypothesis, as in Approach 1.

*Notes on the Paired t Test*

1. The definition of $d_j$ used above is $d_j = x_{2j} - x_{1j}$. Some computer packages (such as R) define $d_j$ as $x_{1j} - x_{2j}$. If a package uses that definition of $d_j$, the value of $t$ so calculated will have the opposite sign to that found when using the formula (13.21). This implies that for a one-sided test, you have to be careful and check which definition of $d_j$ your package uses. A test that is one-sided up using one definition of the $d_j$ values is one-sided down using the other definition of the $d_j$ values.

2. Since the paired two-sample $t$ test reduces to a one-sample $t$ test, a two-sided paired $t$ test is carried out as for a two-sided one-sample $t$ test. Thus if the alternative hypothesis in the blood pressure example discussed above is that the mean blood pressure for men differs from that of women, but in an unspecified direction, we would still calculate $t$ as in (13.22) as the test statistic. Since the test is now two-sided with $\alpha = 0.05$ and 11 degrees of freedom, we would reject the null hypothesis if $t \geq 2.201$ or if $t \leq -2.201$.

3. A far better way of doing the "temperatures" test discussed when considering one-sample $t$ tests would be to take the temperatures of the individuals having the medical procedure before the procedure as well as 24 hours after the procedure. Then there is a natural pairing, within each person, of the temperatures before and after the procedure, so that for person $i$ we calculate $d_i$, that person's temperature after the operation minus that person's temperature before the operation. The subsequent paired $t$ test would eliminate the natural person-to-person differences in temperature. This point is illustrated in Problem 13.9.

## 13.4  $t$ Tests in Regression

The regression procedure that we consider concerns the question: "how does one random quantity depend on some non-random quantity?" In the plant growth example in Sect. 8.6, we asked: "how does the growth height of a plant depend on the amount of water given to the plant in the growing period?"

The amount of water given to any plant is not random: we can choose this for ourselves, and so we denote this in a lower case letter. The growth height of any plant is random: this will depend on various factors such as soil fertility that we might not know much about. The basic linear regression assumptions that are made are that if $Y$ is the (random) growth height for a plant given $x$ units of water, then the mean of $Y$ is of the form $\alpha + \beta x$ and the variance of $Y$ is $\sigma^2$. Here $\alpha$, $\beta$ and $\sigma^2$ are all (unknown) parameters which we previously saw how to estimate from the eventual data.

Once the experiment is completed, the data are the respective amounts of water $x_1, x_2, \ldots, x_n$ given to $n$ plants and the corresponding growth heights $y_1, y_2, \ldots, y_n$. The first thing that we do is to plot the data values on a graph. If the linearity assumption, namely that the mean of $Y$ is of the form $\alpha + \beta x$, is true, these data values should "more or less" lie on a straight line. If the constant variance assumption, namely that the variance of $Y$ is $\sigma^2$, is true, the amount of spread around the line should not vary much as $x$ varies. If either of these assumptions appear violated, the procedure described below should not be carried out. This matter is discussed in Note 2 below.

Assuming that the data do more or less fall on a straight line, we next calculate the five auxiliary quantities referred to in Sect. 8.6, namely $\bar{x}$, $\bar{y}$, $s_{xx}$, $s_{yy}$ and $s_{xy}$. From these, we estimate $\beta$ by $b = s_{xy}/s_{xx}$, $\alpha$ by $a = \bar{y} - b\bar{x}$ and $\sigma^2$ by

$s_r^2 = (s_{yy} - b^2 s_{xx})/(n-2)$. With these estimates in place, we now turn to hypothesis testing questions.

We first consider the question: "is there any effect of the amount of water on the growth height?" This is identical to asking the question: "is $\beta = 0$?". This test is carried out by the regression *t* test, and the estimate *b* of $\beta$ will be the key component in the numerator, or "signal", of the regression *t* statistic.

The details of how the regression *t* test statistic is derived are complex and here we just state that the appropriate test statistic is

$$t = \frac{b}{s_r/\sqrt{s_{xx}}}. \tag{13.24}$$

The key element in the numerator signal is *b*, the estimate of $\beta$, as indicated above. The derivation of the denominator of the *t* statistic (13.24) is complex and is omitted. The number of degrees of freedom for this *t* statistic is $n - 2$, a matter discussed further below.

We now put all of this together to carry out the regression *t* test in the water/growth-heights example, using the data in Sect. 8.6.

Step 1. The null hypothesis is "no effect of the amount of water on the growth height", or equivalently, "$\beta = 0$". Although in general, the alternative hypothesis could be one-sided up ("$\beta > 0$"), one-sided down ("$\beta < 0$"), or two-sided ("$\beta \neq 0$"), in the water/growth-heights example, the natural alternative hypothesis from the context is "$\beta > 0$". This concludes Step 1: we have formulated our null and alternative hypotheses.

Step 2. Here, we choose the numerical value we accept for making a Type I error. In this example, this is the probability that we claim that there is a positive effect of water on growth height when in fact there is no effect. In this example we choose 0.05.

Step 3. The test statistic is *t* as given in Eq. (13.24).

Step 4, Approach 1. What values of *t* will lead us to reject the null hypothesis? For the data in Sect. 8.6, for which $n = 12$, there are $12 - 2 = 10$ degrees of freedom. Because of the nature of the alternative hypothesis in this example, the test is one-sided up, and since we chose $\alpha = 0.05$, the *t* chart shows that we will reject the null hypothesis if the eventually calculated value of *t* is 1.812 or more.

Step 5, Approach 1. From the data in Sect. 8.6 and from the formula for *t* in Eq. (13.24), the numerical value of *t* is

$$\frac{0.6510638}{\sqrt{0.384979}/\sqrt{188}} = 14.39. \tag{13.25}$$

This value clearly exceeds the *t* chart critical point 1.812 found in Step 4, so we reject the null hypothesis and claim that we have significant evidence of a positive effect of the amount of water on the growth height.

Step 4, Approach 2. In this step we calculate *t*, getting the value 14.39 as above.

Step 5, Approach 2. Find the $P$-value corresponding to the calculated value of $t$. This can only be done with a computer package.

In R, we can calculate the $P$-value manually with pt(14.39, df = 10, lower.tail = FALSE). We can also see the desired information from the linear model summary with the code shown below. We find $t$ for the test of $\beta = 0$ in the Coefficients table in the row for x and the column for t value. We find the corresponding $P$-value in the column to the right for Pr(>|t|). Note that this is a **two-sided** $P$-value, so we need to divide by 2 to get the one-sided $P$-value of interest. This is $2.6 \times 10^{-8}$, highly significant and in agreement with the conclusion from Approach 1. We also see a row for (Intercept), which tests the null hypothesis $\alpha = 0$ and is not of interest to us.

```
x <- c(16, 16, 16, 18, 18, 20, 22, 24, 24, 26, 26, 26)
y <- c(76.2, 77.1, 75.7, 78.1, 77.8, 79.2, 80.2, 82.5, 80.7, 83.1, 82.2,
83.6)
model <- lm(y ~ x)
summary(model)
```

*Notes on the Regression t Test*

1. In using a $t$ test, we implicitly assume that the growth heights have a normal distribution. (This assumption was not necessary in the regression estimation activities.) A so-called non-parametric test is available in which the normal distribution assumption is not made, but we do not consider this test in this book.
2. There are formal tests of the linear assumption that the mean of $Y$ is of the linear from $\alpha + \beta x$ and of the homoscedasticity assumption that the variance of $Y$ is equal to $\sigma^2$ for all $x$. These are not discussed in this book. For our purposes, it is sufficient to use judgment and common sense in assessing whether the linear assumption is reasonable, as discussed in Sect. 8.6.
3. A formula equivalent to (13.24) is

$$ t = \frac{b\sqrt{s_{xx}}}{s_r}. \tag{13.26} $$

This is slightly more convenient than (13.24) for purposes of computation.
4. *Generalization.* In the regression examples considered so far, the null hypothesis is "$\beta = 0$". In some cases, the null hypothesis is of the form "$\beta = \beta_0$", where $\beta_0$ is some specified numerical value. The relevant $t$ statistic is then the generalization of (13.26), namely

$$ t = \frac{(b - \beta_0)\sqrt{s_{xx}}}{s_r}. \tag{13.27} $$

In this more general procedure, the alternative hypothesis could be one-sided up ("$\beta > \beta_0$"), one-sided down ("$\beta < \beta_0$"), or two-sided ("$\beta \neq \beta_0$"), depending on the context. There are still $n - 2$ degrees of freedom.
5. *Degrees of freedom.* As stated previously, the numerical value for the number of degrees of freedom is sometimes mysterious. Broadly speaking, the number

of degrees of freedom in any $t$ test is the number of observations minus the number of parameters that were estimated before making the estimate of the relevant variance. In the one-sample $t$ test, we estimate one parameter (the mean, estimated by $\bar{x}$) before we estimate the variance, so we have $n - 1$ degrees of freedom. The same is true in the paired $t$ test. In the two-sample $t$ test, we estimate two means, $\mu_1$ and $\mu_2$ (respectively by $\bar{x}_1$ and $\bar{x}_2$), before estimating the variance, so we have $n + m - 2$ degrees of freedom. In the regression case, we estimate two parameters ($\alpha$ and $\beta$) before we estimate the variance ($\sigma^2$), so we have $n - 2$ degrees of freedom.

Another way of looking at the regression degrees of freedom $n - 2$ is as follows. Suppose that in the plant example we only had two plants ($n = 2$). Then we have no degrees of freedom. Why is this?

With $n = 2$, there are only two data points, $(x_1, y_1)$ and $(x_2, y_2)$. When the data are plotted in the $x$-$y$ plane, the regression line $y = a + bx$ will pass exactly through these two points, and there would be no scatter of data points around the regression line. However, such a scatter is what is needed to estimate a variance, so it is impossible to estimate $\sigma^2$ if $n = 2$. Another way of seeing this is that the variance estimate $s_r^2$ becomes the meaningless quantity $0/0$ when $n = 2$ and this expression in effect states "you cannot estimate the variance when $n = 2$".

The following example illustrates this. Suppose that the first data point has $x = 1$ and $y = 3$ and the second data point has $x = 3$ and $y = 7$. Then $\bar{x} = 2$, $\bar{y} = 5$, $s_{xx} = 2$, $s_{yy} = 8$ and $s_{xy} = 4$. This gives $b = 2$, $a = 1$ and so the regression line is $y = 1 + 2x$. This line passes through the two data points: when $x = 1$, $y = 1 + 2 = 3$ and when $x = 3$, $y = 1 + 2 \times 3 = 7$. Further, $s_r^2 = \frac{8 - 4 \times 2}{2 - 2} = \frac{0}{0}$, which is meaningless.

## 13.5   General Notes on $t$ Statistics

In Sects. 13.1, 13.2, 13.3, and 13.4, we have respectively discussed four $t$ statistics: the one-sample $t$ test statistic (13.3), the two-sample $t$ test statistic (13.14), the two-sample paired $t$ test statistic (13.21) and the $t$ statistic in regression (13.24). It is convenient to think of each of the test statistics used as a signal-to-noise ratio. The numerator in each of these statistics is the signal: it is a measure of the extent to which the data do not support the null hypothesis. For example, the numerator in the one-sample $t$ test statistic measures the extent to which the data average differs from the null hypothesis mean. For a given level of noise, the larger this difference is, the more likely we are to accept the alternative hypothesis. The same general comment applies for the other three $t$ tests.

Sometimes we might wish to test for the equality of more than two means. This leads into the important topic of the Analysis of Variance (ANOVA). The simplest form of ANOVA considers the extension of the two-sample $t$ tests to the case of more than two samples. However, there are many further aspects of the ANOVA concept, and full treatment of ANOVA requires a book of its own.

The form of regression that is described in this book is the simplest one possible. A more complicated situation arises when both the $x$ data values and the $y$ data values are the observed values of random variables. This case is associated with the concept of correlation, the relation between two *random* variables, for example the heights and weights of randomly chosen adult males. Correlation is not considered in this book. A further generalization is to that of multiple regression, in which we ask the question: "how does one random quantity depend on several non-random quantities?" This topic also deserves a book on its own.

Non-parametric alternatives to the one-sample and the two-sample $t$ tests, for which the assumption of a normal distribution is not required, are described in Chap. 14.

## 13.6   Exact Confidence Intervals

It has been stated in previous sections that the confidence intervals (8.14) and (8.15) for a mean are inexact since they take no account of the fact that they involve an estimated standard deviation instead of an exact standard deviation. The same is true of the confidence intervals (8.32) and (8.34) for the difference between two means and the confidence intervals (8.51) and (8.52) for the regression parameter $\beta$. In this section, we see how more precise confidence intervals can be found.

We start with the random variable $T$ discussed in Eq. (13.4) and its null hypothesis distribution given in Eq. (13.5) and illustrate the procedure with an example. Suppose that, in the case of finding the confidence interval for a single mean $\mu$, we have $n = 21$ data values, so that there are $\nu = 20$ degrees of freedom. Assuming that the random variables $X_1, \ldots, X_{21}$ are $iid$, each having a normal distribution with mean $\mu$, the discussion surrounding Eqs. (13.4) and (13.5) together with the $t$ chart (Chart 4) shows that Prob$(-2.086 \leq T \leq +2.086) = 0.95$. Writing $T$ as in Eq. (13.4), this shows that

$$\text{Prob}\left(-2.086 \leq \frac{\bar{X} - \mu}{S/\sqrt{n}} \leq 2.086\right) = 0.95. \tag{13.28}$$

We now reorganize this equation to get

$$\text{Prob}\left(\bar{X} - \frac{2.086S}{\sqrt{n}} \leq \mu \leq \bar{X} + \frac{2.086S}{\sqrt{n}}\right) = 0.95. \tag{13.29}$$

Given data $x_1, \ldots, x_n$, this leads to the exact 95% confidence interval

$$\bar{x} - \frac{2.086s}{\sqrt{n}} \quad \text{to} \quad \bar{x} + \frac{2.086s}{\sqrt{n}} \tag{13.30}$$

for $\mu$.

The general exact 95% confidence interval, of which (13.30) is a special case, is

$$\bar{x} - \frac{(t_{0.025,v})s}{\sqrt{n}} \quad \text{to} \quad \bar{x} + \frac{(t_{0.025,v})s}{\sqrt{n}}, \tag{13.31}$$

where $t_{0.025,v}$ is found from the $\alpha = 0.025$ column of the $t$ chart and $v$ is the appropriate degrees of freedom.

Comparison of the confidence intervals (13.30), (13.32) and (8.14) shows that the approximate "rule of thumb" confidence interval

$$\bar{x} - \frac{2s}{\sqrt{n}} \quad \text{to} \quad \bar{x} + \frac{2s}{\sqrt{n}} \tag{13.32}$$

is often closer to the exact confidence interval (13.30) than is (8.14). More exactly, examination of the $t$ chart shows that this is true whenever the degrees of freedom $v$ is less than 80 and also that (13.32) is reasonably accurate unless $v$ is less than 20. For this reason, it is sometimes preferred to use (13.32) as a convenient simple approximation unless $v$ is very small.

*Example* It was noted at the end of Sect. 8.3 that the confidence interval given below (8.18) is inexact. Since for this example there are 10 degrees of freedom, that confidence interval should be replaced by

$$1877.64 - \frac{2.228\sqrt{26,623.05}}{\sqrt{11}} \quad \text{to} \quad 1877.64 + \frac{2.228\sqrt{26,623.05}}{\sqrt{11}}. \tag{13.33}$$

This is about from 1768 to 1987. This is slightly wider than the confidence interval given below (8.18)

We now consider an exact confidence interval for the regression parameter $\beta$. If there are $n$ data pairs, $v = n - 2$ and the approximate confidence interval (8.51) should be replaced by the exact 95% confidence interval

$$b - \frac{(t_{0.025,v})s_r}{\sqrt{S_{xx}}} \quad \text{to} \quad b + \frac{(t_{0.025,v})s_r}{\sqrt{S_{xx}}}. \tag{13.34}$$

When $v$ is less than 80, a more precise confidence interval than that given by (8.51) is given by (8.53).

The case of the confidence interval for the difference between two means is more difficult. In the notation of Sect. 8.5, if $\sigma_1^2 \neq \sigma_2^2$, there is no random variable having an exact $t$ distribution and we have to use an approximation. Following the discussion in Note 2 of Sect. 13.2, we replace the approximate 95% confidence interval (8.32) by the approximate 95% confidence interval obtained by replacing

1.96 by $t_{0.025,\nu}$, namely

$$\bar{x}_1 - \bar{x}_2 - (t_{0.025,\nu})\sqrt{\frac{s_1^2}{n} + \frac{s_2^2}{m}} \quad \text{to} \quad \bar{x}_1 - \bar{x}_2 + (t_{0.025,\nu})\sqrt{\frac{s_1^2}{n} + \frac{s_2^2}{m}}, \quad (13.35)$$

where the number of degrees of freedom $\nu$ is found from Eq. (13.19) and the discussion following it.

When $\sigma_1^2 = \sigma_2^2$, an exact confidence interval exists. The random variable $T$ analogous to the statistic $t_1$ defined in (13.14), namely $T = \frac{\bar{X}_1 - \bar{X}_2}{s\sqrt{\frac{1}{n} + \frac{1}{m}}}$, has the $t$ distribution with $\nu = n + m - 2$ degrees of freedom when the null hypothesis $(\mu_1 = \mu_2)$ is correct. Following procedures similar to those that led to (13.31), we obtain the following exact 95% confidence interval for $\mu_1 - \mu_2$:

$$\bar{x}_1 - \bar{x}_2 - (t_{0.025,\nu})s\sqrt{\frac{1}{n} + \frac{1}{m}} \quad \text{to} \quad \bar{x}_1 - \bar{x}_2 + (t_{0.025,\nu})s\sqrt{\frac{1}{n} + \frac{1}{m}}, \quad (13.36)$$

where $\nu = n + m - 2$ and $s$ is found from Eq. (13.13).

The comments made about the confidence interval (13.32) for $\mu$ apply equally for the confidence interval for $\mu_1 - \mu_2$. The approximate confidence interval (8.33) is closer to the exact confidence interval than is (8.32) whenever $\nu$ is less than 80.

*Example* It was noted at the end of Sect. 8.5 that the confidence interval given below (8.35) is inexact. Since for this example, there are 20 degrees of freedom, that confidence interval should be replaced by

$$112.50 - 2.086\sqrt{\frac{26{,}623.05}{11} + \frac{21{,}284.42}{11}} \quad \text{to}$$

$$112.50 + 2.086\sqrt{\frac{26{,}623.05}{11} + \frac{21{,}284.42}{11}}, \quad (13.37)$$

that is, about from $-25$ to $250$. This is somewhat wider than the confidence interval given below (8.35).

The above discussion concerns 95% confidence intervals. Similar comments apply for 99% confidence intervals. For example, when $\nu = 15$, the approximate 99% confidence interval (8.15) for $\mu$ should be replaced by

$$\bar{x} - \frac{2.947s}{\sqrt{n}} \quad \text{to} \quad \bar{x} + \frac{2.947s}{\sqrt{n}} \quad (13.38)$$

where 2.947 was found in the $\alpha/2 = 0.005$ column of Chart 4 for 15 degrees of freedom.

## 13.7 Problems

In each problem, assume that the data for that question are the observed values of *iid* random variables, each having a normal distribution.

**13.1** Different people remember a set of instructions for different lengths of time. It is well known from considerable past experience that the mean length of time that a person can remember a certain set of instructions is 6.5 hours.

(a) A group of 8 people was given special training in remembering these instructions. The times that they remembered them were, respectively, 6.39, 6.75, 6.60, 6.43, 6.65, 7.05, 6.47 and 6.71 hours.

Carry out a $t$ test with $\alpha = 0.05$ to test the null hypothesis that the mean length of time that a trained person can remember a certain set of instructions is equal to 6.5 hours against the alternative hypothesis that this mean exceeds 6.5 hours.

Hint: with the above data, $\bar{x} = 6.63125$ and $s^2 = 0.045955354$, so that $s = 0.21437$.

(b) Suppose now that in a different sample, the sample size is 25 and that with the data in this sample, $\bar{x} = 6.65$ and $s^2 = 0.04$, so that $s = 0.2$. Carry out the $t$ test with $\alpha = 0.01$.

**13.2** Items in a manufacturing process must fit to a certain size. Although a small tolerance in size is allowed, too big or too small are equally bad. Suppose that the desired size of a certain component is 15 inches. Each day, the first 25 items manufactured are measured to assess whether the process is in control. With this "too big or too small" concept in mind, we carry out a two-sided $t$ test.

(a) Given the 25 data values $x_1, x_2, \ldots, x_{25}$, we find that $\bar{x} = 14.985$ and $s^2 = 0.0025$. If $\mu$ is the mean item size, carry out the $t$ test of the null hypothesis $\mu = 5$ against the alternative hypothesis $\mu \neq 5$ with $\alpha = 0.05$.
(b) As in part (a), except that now $\bar{x} = 14.975$.
(c) As in part (a), except that now $s^2 = 0.0009$.

**13.3** This question refers to Example 2 at the end of Sect. 13.1.

(a) Suppose that $n = 16$, that $\bar{x} = 4.98$ and $s^2 = 0.0025$ (so that $s = 0.05$). Carry out the relevant $t$ test with numerical value of the Type I error $\alpha = 0.05$. (Recall that the null hypothesis mean is 5 and the alternative hypothesis is one-sided down.)
(b) Except that now $s^2 = 0.0016$ (so that s = 0.04), everything else is the same as in part (a), that is, $\bar{x} = 4.98$, the sample size is 16, and the choice of $\alpha$ is 0.05. Carry out the appropriate $t$ test.
(c) Comment on the difference between the conclusions reached in parts (a) and (b).

**13.4** Water-treatment facilities attempt to keep the pH level in their water close to 8.5. Too small a pH value is undesirable, and too large a pH value is also undesirable. (This implies that we will need a two-sided test.)

(a) A sample of nine pH test results gave an average of $\bar{x} = 8.42$, with an estimated standard deviation value of $s = 0.16$.

(i) Calculate the value of $t$.

(ii) If $\mu_0$ is the mean pH level of the water, test the null hypothesis $\mu_0 = 8.5$ against the alternative hypothesis $\mu_0 \neq 8.5$ with $\alpha = 0.05$.

(b) What would the value of $t$, and the corresponding conclusion, be if now the sample size is 25 (and the values of $\bar{x}$ and $s$ somehow miraculously are the same as in part (a))?

(c) Comment on the difference in your conclusion in parts (a) and (b) (that is, what is the main reason for the different conclusions in the two parts of the problem?).

**13.5** Suppose we want to test the null hypothesis that the mean time for PA residents to commute to work is 26.9 minutes against the alternative hypothesis that the mean time for PA residents to commute to work is greater than 26.9 minutes. We collect six PA residents' commute times: 27.9, 27.5, 30.5, 23.8, 26.4, 28.9. Conduct a hypothesis test with $\alpha = 0.05$ level.

**13.6** With reference to the reaction time example in Sect. 13.2, suppose now that there had been 9 young people and 11 old people. We arbitrarily choose the young people as "group 1" and the old people as "group 2". Suppose that with the data for these two groups, we find that $\bar{x}_1 = 428$, $\bar{x}_2 = 474$, and $s^2$ (as defined in Eq. (13.13)) = 1024, so that s = 32.

(a) Calculate $t_2$ as defined in (13.15) and then carry out the relevant $t$ test with $\alpha = 0.01$.

(b) Calculate $t_1$ as defined in (13.14) and then carry out the relevant $t$ test with $\alpha = 0.01$.

**13.7** We are curious as to whether the mean blood pressure for men is equal to the mean blood pressure for women. We arbitrarily think of men as "group 1" and women as "group 2". The alternative hypothesis, based on physiological grounds, is that the mean blood pressure for women exceeds the mean blood pressure for men. To test the null hypothesis against the alternative we plan to take the blood pressures of a sample of 6 men and of a sample of 7 women.

Having taken the blood pressures, we get the following data in coded units (with men as group 1 and women as group 2): $\bar{x}_1 = 8.75$, $\bar{x}_2 = 9.742857$, $s_1^2 = 0.339$, $s_2^2 = 0.669527$.

(a) We choose the value of $\alpha$ to be 0.05. Calculate $t_2$ and then carry out the test of the null hypothesis against the alternative hypothesis.

(b) Using the value of $t_2$ as calculated in part (a), carry out the test of the null hypothesis against the alternative hypothesis but now with $\alpha = 0.01$.

**13.8** Suppose that we want to test whether the mean time for PA residents to commute to work is equal to the mean time for MA residents. We collect six PA residents' commute times, which are: 27.9, 27.5, 30.5, 23.8, 26.4, 28.9. We also collect seven MA residents' commute times, which are: 30.9, 28.3, 30.7, 26.7, 30.7,

30.6, 31.7. Test the null hypothesis that the mean commute time for PA residents is equal to the mean commute time for MA residents against the alternative hypothesis that these two means are different, with $\alpha = 0.05$ and using $t_1$ as the test statistic.

Hint: With the data values given, the average PA commute time $\bar{x}_1$ is 27.5 and the estimated variance $s_1^2$ is 5.204 and the average MA commute time $\bar{x}_2$ is 29.94 and the estimated variance $s_2^2$ is 3.1329.

**13.9**  This question refers to the temperatures example described in Sect. 13.1.

Suppose that before the operation, the temperatures of the 10 people had been 98.8, 98.4, 99.1, 98.6, 98.5, 98.3, 98.8, 98.3, 98.6, 98.6.

As indicated in Sect. 13.1, after the operation the temperatures of these same 10 people are, respectively, 98.9, 98.6, 99.3, 98.7, 98.7, 98.4, 99.0, 98.5, 98.8, 98.8.

(a) Carry out a paired $t$ test with $\alpha = 0.01$. (The numerical values before the operation were chosen so that their average is 98.6. This then affords a fair comparison with the $t$ test carried out in Sect. 13.1, where the null hypothesis mean was 98.6.)
(b) Carry out the (inappropriate) unpaired two-sample $t$ test, using the same data as in part (a) of this problem. Regard the "after the operation" data set as data set 2, so that $\bar{x}_2 = 98.77$ as calculated in Sect. 13.1. The "before the operation" data set are set 1, for which $\bar{x}_1 = 98.6$. The value of $s^2$ as computed from Eq. (13.13) is 0.0645, so that s=0.25397. Calculate the value of the unpaired two-sample test statistic $t_2$ and then carry out the associated $t$ test with $\alpha = 0.01$.
(c) Discuss the difference between the numerical value of the paired $t$ statistic calculated in part (a) and the numerical value of the unpaired $t$ statistic calculated in part (b) from the point of view of the benefit of using a paired $t$ test.

**13.10**  Suppose that the brother/sister data given in Sect. 13.3 are replaced by

| Family | 1 | 2 | 3 | 4 | 5 | 6 | 7 | 8 | 9 | 10 |
|---|---|---|---|---|---|---|---|---|---|---|
| Sister | 124 | 131 | 109 | 133 | 104 | 137 | 122 | 106 | 153 | 121 |
| Brother | 128 | 137 | 114 | 126 | 116 | 138 | 125 | 110 | 161 | 125 |

The null hypothesis is that the mean blood pressure for men is the same as that for women and the alternative is that the mean blood pressure for men exceeds that for women. Conduct the paired $t$ test with $\alpha = 0.05$. (As an exercise in the relevant computations, you have to evaluate $\bar{d}$ and $s_d^2$ for yourself.)

**13.11**  This question relates to Problem 8.12. The null hypothesis is $\beta = 0$ against the alternative hypothesis $\beta > 0$ with Type I error $\alpha = 0.05$.

(a) Use the values $s_{xx} = 464.9$, $s_r = 1.45878$, $b = 0.2011831$ calculated in Problem 8.12 to calculate the appropriate $t$ statistic. Given your value of $t$, would you accept or reject the null hypothesis?

(b) You will find in part (a) that you will reject the null hypothesis $\beta = 0$ in favor of the alternative hypothesis $\beta > 0$. In other words, we have significant evidence that weight does increase with age.

However, the infant girls in the data set have a feeding disorder and we are concerned that their rate of increase of weight with age is less than the well-known mean rate for this for healthy infant girls in this age group of 3 kg per year, equal to 0.25 kg per month. To address this concern, test the null hypothesis $\beta = \beta_0 = 0.25$ against the alternative hypothesis $\beta < 0.25$, using a Type I error of 0.05.

**13.12** This question is intended to show the effect of the extent of dispersion around a regression line on the value of $s_r^2$, and from that, on the value of t. The numbers are chosen so that the calculations are simple and also so that the values of $a$ and $b$ in the two examples below are equal. This question relates to the "plant and growth height" context discussed throughout Sects. 8.6 and 13.4.

(a) Suppose that we have four plants in the experiment and after the growing season is over, we record the following data:

$$\begin{array}{l|llll} \text{Amount of water (x)} & 1 & 2 & 3 & 4 \\ \text{Growth height (y)} & 5.8 & 6.2 & 8.2 & 11.8 \end{array}$$

First, sketch the data on a graph. Next, calculate $a$ and $b$ and from these, draw the regression line. Does it "skewer through" the data points?
(b) If the chosen value of the Type I error is 0.05, would you reject the null hypothesis $\beta = 0$ in favor of the alternative hypothesis $\beta > 0$?
(c) Suppose now that the data had been:

$$\begin{array}{l|llll} \text{Amount of water (x)} & 1 & 2 & 3 & 4 \\ \text{Growth height (y)} & 6.2 & 5.8 & 7.8 & 12.2 \end{array}$$

Sketch the data on a graph. Then calculate $a$ and $b$ and from these, draw the regression line. Does it "skewer through" the data points?
(d) If the chosen value of the Type I error is 0.05, would you reject the null hypothesis $\beta = 0$ in favor of the alternative hypothesis $\beta > 0$?
(e) Comment on the relation between the scatter of the data points around the regression line in examples (a) and (c) and the effect that this scatter has on the respective values of $s_r^2$ and $t$ and the conclusions reached in (b) and (d).

**13.13 (Degrees of Freedom)** Suppose that we only have two plants in the plant and growth height example and that after the growing season is over, we record the following data:

$$\begin{array}{l|ll} \text{Amount of water (x)} & 1 & 3 \\ \text{Growth height (y)} & 2 & 8 \end{array}$$

(a) Calculate the formula for the regression line and show that it goes through the two data points.
(b) Show that a formal calculation for $s_r^2$ gives 0/0, which is meaningless. (This is the mathematics saying that we can't estimate $\sigma^2$ with only two data points.)

**13.14** Suppose we have observations of town size (in thousands) and total pizza sales for a 1-month period for eight different towns:

| Town | 1 | 2 | 3 | 4 | 5 | 6 | 7 | 8 |
|---|---|---|---|---|---|---|---|---|
| Town size (in thousands) | 5 | 10 | 20 | 8 | 4 | 6 | 12 | 15 |
| Pizza sales (in thousands) | 27 | 46 | 73 | 40 | 30 | 28 | 46 | 59 |

Carry out a two-sided hypothesis test of the null $\beta = 0$ against $\beta \neq 0$ with $\alpha = 0.05$.
  Hint. $\bar{x} = 10$, $\bar{y} = 43.625$, $s_{xx} = 210$, $s_{yy} = 1829.875$, $s_{xy} = 610$.

**13.15** This problem relates to Problem 8.4. Answer that problem in the light of the material in Sect. 13.6.

**13.16** This problem relates to Problem 8.5. Answer that problem in the light of the material in Sect. 13.6.

**13.17** This problem relates to Problem 8.6. Answer that problem in the light of the material in Sect. 13.6.

**13.18** This problem relates to Problem 8.10. Answer that problem in the light of the material in Sect. 13.6.

**13.19** This problem relates to Problem 8.11. Answer part (b) of that problem in the light of the material in Sect. 13.6.

**13.20** This problem relates to Problem 8.12. Answer part (c) of that problem in the light of the material in Sect. 13.6.

**13.21** This problem relates to Problem 8.13. Answer part (b) of that problem in the light of the material in Sect. 13.6.

**13.22** This problem relates to Problem 8.14. Answer part (b) of that problem in the light of the material in Sect. 13.6.

# Chapter 14
# Non-parametric Tests

## 14.1  Introduction

So far, most of the tests of hypotheses described in this book have concerned the values of one or more parameters. For example, a one-sample $t$ test concerns the numerical value of some parameter, in this case a mean $\mu$. The two-sample $t$ test concerns the equality (or otherwise) of two parameters, $\mu_1$ and $\mu_2$, both unknown means. Two-by-two table tests concern the equality (or otherwise) of two binomial parameters, $\theta_1$ and $\theta_2$. And so on.

By way of contrast, the hypotheses discussed in the following sections are not tests concerning parameters. Thus they are called *non-parametric* tests. An alternative name for these tests is *distribution-free* tests. Any time that we use a $t$ test, we implicitly assume that the data are the observed values of random variables having a normal distribution: the values in the $t$ chart were found making this assumption. The alternative to $t$ tests discussed in this chapter do not make this normal distribution assumption, hence the alternative expression "distribution-free".

There are several non-parametric alternatives to the one-sample $t$ test and also several alternatives to the two-sample $t$ test. In this chapter we consider one non-parametric alternative for each of these tests, and also some other non-parametric procedures.

## 14.2  Non-parametric Alternative to the One-Sample $t$ Test: The Wilcoxon Signed-Rank Test

The Wilcoxon signed-rank test is an alternative to the one-sample $t$ test in which it is not assumed that the data are the observed values of random variables having a normal distribution. There are two situations to consider. The first arises when we are willing to make the assumption that the data $x_1, x_2, \ldots, x_n$ are the

© The Author(s), under exclusive license to Springer Nature Switzerland AG 2023
W. J. Ewens, K. Brumberg, *Introductory Statistics for Data Analysis*,
https://doi.org/10.1007/978-3-031-28189-1_14

observed values of $n$ $iid$ random variables $X_1, X_2, \ldots, X_n$, each $X$ having the same *symmetric* probability distribution. We denote the point of symmetry of this distribution by $\mu$, the symbol for a mean, since if a probability distribution is symmetric, the point of symmetry is also the mean of the distribution. We first describe the hypothesis testing procedure if we are willing to make this assumption, and later consider the case where we are not willing to make this assumption.

Step 1. The null hypothesis claims that $\mu = \mu_0$, where $\mu_0$ is some prescribed numerical value. The alternative hypothesis will be one-sided up ($\mu > \mu_0$), one-sided down ($\mu < \mu_0$), or two-sided ($\mu \neq \mu_0$), depending on the context.

Step 2. As always, in this step we choose the value of $\alpha$, the numerical value we accept for the probability of making a Type I error.

Step 3. Suppose that we have carried out our experiment and thus have data values $x_1, x_2, \ldots, x_n$. We first construct the differences $x_1 - \mu_0, x_2 - \mu_0, \ldots, x_n - \mu_0$. Some of these differences will probably be negative, some positive. Next, we ignore the signs of these differences and construct the absolute values $|x_1 - \mu_0|, |x_2 - \mu_0|, \ldots, |x_n - \mu_0|$. These absolute values are then put in order from smallest to largest, and ranks are then assigned to these absolute differences, the smallest getting rank 1, ..., the largest getting rank $n$. The test statistic is $t^+$, the sum of the ranks of the *originally positive* differences. (Other test statistics are possible and frequently used, for example $t^+ - t^-$, the difference between the sum of the ranks corresponding to the originally positive $x_i - \mu_0$ values minus the sum of the ranks corresponding to the originally negative $x_i - \mu_0$ values. The conclusion reached when that test statistic is used will be identical to that reached using the test described here.)

Step 4, Approach 1. What values of $t^+$ lead us to reject the null hypothesis? If the alternative hypothesis is one-sided up ($\mu > \mu_0$), and this alternative hypothesis is true, we expect that many of the differences will tend to be positive so that $t^+$ would tend to be large. Hence sufficiently large values of $t^+$ lead us to reject the null hypothesis. If the alternative hypothesis is one-sided down ($\mu < \mu_0$), and this alternative hypothesis is true, we will expect that few of the differences will be positive and thus $t^+$ would tend to be small. Thus in this case, sufficiently small values of $t^+$ lead us to reject the null hypothesis.

If the alternative hypothesis is two-sided ($\mu \neq \mu_0$), sufficiently large or sufficiently small values of $t^+$ would lead us to reject the null hypothesis.

For small sample sizes, charts are available that indicate how large or small $t^+$ has to be for us to reject the null hypothesis. The calculation of the values in this chart is complicated and we do not describe it here. Our focus is on the accuracy of the following approximate procedure.

We consider the "before the experiment" random variable $T^+$ corresponding to $t^+$. With $n$ data values, the sum of *all* the ranks is $1 + 2 + \cdots + n = n(n+1)/2$. Under the null hypothesis, the probability that any given $X$ value is greater than $\mu_0$ is $1/2$: this is where the assumption of symmetry of the distribution of each $X$ is relevant. This implies that if the null hypothesis is true, the mean of $T^+$ is half of $n(n+1)/2$, that is, $n(n+1)/4$. Thus for a one-sided up test, values of $t^+$ sufficiently larger than $n(n+1)/4$ lead us to reject the null hypothesis. For a one-sided down test, values of $t^+$ sufficiently smaller than $n(n+1)/4$ lead us to reject the null hypothesis. For a two-sided test, values of $t^+$ sufficiently larger or sufficiently smaller than $n(n+1)/4$ lead us to reject the null hypothesis.

How much larger or smaller? This depends on the variance of $T^+$ when the null hypothesis is true. It is not straightforward to calculate this variance, so here we just give the result: When the null hypothesis is true and if there are no ties in the ranks, the variance of $T^+$ is $n(n+1)(2n+1)/24$. (If there are ties in the data, a slightly different formula applies. We will ignore this possibility and use $n(n+1)(2n+1)/24$ as a reasonable approximation.)

We give examples below that suggest that $T^+$ has approximately a normal distribution when $n$ is large, in practice 20 or more. The Central Limit Theorem helps with this assertion, since $T^+$ is a sum. This implies that we can calculate $z$, defined by

$$z = \frac{t^+ - \frac{n(n+1)}{4}}{\sqrt{\frac{n(n+1)(2n+1)}{24}}}, \tag{14.1}$$

and then use the $Z$ chart to carry out the test as a reasonably accurate procedure.

A more accurate calculation uses a continuity correction. We illustrate this with a one-sided up test. In this case, we replace the calculation of $z$ by the continuity-corrected value of $z$, defined by

$$z = \frac{t^+ - \frac{1}{2} - \frac{n(n+1)}{4}}{\sqrt{\frac{n(n+1)(2n+1)}{24}}}, \tag{14.2}$$

Suppose that we choose $\alpha = 0.05$. Then under the approximating procedure using a continuity correction, we would reject the null hypothesis if $z$, as defined in (14.2), is 1.645 or more. This value can be found from Chart 3 or Eq. (6.12). This is equivalent to rejecting the null hypothesis if

$$t^+ \geq \frac{n(n+1)}{4} + \frac{1}{2} + 1.645\sqrt{\frac{n(n+1)(2n+1)}{24}}. \tag{14.3}$$

The right-hand side in (14.3) is the critical point under this approximating procedure.

Step 5, Approach 1. Get the data, do the test.

The following example provides a comparison with exact critical points.

*Example* We are interested in whether students given special training score higher on a test than students not given special training. It can be assumed, from much previous experience, that the mean score for students not given special training is 69. Suppose that while we are not willing to believe that the probability distribution for scores for students given special training is a normal distribution, we are willing to believe that it has a symmetric distribution about its mean, so we plan to use the Wilcoxon one-sample test.

Step 1. Let $\mu$ be the mean score for students given special training. The null hypothesis is that this mean score is the same as that for students not given special training, that is, $\mu = 69$. The natural alternative hypothesis for this example is that $\mu > 69$. This concludes Step 1.

Step 2. Suppose that we choose $\alpha$ to be 0.05.

Step 3 The test statistic will be $t^+$.

Step 4, Approach 1. Since $\alpha$ was chosen to be 0.05 and the test is one-sided up, we will reject the null hypothesis if the inequality (14.3) holds. Suppose that $n = 7$. Then the right-hand side in (14.3) is

$$\frac{7 \times 8}{4} + \frac{1}{2} + 1.645\sqrt{\frac{7 \times 8 \times 15}{24}} = 24.23. \tag{14.4}$$

Since $t^+$ is necessarily a whole number, in practice we would reject the null hypothesis if $t^+ \geq 25$.

Step 5, Approach 1. Suppose that the scores for the $n = 7$ randomly chosen students given special training are as given in the table below. From these scores, we can calculate the various quantities needed for the test. They are:

| Scores: | 67.2 | 69.3 | 69.7 | 68.5 | 69.8 | 68.9 | 69.4 |
|---|---|---|---|---|---|---|---|
| Differences from 69: | −1.8 | 0.3 | 0.7 | −0.5 | 0.8 | −0.1 | 0.4 |
| Absolute differences: | 1.8 | 0.3 | 0.7 | 0.5 | 0.8 | 0.1 | 0.4 |
| Ranks: | 7 | 2 | 5 | 4 | 6 | 1 | 3 |

The sum $t^+$ of the ranks of the originally positive differences is $2+5+6+3 = 16$. Since the observed value (16) of $t^+$ is less than 25 we do not have enough evidence to reject the null hypothesis.

How accurate is this procedure? An exact procedure shows that if the null hypothesis is true, $\mathrm{Prob}(T^+ \geq 16) = 0.406$. If $t^+$ is 16, the value of $z$ defined by (14.2) is 0.2535. Since $\mathrm{Prob}(Z \geq 0.2535)$ is about 0.400, the normal distribution approximation with a continuity correction is quite accurate.

In R, we can use the `wilcox.test()` function to conduct the Wilcoxon signed-rank test:
`wilcox.test(x = c(67.2, 69.3, 69.7, 68.5, 69.8, 68.9, 69.4),`
`alternative = "greater", mu = 69)`. This will perform the exact procedure when reasonable and the normal approximation otherwise.

As a further check on the accuracy of the approximating procedure, suppose that $\alpha = 0.05$. If $n = 10$, the critical point calculated from (14.3) is the smallest whole number greater than $\frac{10 \times 11}{4} + \frac{1}{2} + 1.645\sqrt{\frac{10 \times 11 \times 21}{24}}$, which is 45. The exact critical point, found by extensive enumeration of all possibilities of rank assignments, is also 45. If $n = 20$, the critical point calculated from (14.3) is 150, as is the exact critical point. Clearly, the approximating procedure is sufficiently accurate for all practical purposes if $n \geq 20$, and is quite accurate even for $n = 10$.

*A Note on the Symmetry Assumption* In carrying out the test described above, we assumed that the probability distribution for scores for students given special training is symmetric about its mean. The most frequent situation when this assumption is justified is when we have two groups of observations with the observations in the two groups being paired, as in a paired $t$ test. The test is based on the paired differences of the data values in the two groups, as in the paired $t$ test. If the null hypothesis of no difference between the groups is true, these differences are the observed values of random variables having a symmetric distribution (around 0), so the requirements for the Wilcoxon signed-rank test apply. The alternative hypothesis comes from the context.

To illustrate this, we consider an example similar to the "brother-sister blood pressure" example in Sect. 13.3. As in that example, the null hypothesis now is that the probability distribution of blood pressures among men is the same as that among women. The alternative hypothesis, similar to that in Sect. 13.3, is that these distributions are the same except that the brother distribution is moved to higher values than the sister values. We choose $\alpha = 0.05$.

The differences, absolute differences, and the rankings of the absolute differences in the brother-sister blood pressure values in this example are as follows:

| Family | 1 | 2 | 3 | 4 | 5 | 6 | 7 | 8 | 9 | 10 |
|---|---|---|---|---|---|---|---|---|---|---|
| Difference | 9 | −2 | 5 | −6 | 11 | −4 | 3 | 7 | 8 | 1 |
| Absolute difference | 9 | 2 | 5 | 6 | 11 | 4 | 3 | 7 | 8 | 1 |
| Ranking | 9 | 2 | 5 | 6 | 10 | 4 | 3 | 7 | 8 | 1 |

The sum $t^+$ of the ranks of the originally positive differences is $9 + 5 + 10 + 3 + 7 + 8 + 1 = 43$. The critical point found by enumeration is 45, as is also the approximating critical point as found from (14.3), so we do not quite have enough evidence to reject the null hypothesis.

In R, to conduct this test, we use
```
wilcox.test(x = c(9, -2, 5, -6, 11, -4, 3, 7, 8, 1),
alternative = "greater", mu = 0).
```
If we are not willing to make the symmetry assumption, the test concerns the *median* of the probability distribution of each $X$. The procedure follows as above, but now $\mu$ is to be regarded as the median of the distribution of each $X$ and $\mu_0$ is the null hypothesis median value.

## 14.3    Non-parametric Alternative to the Two-Sample $t$ Test: The Wilcoxon Rank-Sum Test

The Wilcoxon rank-sum test (also known as the Mann-Whitney test) is a non-parametric alternative to the two-sample $t$ test. As with the two-sample $t$ test, there are two groups of observations, Group 1 with $n$ data values and Group 2 with $m$ data values. We label the groups so that $n \le m$.

Step 1. The null hypothesis is that these $n + m$ observations are the observed values of random variables all having the same probability distribution. The alternative hypothesis might be that the probability distribution corresponding to the observations in Group 2 is of the same shape as that corresponding to the observations in Group 1 except that it is moved to the left. It might be that the probability distribution corresponding to the observations in Group 2 is of the same shape as that corresponding to the observations in Group 1 except that it is moved to the right. Finally, it might be that the probability distribution corresponding to the observations in Group 1 is of the same shape as that corresponding to the observations in Group 2 except that it is moved either to the left or to the right. One of these three possibilities will be relevant for any given situation, and we declare which of these is appropriate for the situation at hand as the alternative hypothesis.

To give a specific example, suppose that the data values will be the respective blood pressures of $n$ women (Group 1) and $m$ men (Group 2), with $n \le m$, that the null hypothesis is that the groups come from the same probability distribution, and that the alternative hypothesis is that the probability distribution corresponding to the observations in Group 2 (men) is moved to the right relative to the probability distribution for Group 1 (women): that is, the alternative hypothesis is that men tend to have higher blood pressures than women.

Step 2. As always, in this step, we choose the numerical value of $\alpha$. Suppose that for the blood pressure example, we choose $\alpha = 0.05$.

Step 3. In this step, we determine the form of the test statistic. This is done as follows. All the $n + m$ data values are put into one sequence, ordered from lowest to highest. As a simple example, suppose that we have the blood pressures of $n = 4$ women (labelled as "$x$" values) and the blood pressures of $m = 3$ men (labelled as "$y$" values) in our sample, and that when these are put into one sequence and ordered from lowest to highest, we get

$$x_3, y_1, x_4, x_2, x_1, y_2, y_3. \tag{14.5}$$

That is, the person with the lowest blood pressure was woman number 3, the person with the next to lowest blood pressure was man number 1, and so on.

Having done this, we assign the ranks $1, 2, \ldots, n + m$ to the data values, with the smallest data value getting rank 1, the next smallest getting rank 2, $\ldots$, the largest getting rank $n + m$ ($n + m = 7$ in the above example). If there are ties, we share out the ranks in any set of tied data values: this leads to minor complications that we do not consider in this book. The test statistic is then $w$, the sum of the ranks of the data values in Group 2 (the smaller group). This test statistic is the observed value of the random variable $W$, the random value of the sum of the ranks in Group 2 before the data are found. This is the end of Step 3.

Step 4. There are two methods available for carrying out the test. The first uses exact calculations, but because of computational problems, this is possible in practice only when $n$ and $m$ are quite small, say $n \leq 20$, $m \leq 20$. The second method is approximate. Both are discussed briefly below.

*Method 1* This method is exact, but in practice only possible when $n$ and $m$ are both small. To assess whether the eventually observed value of $w$ will lead us to reject the null hypothesis, it is necessary to find the null hypothesis distribution of $W$. To do this, we observe that the actual labeling of the various women and the various men in (14.5) is irrelevant, since the statistic $w$ adds up the ranks of the individuals in Group 2 (men, in this example) and takes no account of the labeling of the individual women or of the individual men. This means that we can simplify (14.5) by re-writing it as $xyxxxyy$. Under the null hypothesis, all the possible re-orderings of the $x$'s and $y$'s have the same probability. In general, the number of possible re-orderings is $\binom{n+m}{m}$, and under the null hypothesis, each re-ordering has probability $\dfrac{1}{\binom{n+m}{m}}$. From this, it follows that if the null hypothesis is true,

$$\text{Prob}(W = w) = \frac{\text{number of orderings for which } W = w}{\binom{n+m}{m}}. \tag{14.6}$$

If the test is one sided up, then given the observed value $w_{obs}$, the $P$-value is

$$P\text{-value} = \frac{1}{\binom{n+m}{m}}(\text{sum of the number of orderings for which } w \geq w_{obs}).$$
$$\tag{14.7}$$

In the blood pressure example, the largest possible value for $w$ is $5 + 6 + 7 = 18$, arising only for the ordering $xxxxyyy$. Under the null hypothesis, this value has probability $\dfrac{1}{\binom{7}{3}} = \frac{1}{35}$. The next to highest possible value is 17, arising only for the ordering $xxxyxyy$, and also having null hypothesis probability $\frac{1}{35}$. Therefore, the null hypothesis probability of getting a value of $w$ 17 or larger is $\frac{2}{35} \approx 0.0571$. Thus if the observed value of $w$ is 17, the $P$-value is $\frac{2}{35}$.

For larger values of $n$ and $m$, the $P$-value calculations become tedious. Even for the case $n = m = 10$, there are $\binom{20}{10} = 2,628,800$ different re-orderings of the $x$'s and the $y$'s and clearly a computer is needed to consider all of these, evaluate the value of $w$ for each, and thus arrive at the exact null hypothesis distribution of $W$. In the case $n = m = 20$, there are $\binom{40}{20} \approx 2.43 \times 10^{18}$ different re-orderings, and it would take a long time even for a powerful computer to consider all of these, evaluate the value of $w$ for each, and thus arrive at an exact null hypothesis distribution of $W$. Fortunately, as shown below, a sufficiently accurate approximation is available when $n \geq 10, m \geq 10$.

*Method 2* The method is not exact, and is used for larger sample sizes. Steps 1, 2 and 3 are as described above, so we now consider Step 4.

Step 4, Approach 1. To find values of $w$ that lead us to reject the null hypothesis, we approximate the distribution of $W$ by a normal distribution. To do this, we need to find the null hypothesis mean and variance of $W$.

The sum of the ranks of all $n + m$ observations is $1 + 2 + \cdots + (n + m)$, and this simplifies to $(n + m)(n + m + 1)/2$. We next use a proportionality argument to say that since Group 2 comprises a proportion $m/(n + m)$ of all the data values, then if the null hypothesis is true, the mean of $W$ is the fraction $m/(n + m)$ multiplied by the sum $(n + m)(n + m + 1)/2$, and this gives $m(n + m + 1)/2$. Thus if the null hypothesis is true, the mean of $W$ is $m(n + m + 1)/2$.

How far from $m(n + m + 1)/2$ does $w$ have to get for us to reject the null hypothesis? This depends on the null hypothesis variance of $W$. This variance is much harder to establish, so here we just provide the result. If there are no ties in the data, the null hypothesis variance of $W$ is $nm(n + m + 1)/12$. If there are ties, a slightly different formula applies, but we do not consider this complication in this book. In summary, when the null hypothesis is true,

$$\text{mean   of } W = \frac{m(n + m + 1)}{2}, \quad \text{variance   of } W = \frac{nm(n + m + 1)}{12}. \quad (14.8)$$

In using a normal distribution to approximate the distribution of $W$, we are approximating a discrete distribution by a continuous distribution, so that a more accurate approximation will be found by introducing a continuity correction. Because of this, it is easiest to carry out the test using Approach 2 and a $P$-value calculation. An illustration of this is given in the example below.

Step 5. Under both methods described, Step 5 is straightforward: get the data and do the test.

*Example* We are interested in assessing whether special training tends to increase the test scores of school children. The null hypothesis is that the special training has no effect and the alternative hypothesis is that it does tend to increase the test scores of school children. This in effect completes Step 1 of the testing procedure.

Step 2. We choose the value of $\alpha$. In this example we choose $\alpha = 0.05$.

Step 3. The data consist of the test scores of a control group of $n = 10$ students (Group 1) not given special training as well as test scores of $m = 10$ students (Group 2) who were given special training. From these, the value of the test statistic $w$, the sum of the ranks of the students given special training, can be computed.

Steps 4 and 5. If the null hypothesis is true, the mean and variance of $W$ are, respectively, 105 and 175 (from Eqs. (14.8)). Suppose that $w$, the sum of the ranks of Group 2 (the students given special training) is 131. Use of a continuity correction shows that, to a close approximation, the $P$-value is $\text{Prob}(X \geq 130.5)$, where $X$ has a normal distribution with this mean and this variance. A standardization procedure shows that the approximating $P$-value is $\text{Prob}(Z \geq 1.9276) \approx 0.027$, and since this is less than 0.05, we reject the null hypothesis and claim that we have evidence that the special training does tend to increase the test scores.

In R, we can use the `wilcox.test()` function again, inputting two samples as x and y. However, R's calculations differ a bit from those presented here, in that the ranks will be summed for the first group inputted (as the x argument) instead of the second group, and that the minimum sum will be subtracted, meaning the value it gives for W is $m(m + 1)/2$ smaller than what we calculate here. However, the P-value and conclusion will not differ between this book and R's calculations. R will perform the exact test when feasible and the normal approximation otherwise.

How accurate is the normal distribution approximation? When $n = m = 10$ it can be shown by enumeration that when the null hypothesis is true, $\text{Prob}(W \geq 131) \approx 0.026$. The approximate $P$-value found in the example above is therefore quite accurate. The answer to Problem 14.5 also supports the claim that the normal distribution approximation is sufficiently accurate when $n \geq 10, m \geq 10$ if a continuity correction is used.

## 14.4 Other Non-parametric Procedures

The two Wilcoxon tests described above can be regarded as tests of location. In the signed-rank test, they are sensitive to changes in location of the mean in the symmetric case, otherwise the median, from a null hypothesis value $\mu$. In the rank-sum test, they are sensitive to a difference in location of the two distributions involved. There are many further non-parametric tests that are sensitive to other aspects of a distribution or two distributions, for example a difference in the variances of two distributions. There are non-parametric tests in the context of regression, and indeed there are non-parametric alternatives to many parametric tests. We do not consider any of these in this book.

## 14.5 Permutation Methods

### 14.5.1 The Permutation Alternative to the Signed-Rank Test

The permutation analogue of the signed-rank test in the "symmetric distribution" case in Sect. 14.2 is to consider all possible $2^n$ assignments of $+$ and $-$ to the values of $|x_1 - \mu_0|, |x_2 - \mu_0|, \ldots, |x_n - \mu_0|$, to calculate the value of $t^+$ for each assignment, and to reject the null hypothesis (for example) in the one-sided up case if the observed value of $t^+$ is among the largest $100 \times \alpha\%$ of the $2^n$ permutation values. For example, if $n = 10$ and the various values of the $|x_i - \mu_0|$ quantities, arbitrarily but conveniently sorted by magnitude, are 1, 2, 2, 3, 3, 4, 4, 6, 7, and 9, the first possible assignment is +1, +2, +2, +3, +3, +4, +4, +6, +7, and +9 ($t^+ = 1 + \ldots + 10 = 55$), the next possible assignment is +1, +2, +2, +3, +3, +4, +4, +6, +7, and -9 ($t^+ = 1 + \ldots + 9 = 45$), and the final possible assignment is $-1, -2, -2, -3, -3, -4, -4, -6, -7$, and $-9$ ($t+ = 0$). If $\alpha = 0.05$ and the test is one-sided up, the null hypothesis is rejected if the observed value of $t^+$ is among the $0.05 \times 2^{10} = 0.05 \times 1024 = 51.2$ (in practice, 51) largest of the 1024 values of $t^+$ calculated for the permuted values.

The Wilcoxon signed-rank procedure is identical to the permutation procedure on the ranking values, and thus can be regarded as a permutation procedure. This is illustrated in the simple case $n = 3$ where $\mu_0 = 10$ and $x_1 = 12$, $x_2 = 6$ and $x_3 = 17$. The absolute differences $|x_i - \mu_0|$ are 2, 4 and 7. There are $2^3 = 8$ allocations of $+$ and $-$ to these the absolute differences. These are as follows, with the respective associated values of $t^+$ given.

| Permutation | Ranks of positive values | $t^+$ |
|---|---|---|
| +2, +4, +7 | 1, 2, 3 | 6 |
| −2, +4, +7 | 2, 3 | 5 |
| +2, −4, +7 | 1, 3 | 4 |
| +2, +4, −7 | 1, 2 | 3 |
| −2, −4, +7 | 3 | 3 |
| −2, +4, −7 | 2 | 2 |
| +2, −4, −7 | 1 | 1 |
| −2, −4, −7 | None | 0 |

Under the null hypothesis, each assignment has probability 1/8. This distribution is identical to that found under the procedure described in Sect. 14.2. This is confirmed by the fact that the mean of the distribution of the $t^+$ permutation values is 3 and the variance is 3.5, which agree with the mean and variance given in Sect. 14.2 for the case $n = 3$.

## 14.5.2  The Permutation Alternative to the Rank-Sum Test

The permutation analogue of the rank-sum test in Sect. 14.3 is to permute the data in all possible ways and calculate the two-sample $t_1$ (or $t_2$) statistic as defined in Eq. (13.14) (or Eq. (13.15)) for each permutation. One of these permutations will correspond to the actual data. The null hypothesis is rejected if the value of $t_1$ as calculated from the actual data is a significantly extreme one of all the values of $t_1$ found under permutation. This is demonstrated with an example.

Suppose that the null hypothesis is that men (Group 1) and women (Group 2) have the same distribution of blood pressure, and that we plan to test this null hypothesis by taking the blood pressures of $n = 5$ men and $m = 5$ women. The blood pressures of the five men are 122, 131, 98, 114, 132 and the blood pressures of the five women are 113, 110, 127, 99, 119. There are $\binom{10}{5} = 252$ permutations of the data such that five of the data values are for men and the remaining five are for women. Each will lead to a value of $t_1$. Here are some of the 252 permutations with the corresponding values of $t_1$:

| Permutation | Men data values | Women data values | $t_1$ value |
|---|---|---|---|
| 1 (the real data) | 122, 131, 98, 114, 132 | 113, 110, 127, 99, 119 | 0.74 |
| 2 | 127, 114, 132, 99, 113 | 110, 122, 131, 119, 98 | 0.12 |
| ⋮ | | | |
| 252 | 132, 99, 113, 127, 131 | 110, 119, 122, 98, 114 | 1.03 |

Suppose that the alternative hypothesis is that the blood pressure for men tends to exceed that for women. If we had chosen $\alpha = 0.05$, we reject the null hypothesis (that men and women have the same probability distribution of blood pressure) if the observed value of $t_1$, here 0.74, is among the highest $0.05 \times 252 = 12.6$, or conservatively in practice 13, of these 252 permutation $t_1$ values. The logic behind this is that if the null hypothesis is true, then given the 10 data values, but without any labeling as to gender, all of the 252 permutation values of $t_1$ are equally likely. Thus if the null hypothesis is true, the probability that the actual value of $t_1$ is among the 13 largest permutation values of $t_1$ is slightly less than 0.05, so that if the null hypothesis is true, the probability that we will incorrectly reject the null hypothesis is slightly less than the chosen value of $\alpha$.

From the computational point of view it is not necessary to compute the value of $t_1$ for each permutation. We demonstrate this in the case of a two-sided test, in which the test statistic can be taken as $t_1^2$.

Standard algebra shows that the numerator of the joint variance estimate $s^2$ given in (13.13) can equivalently be written as

$$\sum_{i=1}^{n} x_{1i}^2 + \sum_{i=1}^{m} x_{2i}^2 - (n+m)\bar{\bar{x}}^2 - \frac{nm}{n+m}d^2, \tag{14.9}$$

where $\bar{\bar{x}} = (\sum_{i=1}^{n} x_{1i} + \sum_{i=1}^{m} x_{2i})/(n+m)$ and $d = \bar{x}_1 - \bar{x}_2$. The sum of the first three terms in (14.9) is invariant under permutation, and we write it as $C$. This means that $t_1^2$ (the square of (13.14)) can equivalently be written as

$$t_1^2 = \frac{d^2}{(C - \frac{nm}{n+m}d^2)(\frac{1}{n} + \frac{1}{m})}. \tag{14.10}$$

This is a monotonic increasing function of $d^2$, and this implies that under permutation, it is equivalent to compute $d^2$ instead of $t_1^2$ for each permutation and to reject the null hypothesis if the observed value of $d^2$ is among the largest $100 \times \alpha\%$ of all the permutation values. This reduces the amount of computing involved.

The permutation procedure clearly involves substantial computation unless both $n$ and $m$ are small, since the number of different permutations is extremely large even for relatively small values of $n$ and $m$. Modern computing power makes this an increasingly unimportant problem. When $m$ and $n$ are jointly so large that computation of all possible permutations is not feasible, close approximations to $P$-values and other quantities may be found from a random sample of a large number of permutations.

The rank-sum test described in Sect. 14.3 is also a permutation procedure, but now as applied to the ranks and not the original data. This is illustrated in the simple case $n = m = 2$. There are $\binom{4}{2} = 6$ permutation allocations of the ranks to group 1, resulting in the six possible values $1 + 2 = 3$, $1 + 3 = 4$, $1 + 4 = 5$, $2 + 3 = 5$, $2 + 4 = 6$ and $3 + 4 = 7$ of $W$. Under the null hypothesis, each of these allocations has probability 1/6. This permutation distribution of $W$ is identical to the distribution of $W$ found under the procedures of Sect. 14.3. This is confirmed by the fact that the mean of the permutation distribution of $W$ is 5 and the variance is 5/3 and these agree with the values found in (14.8) for the case $n = m = 2$. Thus the rank-sum procedure of Sect. 14.3 is identical to the permutation procedure applied to the ranks of the observations rather than to the observations themselves.

## 14.6   Problems

**14.1** In this problem, assume that the probability distribution of the original random variables is symmetric (around some mean $\mu$). The possible values of $T^+$ are 0, 1, $\ldots$, $\frac{n(n-1)}{2}$. Show that if the null hypothesis is true, $\text{Prob}(T^+ = 0)$, $\text{Prob}(T^+ = 1)$, $\text{Prob}(T^+ = \frac{n(n-1)}{2} - 1)$ and $\text{Prob}(T^+ = \frac{n(n-1)}{2})$ are all equal.

**14.2** In this problem, assume that the probability distribution of the original random variables is symmetric (around some mean $\mu$). Suppose that $n = 2$. Find the null hypothesis distribution of $T^+$. From this, find the mean and variance of $T^+$ and check that they agree with the values given in Sect. 14.2 for the case $n = 2$.

**14.3** (a) Suppose that in the Wilcoxon rank-sum test, $n = m = 3$. Find all possible values of $W$ and their null hypothesis probabilities. Check that these probabilities add to 1.

(b) Use the probabilities found in part (a) of this question to find the null hypothesis mean and variance of $W$ and check that the values that you obtain agree with those given in Eqs. (14.8).

**14.4** In the simple "blood pressure" example considered in Sect. 14.3, $n = 4$, $m = 3$. It was shown that if the null hypothesis is true, $\text{Prob}(W \geq 17) = \frac{2}{35} \approx 0.0571$. Find the normal distribution approximation to this probability, both using and not using a continuity correction, and comment on your answers.

**14.5**  Suppose that in the Wilcoxon rank-sum test, $n = m = 6$. Exact enumeration shows that if the null hypothesis is true, Prob($W \geq 50$) = 0.047 (to three decimal place accuracy). Find the normal distribution approximation to this probability, both using and not using a continuity correction, and comment on your answer.

**14.6**  Suppose that in the Wilcoxon rank-sum test, $n = 8$, $m = 4$. Exact enumeration shows that if the null hypothesis is true, Prob($W \geq 36$) = 0.055 (to three decimal place accuracy). Find the normal distribution approximation to this probability, both using and not using a continuity correction and comment on your answer.

**14.7**  Suppose that in the Wilcoxon rank-sum test, $n = m = 10$. Exact enumeration shows that if the null hypothesis is true, Prob($W \geq 127$) = 0.053 (to three decimal place accuracy). Find the normal distribution approximation to this probability, both using and not using a continuity correction and comment on your answer.

# Useful Charts

**Chart 1** A chart of binomial probabilities $\text{Prob}(X = x)$ for specified indices $n$ and success probabilities $\theta$

| n | x | $\theta$ | | | | | | | | | |
|---|---|--------|--------|--------|--------|--------|--------|--------|--------|--------|--------|
|   |   | 0.05 | 0.1 | 0.15 | 0.2 | 0.25 | 0.3 | 0.35 | 0.4 | 0.45 | 0.5 |
| 2 | 0 | 0.9025 | 0.8100 | 0.7225 | 0.6400 | 0.5625 | 0.4900 | 0.4225 | 0.3600 | 0.3025 | 0.2500 |
|   | 1 | 0.0950 | 0.1800 | 0.2550 | 0.3200 | 0.3750 | 0.4200 | 0.4550 | 0.4800 | 0.4950 | 0.5000 |
|   | 2 | 0.0025 | 0.0100 | 0.0225 | 0.0400 | 0.0625 | 0.0900 | 0.1225 | 0.1600 | 0.2025 | 0.2500 |
| 3 | 0 | 0.8574 | 0.7290 | 0.6141 | 0.5120 | 0.4219 | 0.3430 | 0.2746 | 0.2160 | 0.1664 | 0.1250 |
|   | 1 | 0.1354 | 0.2430 | 0.3251 | 0.3840 | 0.4219 | 0.4410 | 0.4436 | 0.4320 | 0.4084 | 0.3750 |
|   | 2 | 0.0071 | 0.0270 | 0.0574 | 0.0960 | 0.1406 | 0.1890 | 0.2389 | 0.2880 | 0.3341 | 0.3750 |
|   | 3 | 0.0001 | 0.0010 | 0.0034 | 0.0080 | 0.0156 | 0.0270 | 0.0429 | 0.0640 | 0.0911 | 0.1250 |
| 4 | 0 | 0.8145 | 0.6561 | 0.5220 | 0.4096 | 0.3164 | 0.2401 | 0.1785 | 0.1296 | 0.0915 | 0.0625 |
|   | 1 | 0.1715 | 0.2916 | 0.3685 | 0.4096 | 0.4219 | 0.4116 | 0.3845 | 0.3456 | 0.2995 | 0.2500 |
|   | 2 | 0.0135 | 0.0486 | 0.0975 | 0.1536 | 0.2109 | 0.2646 | 0.3105 | 0.3456 | 0.3675 | 0.3750 |
|   | 3 | 0.0005 | 0.0036 | 0.0115 | 0.0256 | 0.0469 | 0.0756 | 0.1115 | 0.1536 | 0.2005 | 0.2500 |
|   | 4 | 0.0000 | 0.0001 | 0.0005 | 0.0016 | 0.0039 | 0.0081 | 0.0150 | 0.0256 | 0.0410 | 0.0625 |
| 5 | 0 | 0.7738 | 0.5905 | 0.4437 | 0.3277 | 0.2373 | 0.1681 | 0.1160 | 0.0778 | 0.0503 | 0.0312 |
|   | 1 | 0.2036 | 0.3280 | 0.3915 | 0.4096 | 0.3955 | 0.3601 | 0.3124 | 0.2592 | 0.2059 | 0.1562 |
|   | 2 | 0.0214 | 0.0729 | 0.1382 | 0.2048 | 0.2637 | 0.3087 | 0.3364 | 0.3456 | 0.3369 | 0.3125 |
|   | 3 | 0.0011 | 0.0081 | 0.0244 | 0.0512 | 0.0879 | 0.1323 | 0.1811 | 0.2304 | 0.2757 | 0.3125 |
|   | 4 | 0.0000 | 0.0005 | 0.0022 | 0.0064 | 0.0146 | 0.0284 | 0.0488 | 0.0768 | 0.1128 | 0.1562 |
|   | 5 | 0.0000 | 0.0000 | 0.0001 | 0.0003 | 0.0010 | 0.0024 | 0.0053 | 0.0102 | 0.0185 | 0.0312 |
| 6 | 0 | 0.7351 | 0.5314 | 0.3771 | 0.2621 | 0.1780 | 0.1176 | 0.0754 | 0.0467 | 0.0277 | 0.0156 |
|   | 1 | 0.2321 | 0.3543 | 0.3993 | 0.3932 | 0.3560 | 0.3025 | 0.2437 | 0.1866 | 0.1359 | 0.0937 |
|   | 2 | 0.0305 | 0.0984 | 0.1762 | 0.2458 | 0.2966 | 0.3241 | 0.3280 | 0.3110 | 0.2780 | 0.2344 |
|   | 3 | 0.0021 | 0.0146 | 0.0415 | 0.0819 | 0.1318 | 0.1852 | 0.2355 | 0.2765 | 0.3032 | 0.3125 |

(continued)

© The Author(s), under exclusive license to Springer Nature Switzerland AG 2023
W. J. Ewens, K. Brumberg, *Introductory Statistics for Data Analysis*,
https://doi.org/10.1007/978-3-031-28189-1

**Chart 1** (continued)

| n | x | θ | | | | | | | | | |
|---|---|------|-----|------|-----|------|-----|------|-----|------|-----|
| | | 0.05 | 0.1 | 0.15 | 0.2 | 0.25 | 0.3 | 0.35 | 0.4 | 0.45 | 0.5 |
| | 4 | 0.0001 | 0.0012 | 0.0055 | 0.0154 | 0.0330 | 0.0595 | 0.0951 | 0.1382 | 0.1861 | 0.2344 |
| | 5 | 0.0000 | 0.0001 | 0.0004 | 0.0015 | 0.0044 | 0.0102 | 0.0205 | 0.0369 | 0.0609 | 0.0938 |
| | 6 | 0.0000 | 0.0000 | 0.0000 | 0.0001 | 0.0002 | 0.0007 | 0.0018 | 0.0041 | 0.0083 | 0.0156 |
| 7 | 0 | 0.6983 | 0.4783 | 0.3206 | 0.2097 | 0.1335 | 0.0824 | 0.0490 | 0.0280 | 0.0152 | 0.0078 |
| | 1 | 0.2573 | 0.3720 | 0.3960 | 0.3670 | 0.3115 | 0.2471 | 0.1848 | 0.1306 | 0.0872 | 0.0547 |
| | 2 | 0.0406 | 0.1240 | 0.2097 | 0.2753 | 0.3115 | 0.3177 | 0.2985 | 0.2613 | 0.2140 | 0.1641 |
| | 3 | 0.0036 | 0.0230 | 0.0617 | 0.1147 | 0.1730 | 0.2269 | 0.2679 | 0.2903 | 0.2918 | 0.2734 |
| | 4 | 0.0002 | 0.0026 | 0.0109 | 0.0287 | 0.0577 | 0.0972 | 0.1442 | 0.1935 | 0.2388 | 0.2734 |
| | 5 | 0.0000 | 0.0002 | 0.0012 | 0.0043 | 0.0115 | 0.0250 | 0.0466 | 0.0774 | 0.1172 | 0.1641 |
| | 6 | 0.0000 | 0.0000 | 0.0001 | 0.0004 | 0.0013 | 0.0036 | 0.0084 | 0.0172 | 0.0320 | 0.0547 |
| | 7 | 0.0000 | 0.0000 | 0.0000 | 0.0000 | 0.0001 | 0.0002 | 0.0006 | 0.0016 | 0.0037 | 0.0078 |
| 8 | 0 | 0.6634 | 0.4305 | 0.2725 | 0.1678 | 0.1001 | 0.0576 | 0.0319 | 0.0168 | 0.0084 | 0.0039 |
| | 1 | 0.2793 | 0.3826 | 0.3847 | 0.3355 | 0.2670 | 0.1977 | 0.1373 | 0.0896 | 0.0548 | 0.0313 |
| | 2 | 0.0515 | 0.1488 | 0.2376 | 0.2936 | 0.3115 | 0.2965 | 0.2587 | 0.2090 | 0.1569 | 0.1094 |
| | 3 | 0.0054 | 0.0331 | 0.0839 | 0.1468 | 0.2076 | 0.2541 | 0.2786 | 0.2787 | 0.2568 | 0.2188 |
| | 4 | 0.0004 | 0.0046 | 0.0185 | 0.0459 | 0.0865 | 0.1361 | 0.1875 | 0.2322 | 0.2627 | 0.2734 |
| | 5 | 0.0000 | 0.0004 | 0.0026 | 0.0092 | 0.0231 | 0.0467 | 0.0808 | 0.1239 | 0.1719 | 0.2188 |
| | 6 | 0.0000 | 0.0000 | 0.0002 | 0.0011 | 0.0038 | 0.0100 | 0.0217 | 0.0413 | 0.0703 | 0.1094 |
| | 7 | 0.0000 | 0.0000 | 0.0000 | 0.0001 | 0.0004 | 0.0012 | 0.0033 | 0.0079 | 0.0164 | 0.0313 |
| | 8 | 0.0000 | 0.0000 | 0.0000 | 0.0000 | 0.0000 | 0.0001 | 0.0002 | 0.0007 | 0.0017 | 0.0039 |
| 9 | 0 | 0.6302 | 0.3874 | 0.2316 | 0.1342 | 0.0751 | 0.0404 | 0.0207 | 0.0101 | 0.0046 | 0.0020 |
| | 1 | 0.2985 | 0.3874 | 0.3679 | 0.3020 | 0.2253 | 0.1556 | 0.1004 | 0.0605 | 0.0339 | 0.0176 |
| | 2 | 0.0629 | 0.1722 | 0.2597 | 0.3020 | 0.3003 | 0.2668 | 0.2162 | 0.1612 | 0.1110 | 0.0703 |
| | 3 | 0.0077 | 0.0446 | 0.1069 | 0.1762 | 0.2336 | 0.2668 | 0.2716 | 0.2508 | 0.2119 | 0.1641 |
| | 4 | 0.0006 | 0.0074 | 0.0283 | 0.0661 | 0.1168 | 0.1715 | 0.2194 | 0.2508 | 0.2600 | 0.2461 |
| | 5 | 0.0000 | 0.0008 | 0.0050 | 0.0165 | 0.0389 | 0.0735 | 0.1181 | 0.1672 | 0.2128 | 0.2461 |
| | 6 | 0.0000 | 0.0001 | 0.0006 | 0.0028 | 0.0087 | 0.0210 | 0.0424 | 0.0743 | 0.1160 | 0.1641 |
| | 7 | 0.0000 | 0.0000 | 0.0000 | 0.0003 | 0.0012 | 0.0039 | 0.0098 | 0.0212 | 0.0407 | 0.0703 |
| | 8 | 0.0000 | 0.0000 | 0.0000 | 0.0000 | 0.0001 | 0.0004 | 0.0013 | 0.0035 | 0.0083 | 0.0176 |
| | 9 | 0.0000 | 0.0000 | 0.0000 | 0.0000 | 0.0000 | 0.0000 | 0.0001 | 0.0003 | 0.0008 | 0.0020 |
| 10 | 0 | 0.5987 | 0.3487 | 0.1969 | 0.1074 | 0.0563 | 0.0282 | 0.0135 | 0.0060 | 0.0025 | 0.0010 |
| | 1 | 0.3151 | 0.3874 | 0.3474 | 0.2684 | 0.1877 | 0.1211 | 0.0725 | 0.0403 | 0.0207 | 0.0098 |
| | 2 | 0.0746 | 0.1937 | 0.2759 | 0.3020 | 0.2816 | 0.2335 | 0.1757 | 0.1209 | 0.0763 | 0.0439 |
| | 3 | 0.0105 | 0.0574 | 0.1298 | 0.2013 | 0.2503 | 0.2668 | 0.2522 | 0.2150 | 0.1665 | 0.1172 |
| | 4 | 0.0010 | 0.0112 | 0.0401 | 0.0881 | 0.1460 | 0.2001 | 0.2377 | 0.2508 | 0.2384 | 0.2051 |
| | 5 | 0.0001 | 0.0015 | 0.0085 | 0.0264 | 0.0584 | 0.1029 | 0.1536 | 0.2007 | 0.2340 | 0.2461 |
| | 6 | 0.0000 | 0.0001 | 0.0012 | 0.0055 | 0.0162 | 0.0368 | 0.0689 | 0.1115 | 0.1596 | 0.2051 |
| | 7 | 0.0000 | 0.0000 | 0.0001 | 0.0008 | 0.0031 | 0.0090 | 0.0212 | 0.0425 | 0.0746 | 0.1172 |
| | 8 | 0.0000 | 0.0000 | 0.0000 | 0.0001 | 0.0004 | 0.0014 | 0.0043 | 0.0106 | 0.0229 | 0.0439 |
| | 9 | 0.0000 | 0.0000 | 0.0000 | 0.0000 | 0.0000 | 0.0001 | 0.0005 | 0.0016 | 0.0042 | 0.0098 |
| | 10 | 0.0000 | 0.0000 | 0.0000 | 0.0000 | 0.0000 | 0.0000 | 0.0000 | 0.0001 | 0.0003 | 0.0010 |

(continued)

**Chart 1** (continued)

| n | x | $\theta$ | | | | | | | | | |
|---|---|--------|------|------|-----|------|-----|------|-----|------|-----|
| | | 0.05 | 0.1 | 0.15 | 0.2 | 0.25 | 0.3 | 0.35 | 0.4 | 0.45 | 0.5 |
| 11 | 0 | 0.5688 | 0.3138 | 0.1673 | 0.0859 | 0.0422 | 0.0198 | 0.0088 | 0.0036 | 0.0014 | 0.0005 |
| | 1 | 0.3293 | 0.3835 | 0.3248 | 0.2362 | 0.1549 | 0.0932 | 0.0518 | 0.0266 | 0.0125 | 0.0054 |
| | 2 | 0.0867 | 0.2131 | 0.2866 | 0.2953 | 0.2581 | 0.1998 | 0.1395 | 0.0887 | 0.0513 | 0.0269 |
| | 3 | 0.0137 | 0.0710 | 0.1517 | 0.2215 | 0.2581 | 0.2568 | 0.2254 | 0.1774 | 0.1259 | 0.0806 |
| | 4 | 0.0014 | 0.0158 | 0.0536 | 0.1107 | 0.1721 | 0.2201 | 0.2428 | 0.2365 | 0.2060 | 0.1611 |
| | 5 | 0.0001 | 0.0025 | 0.0132 | 0.0388 | 0.0803 | 0.1321 | 0.1830 | 0.2207 | 0.2360 | 0.2256 |
| | 6 | 0.0000 | 0.0003 | 0.0023 | 0.0097 | 0.0268 | 0.0566 | 0.0985 | 0.1471 | 0.1931 | 0.2256 |
| | 7 | 0.0000 | 0.0000 | 0.0003 | 0.0017 | 0.0064 | 0.0173 | 0.0379 | 0.0701 | 0.1128 | 0.1611 |
| | 8 | 0.0000 | 0.0000 | 0.0000 | 0.0002 | 0.0011 | 0.0037 | 0.0102 | 0.0234 | 0.0462 | 0.0806 |
| | 9 | 0.0000 | 0.0000 | 0.0000 | 0.0000 | 0.0001 | 0.0005 | 0.0018 | 0.0052 | 0.0126 | 0.0269 |
| | 10 | 0.0000 | 0.0000 | 0.0000 | 0.0000 | 0.0000 | 0.0000 | 0.0002 | 0.0007 | 0.0021 | 0.0054 |
| | 11 | 0.0000 | 0.0000 | 0.0000 | 0.0000 | 0.0000 | 0.0000 | 0.0000 | 0.0000 | 0.0002 | 0.0005 |
| 12 | 0 | 0.5404 | 0.2824 | 0.1422 | 0.0687 | 0.0317 | 0.0138 | 0.0057 | 0.0022 | 0.0008 | 0.0002 |
| | 1 | 0.3413 | 0.3766 | 0.3012 | 0.2062 | 0.1267 | 0.0712 | 0.0368 | 0.0174 | 0.0075 | 0.0029 |
| | 2 | 0.0988 | 0.2301 | 0.2924 | 0.2835 | 0.2323 | 0.1678 | 0.1088 | 0.0639 | 0.0339 | 0.0161 |
| | 3 | 0.0173 | 0.0852 | 0.1720 | 0.2362 | 0.2581 | 0.2397 | 0.1954 | 0.1419 | 0.0923 | 0.0537 |
| | 4 | 0.0021 | 0.0213 | 0.0683 | 0.1329 | 0.1936 | 0.2311 | 0.2367 | 0.2128 | 0.1700 | 0.1208 |
| | 5 | 0.0002 | 0.0038 | 0.0193 | 0.0532 | 0.1032 | 0.1585 | 0.2039 | 0.2270 | 0.2225 | 0.1934 |
| | 6 | 0.0000 | 0.0005 | 0.0040 | 0.0155 | 0.0401 | 0.0792 | 0.1281 | 0.1766 | 0.2124 | 0.2256 |
| | 7 | 0.0000 | 0.0000 | 0.0006 | 0.0033 | 0.0115 | 0.0291 | 0.0591 | 0.1009 | 0.1489 | 0.1934 |
| | 8 | 0.0000 | 0.0000 | 0.0001 | 0.0005 | 0.0024 | 0.0078 | 0.0199 | 0.0420 | 0.0762 | 0.1208 |
| | 9 | 0.0000 | 0.0000 | 0.0000 | 0.0001 | 0.0004 | 0.0015 | 0.0048 | 0.0125 | 0.0277 | 0.0537 |
| | 10 | 0.0000 | 0.0000 | 0.0000 | 0.0000 | 0.0000 | 0.0002 | 0.0008 | 0.0025 | 0.0068 | 0.0161 |
| | 11 | 0.0000 | 0.0000 | 0.0000 | 0.0000 | 0.0000 | 0.0000 | 0.0001 | 0.0003 | 0.0010 | 0.0029 |
| | 12 | 0.0000 | 0.0000 | 0.0000 | 0.0000 | 0.0000 | 0.0000 | 0.0000 | 0.0000 | 0.0001 | 0.0002 |
| 13 | 0 | 0.5133 | 0.2542 | 0.1209 | 0.0550 | 0.0238 | 0.0097 | 0.0037 | 0.0013 | 0.0004 | 0.0001 |
| | 1 | 0.3512 | 0.3672 | 0.2774 | 0.1787 | 0.1029 | 0.0540 | 0.0259 | 0.0113 | 0.0045 | 0.0016 |
| | 2 | 0.1109 | 0.2448 | 0.2937 | 0.2680 | 0.2059 | 0.1388 | 0.0836 | 0.0453 | 0.0220 | 0.0095 |
| | 3 | 0.0214 | 0.0997 | 0.1900 | 0.2457 | 0.2517 | 0.2181 | 0.1651 | 0.1107 | 0.0660 | 0.0349 |
| | 4 | 0.0028 | 0.0277 | 0.0838 | 0.1535 | 0.2097 | 0.2337 | 0.2222 | 0.1845 | 0.1350 | 0.0873 |
| | 5 | 0.0003 | 0.0055 | 0.0266 | 0.0691 | 0.1258 | 0.1803 | 0.2154 | 0.2214 | 0.1989 | 0.1571 |
| | 6 | 0.0000 | 0.0008 | 0.0063 | 0.0230 | 0.0559 | 0.1030 | 0.1546 | 0.1968 | 0.2169 | 0.2095 |
| | 7 | 0.0000 | 0.0001 | 0.0011 | 0.0058 | 0.0186 | 0.0442 | 0.0833 | 0.1312 | 0.1775 | 0.2095 |
| | 8 | 0.0000 | 0.0000 | 0.0001 | 0.0011 | 0.0047 | 0.0142 | 0.0336 | 0.0656 | 0.1089 | 0.1571 |
| | 9 | 0.0000 | 0.0000 | 0.0000 | 0.0001 | 0.0009 | 0.0034 | 0.0101 | 0.0243 | 0.0495 | 0.0873 |
| | 10 | 0.0000 | 0.0000 | 0.0000 | 0.0000 | 0.0001 | 0.0006 | 0.0022 | 0.0065 | 0.0162 | 0.0349 |
| | 11 | 0.0000 | 0.0000 | 0.0000 | 0.0000 | 0.0000 | 0.0001 | 0.0003 | 0.0012 | 0.0036 | 0.0095 |
| | 12 | 0.0000 | 0.0000 | 0.0000 | 0.0000 | 0.0000 | 0.0000 | 0.0000 | 0.0001 | 0.0005 | 0.0016 |
| | 13 | 0.0000 | 0.0000 | 0.0000 | 0.0000 | 0.0000 | 0.0000 | 0.0000 | 0.0000 | 0.0000 | 0.0001 |
| 14 | 0 | 0.4877 | 0.2288 | 0.1028 | 0.0440 | 0.0178 | 0.0068 | 0.0024 | 0.0008 | 0.0002 | 0.0001 |
| | 1 | 0.3593 | 0.3559 | 0.2539 | 0.1539 | 0.0832 | 0.0407 | 0.0181 | 0.0073 | 0.0027 | 0.0009 |
| | 2 | 0.1229 | 0.2570 | 0.2912 | 0.2501 | 0.1802 | 0.1134 | 0.0634 | 0.0317 | 0.0141 | 0.0056 |

(continued)

**Chart 1** (continued)

| n | x | θ | | | | | | | | | |
|---|---|--------|--------|--------|--------|--------|--------|--------|--------|--------|--------|
| | | 0.05 | 0.1 | 0.15 | 0.2 | 0.25 | 0.3 | 0.35 | 0.4 | 0.45 | 0.5 |
| | 3 | 0.0259 | 0.1142 | 0.2056 | 0.2501 | 0.2402 | 0.1943 | 0.1366 | 0.0845 | 0.0462 | 0.0222 |
| | 4 | 0.0037 | 0.0349 | 0.0998 | 0.1720 | 0.2202 | 0.2290 | 0.2022 | 0.1549 | 0.1040 | 0.0611 |
| | 5 | 0.0004 | 0.0078 | 0.0352 | 0.0860 | 0.1468 | 0.1963 | 0.2178 | 0.2066 | 0.1701 | 0.1222 |
| | 6 | 0.0000 | 0.0013 | 0.0093 | 0.0322 | 0.0734 | 0.1262 | 0.1759 | 0.2066 | 0.2088 | 0.1833 |
| | 7 | 0.0000 | 0.0002 | 0.0019 | 0.0092 | 0.0280 | 0.0618 | 0.1082 | 0.1574 | 0.1952 | 0.2095 |
| | 8 | 0.0000 | 0.0000 | 0.0003 | 0.0020 | 0.0082 | 0.0232 | 0.0510 | 0.0918 | 0.1398 | 0.1833 |
| | 9 | 0.0000 | 0.0000 | 0.0000 | 0.0003 | 0.0018 | 0.0066 | 0.0183 | 0.0408 | 0.0762 | 0.1222 |
| | 10 | 0.0000 | 0.0000 | 0.0000 | 0.0000 | 0.0003 | 0.0014 | 0.0049 | 0.0136 | 0.0312 | 0.0611 |
| | 11 | 0.0000 | 0.0000 | 0.0000 | 0.0000 | 0.0000 | 0.0002 | 0.0010 | 0.0033 | 0.0093 | 0.0222 |
| | 12 | 0.0000 | 0.0000 | 0.0000 | 0.0000 | 0.0000 | 0.0000 | 0.0001 | 0.0005 | 0.0019 | 0.0056 |
| | 13 | 0.0000 | 0.0000 | 0.0000 | 0.0000 | 0.0000 | 0.0000 | 0.0000 | 0.0001 | 0.0002 | 0.0009 |
| | 14 | 0.0000 | 0.0000 | 0.0000 | 0.0000 | 0.0000 | 0.0000 | 0.0000 | 0.0000 | 0.0000 | 0.0001 |
| 15 | 0 | 0.4633 | 0.2059 | 0.0874 | 0.0352 | 0.0134 | 0.0047 | 0.0016 | 0.0005 | 0.0001 | 0.0000 |
| | 1 | 0.3658 | 0.3432 | 0.2312 | 0.1319 | 0.0668 | 0.0305 | 0.0126 | 0.0047 | 0.0016 | 0.0005 |
| | 2 | 0.1348 | 0.2669 | 0.2856 | 0.2309 | 0.1559 | 0.0916 | 0.0476 | 0.0219 | 0.0090 | 0.0032 |
| | 3 | 0.0307 | 0.1285 | 0.2184 | 0.2501 | 0.2252 | 0.1700 | 0.1110 | 0.0634 | 0.0318 | 0.0139 |
| | 4 | 0.0049 | 0.0428 | 0.1156 | 0.1876 | 0.2252 | 0.2186 | 0.1792 | 0.1268 | 0.0780 | 0.0417 |
| | 5 | 0.0006 | 0.0105 | 0.0449 | 0.1032 | 0.1651 | 0.2061 | 0.2123 | 0.1859 | 0.1404 | 0.0916 |
| | 6 | 0.0000 | 0.0019 | 0.0132 | 0.0430 | 0.0917 | 0.1472 | 0.1906 | 0.2066 | 0.1914 | 0.1527 |
| | 7 | 0.0000 | 0.0003 | 0.0030 | 0.0138 | 0.0393 | 0.0811 | 0.1319 | 0.1771 | 0.2013 | 0.1964 |
| | 8 | 0.0000 | 0.0000 | 0.0005 | 0.0035 | 0.0131 | 0.0348 | 0.0710 | 0.1181 | 0.1647 | 0.1964 |
| | 9 | 0.0000 | 0.0000 | 0.0001 | 0.0007 | 0.0034 | 0.0116 | 0.0298 | 0.0612 | 0.1048 | 0.1527 |
| | 10 | 0.0000 | 0.0000 | 0.0000 | 0.0001 | 0.0007 | 0.0030 | 0.0096 | 0.0245 | 0.0515 | 0.0916 |
| | 11 | 0.0000 | 0.0000 | 0.0000 | 0.0000 | 0.0001 | 0.0006 | 0.0024 | 0.0074 | 0.0191 | 0.0417 |
| | 12 | 0.0000 | 0.0000 | 0.0000 | 0.0000 | 0.0000 | 0.0001 | 0.0004 | 0.0016 | 0.0052 | 0.0139 |
| | 13 | 0.0000 | 0.0000 | 0.0000 | 0.0000 | 0.0000 | 0.0000 | 0.0001 | 0.0003 | 0.0010 | 0.0032 |
| | 14 | 0.0000 | 0.0000 | 0.0000 | 0.0000 | 0.0000 | 0.0000 | 0.0000 | 0.0000 | 0.0001 | 0.0005 |
| | 15 | 0.0000 | 0.0000 | 0.0000 | 0.0000 | 0.0000 | 0.0000 | 0.0000 | 0.0000 | 0.0000 | 0.0000 |
| 16 | 0 | 0.4401 | 0.1853 | 0.0743 | 0.0281 | 0.0100 | 0.0033 | 0.0010 | 0.0003 | 0.0001 | 0.0000 |
| | 1 | 0.3706 | 0.3294 | 0.2097 | 0.1126 | 0.0535 | 0.0228 | 0.0087 | 0.0030 | 0.0009 | 0.0002 |
| | 2 | 0.1463 | 0.2745 | 0.2775 | 0.2111 | 0.1336 | 0.0732 | 0.0353 | 0.0150 | 0.0056 | 0.0018 |
| | 3 | 0.0359 | 0.1423 | 0.2285 | 0.2463 | 0.2079 | 0.1465 | 0.0888 | 0.0468 | 0.0215 | 0.0085 |
| | 4 | 0.0061 | 0.0514 | 0.1311 | 0.2001 | 0.2252 | 0.2040 | 0.1553 | 0.1014 | 0.0572 | 0.0278 |
| | 5 | 0.0008 | 0.0137 | 0.0555 | 0.1201 | 0.1802 | 0.2099 | 0.2008 | 0.1623 | 0.1123 | 0.0667 |
| | 6 | 0.0001 | 0.0028 | 0.0180 | 0.0550 | 0.1101 | 0.1649 | 0.1982 | 0.1983 | 0.1684 | 0.1222 |
| | 7 | 0.0000 | 0.0004 | 0.0045 | 0.0197 | 0.0524 | 0.1010 | 0.1524 | 0.1889 | 0.1969 | 0.1746 |
| | 8 | 0.0000 | 0.0001 | 0.0009 | 0.0055 | 0.0197 | 0.0487 | 0.0923 | 0.1417 | 0.1812 | 0.1964 |
| | 9 | 0.0000 | 0.0000 | 0.0001 | 0.0012 | 0.0058 | 0.0185 | 0.0442 | 0.0840 | 0.1318 | 0.1746 |
| | 10 | 0.0000 | 0.0000 | 0.0000 | 0.0002 | 0.0014 | 0.0056 | 0.0167 | 0.0392 | 0.0755 | 0.1222 |
| | 11 | 0.0000 | 0.0000 | 0.0000 | 0.0000 | 0.0002 | 0.0013 | 0.0049 | 0.0142 | 0.0337 | 0.0667 |
| | 12 | 0.0000 | 0.0000 | 0.0000 | 0.0000 | 0.0000 | 0.0002 | 0.0011 | 0.0040 | 0.0115 | 0.0278 |

(continued)

**Chart 1** (continued)

| n | x | θ | | | | | | | | | |
|---|---|------|------|------|------|------|------|------|------|------|------|
| | | 0.05 | 0.1 | 0.15 | 0.2 | 0.25 | 0.3 | 0.35 | 0.4 | 0.45 | 0.5 |
| | 13 | 0.0000 | 0.0000 | 0.0000 | 0.0000 | 0.0000 | 0.0000 | 0.0002 | 0.0008 | 0.0029 | 0.0085 |
| | 14 | 0.0000 | 0.0000 | 0.0000 | 0.0000 | 0.0000 | 0.0000 | 0.0000 | 0.0001 | 0.0005 | 0.0018 |
| | 15 | 0.0000 | 0.0000 | 0.0000 | 0.0000 | 0.0000 | 0.0000 | 0.0000 | 0.0000 | 0.0001 | 0.0002 |
| | 16 | 0.0000 | 0.0000 | 0.0000 | 0.0000 | 0.0000 | 0.0000 | 0.0000 | 0.0000 | 0.0000 | 0.0000 |
| 17 | 0 | 0.4181 | 0.1668 | 0.0631 | 0.0225 | 0.0075 | 0.0023 | 0.0007 | 0.0002 | 0.0000 | 0.0000 |
| | 1 | 0.3741 | 0.3150 | 0.1893 | 0.0957 | 0.0426 | 0.0169 | 0.0060 | 0.0019 | 0.0005 | 0.0001 |
| | 2 | 0.1575 | 0.2800 | 0.2673 | 0.1914 | 0.1136 | 0.0581 | 0.0260 | 0.0102 | 0.0035 | 0.0010 |
| | 3 | 0.0415 | 0.1556 | 0.2359 | 0.2393 | 0.1893 | 0.1245 | 0.0701 | 0.0341 | 0.0144 | 0.0052 |
| | 4 | 0.0076 | 0.0605 | 0.1457 | 0.2093 | 0.2209 | 0.1868 | 0.1320 | 0.0796 | 0.0411 | 0.0182 |
| | 5 | 0.0010 | 0.0175 | 0.0668 | 0.1361 | 0.1914 | 0.2081 | 0.1849 | 0.1379 | 0.0875 | 0.0472 |
| | 6 | 0.0001 | 0.0039 | 0.0236 | 0.0680 | 0.1276 | 0.1784 | 0.1991 | 0.1839 | 0.1432 | 0.0944 |
| | 7 | 0.0000 | 0.0007 | 0.0065 | 0.0267 | 0.0668 | 0.1201 | 0.1685 | 0.1927 | 0.1841 | 0.1484 |
| | 8 | 0.0000 | 0.0001 | 0.0014 | 0.0084 | 0.0279 | 0.0644 | 0.1134 | 0.1606 | 0.1883 | 0.1855 |
| | 9 | 0.0000 | 0.0000 | 0.0003 | 0.0021 | 0.0093 | 0.0276 | 0.0611 | 0.1070 | 0.1540 | 0.1855 |
| | 10 | 0.0000 | 0.0000 | 0.0000 | 0.0004 | 0.0025 | 0.0095 | 0.0263 | 0.0571 | 0.1008 | 0.1484 |
| | 11 | 0.0000 | 0.0000 | 0.0000 | 0.0001 | 0.0005 | 0.0026 | 0.0090 | 0.0242 | 0.0525 | 0.0944 |
| | 12 | 0.0000 | 0.0000 | 0.0000 | 0.0000 | 0.0001 | 0.0006 | 0.0024 | 0.0081 | 0.0215 | 0.0472 |
| | 13 | 0.0000 | 0.0000 | 0.0000 | 0.0000 | 0.0000 | 0.0001 | 0.0005 | 0.0021 | 0.0068 | 0.0182 |
| | 14 | 0.0000 | 0.0000 | 0.0000 | 0.0000 | 0.0000 | 0.0000 | 0.0001 | 0.0004 | 0.0016 | 0.0052 |
| | 15 | 0.0000 | 0.0000 | 0.0000 | 0.0000 | 0.0000 | 0.0000 | 0.0000 | 0.0001 | 0.0003 | 0.0010 |
| | 16 | 0.0000 | 0.0000 | 0.0000 | 0.0000 | 0.0000 | 0.0000 | 0.0000 | 0.0000 | 0.0000 | 0.0001 |
| | 17 | 0.0000 | 0.0000 | 0.0000 | 0.0000 | 0.0000 | 0.0000 | 0.0000 | 0.0000 | 0.0000 | 0.0000 |
| 18 | 0 | 0.3972 | 0.1501 | 0.0536 | 0.0180 | 0.0056 | 0.0016 | 0.0004 | 0.0001 | 0.0000 | 0.0000 |
| | 1 | 0.3763 | 0.3002 | 0.1704 | 0.0811 | 0.0338 | 0.0126 | 0.0042 | 0.0012 | 0.0003 | 0.0001 |
| | 2 | 0.1683 | 0.2835 | 0.2556 | 0.1723 | 0.0958 | 0.0458 | 0.0190 | 0.0069 | 0.0022 | 0.0006 |
| | 3 | 0.0473 | 0.1680 | 0.2406 | 0.2297 | 0.1704 | 0.1046 | 0.0547 | 0.0246 | 0.0095 | 0.0031 |
| | 4 | 0.0093 | 0.0700 | 0.1592 | 0.2153 | 0.2130 | 0.1681 | 0.1104 | 0.0614 | 0.0291 | 0.0117 |
| | 5 | 0.0014 | 0.0218 | 0.0787 | 0.1507 | 0.1988 | 0.2017 | 0.1664 | 0.1146 | 0.0666 | 0.0327 |
| | 6 | 0.0002 | 0.0052 | 0.0301 | 0.0816 | 0.1436 | 0.1873 | 0.1941 | 0.1655 | 0.1181 | 0.0708 |
| | 7 | 0.0000 | 0.0010 | 0.0091 | 0.0350 | 0.0820 | 0.1376 | 0.1792 | 0.1892 | 0.1657 | 0.1214 |
| | 8 | 0.0000 | 0.0002 | 0.0022 | 0.0120 | 0.0376 | 0.0811 | 0.1327 | 0.1734 | 0.1864 | 0.1669 |
| | 9 | 0.0000 | 0.0000 | 0.0004 | 0.0033 | 0.0139 | 0.0386 | 0.0794 | 0.1284 | 0.1694 | 0.1855 |
| | 10 | 0.0000 | 0.0000 | 0.0001 | 0.0008 | 0.0042 | 0.0149 | 0.0385 | 0.0771 | 0.1248 | 0.1669 |
| | 11 | 0.0000 | 0.0000 | 0.0000 | 0.0001 | 0.0010 | 0.0046 | 0.0151 | 0.0374 | 0.0742 | 0.1214 |
| | 12 | 0.0000 | 0.0000 | 0.0000 | 0.0000 | 0.0002 | 0.0012 | 0.0047 | 0.0145 | 0.0354 | 0.0708 |
| | 13 | 0.0000 | 0.0000 | 0.0000 | 0.0000 | 0.0000 | 0.0002 | 0.0012 | 0.0045 | 0.0134 | 0.0327 |
| | 14 | 0.0000 | 0.0000 | 0.0000 | 0.0000 | 0.0000 | 0.0000 | 0.0002 | 0.0011 | 0.0039 | 0.0117 |
| | 15 | 0.0000 | 0.0000 | 0.0000 | 0.0000 | 0.0000 | 0.0000 | 0.0000 | 0.0002 | 0.0009 | 0.0031 |
| | 16 | 0.0000 | 0.0000 | 0.0000 | 0.0000 | 0.0000 | 0.0000 | 0.0000 | 0.0000 | 0.0001 | 0.0006 |
| | 17 | 0.0000 | 0.0000 | 0.0000 | 0.0000 | 0.0000 | 0.0000 | 0.0000 | 0.0000 | 0.0000 | 0.0001 |
| | 18 | 0.0000 | 0.0000 | 0.0000 | 0.0000 | 0.0000 | 0.0000 | 0.0000 | 0.0000 | 0.0000 | 0.0000 |

(continued)

**Chart 1** (continued)

| n | x | θ | | | | | | | | | |
|---|---|------|-----|------|-----|------|-----|------|-----|------|-----|
| | | 0.05 | 0.1 | 0.15 | 0.2 | 0.25 | 0.3 | 0.35 | 0.4 | 0.45 | 0.5 |
| 19 | 0 | 0.3774 | 0.1351 | 0.0456 | 0.0144 | 0.0042 | 0.0011 | 0.0003 | 0.0001 | 0.0000 | 0.0000 |
| | 1 | 0.3774 | 0.2852 | 0.1529 | 0.0685 | 0.0268 | 0.0093 | 0.0029 | 0.0008 | 0.0002 | 0.0000 |
| | 2 | 0.1787 | 0.2852 | 0.2428 | 0.1540 | 0.0803 | 0.0358 | 0.0138 | 0.0046 | 0.0013 | 0.0003 |
| | 3 | 0.0533 | 0.1796 | 0.2428 | 0.2182 | 0.1517 | 0.0869 | 0.0422 | 0.0175 | 0.0062 | 0.0018 |
| | 4 | 0.0112 | 0.0798 | 0.1714 | 0.2182 | 0.2023 | 0.1491 | 0.0909 | 0.0467 | 0.0203 | 0.0074 |
| | 5 | 0.0018 | 0.0266 | 0.0907 | 0.1636 | 0.2023 | 0.1916 | 0.1468 | 0.0933 | 0.0497 | 0.0222 |
| | 6 | 0.0002 | 0.0069 | 0.0374 | 0.0955 | 0.1574 | 0.1916 | 0.1844 | 0.1451 | 0.0949 | 0.0518 |
| | 7 | 0.0000 | 0.0014 | 0.0122 | 0.0443 | 0.0974 | 0.1525 | 0.1844 | 0.1797 | 0.1443 | 0.0961 |
| | 8 | 0.0000 | 0.0002 | 0.0032 | 0.0166 | 0.0487 | 0.0981 | 0.1489 | 0.1797 | 0.1771 | 0.1442 |
| | 9 | 0.0000 | 0.0000 | 0.0007 | 0.0051 | 0.0198 | 0.0514 | 0.0980 | 0.1464 | 0.1771 | 0.1762 |
| | 10 | 0.0000 | 0.0000 | 0.0001 | 0.0013 | 0.0066 | 0.0220 | 0.0528 | 0.0976 | 0.1449 | 0.1762 |
| | 11 | 0.0000 | 0.0000 | 0.0000 | 0.0003 | 0.0018 | 0.0077 | 0.0233 | 0.0532 | 0.0970 | 0.1442 |
| | 12 | 0.0000 | 0.0000 | 0.0000 | 0.0000 | 0.0004 | 0.0022 | 0.0083 | 0.0237 | 0.0529 | 0.0961 |
| | 13 | 0.0000 | 0.0000 | 0.0000 | 0.0000 | 0.0001 | 0.0005 | 0.0024 | 0.0085 | 0.0233 | 0.0518 |
| | 14 | 0.0000 | 0.0000 | 0.0000 | 0.0000 | 0.0000 | 0.0001 | 0.0006 | 0.0024 | 0.0082 | 0.0222 |
| | 15 | 0.0000 | 0.0000 | 0.0000 | 0.0000 | 0.0000 | 0.0000 | 0.0001 | 0.0005 | 0.0022 | 0.0074 |
| | 16 | 0.0000 | 0.0000 | 0.0000 | 0.0000 | 0.0000 | 0.0000 | 0.0000 | 0.0001 | 0.0005 | 0.0018 |
| | 17 | 0.0000 | 0.0000 | 0.0000 | 0.0000 | 0.0000 | 0.0000 | 0.0000 | 0.0000 | 0.0001 | 0.0003 |
| | 18 | 0.0000 | 0.0000 | 0.0000 | 0.0000 | 0.0000 | 0.0000 | 0.0000 | 0.0000 | 0.0000 | 0.0000 |
| | 19 | 0.0000 | 0.0000 | 0.0000 | 0.0000 | 0.0000 | 0.0000 | 0.0000 | 0.0000 | 0.0000 | 0.0000 |
| 20 | 0 | 0.3585 | 0.1216 | 0.0388 | 0.0115 | 0.0032 | 0.0008 | 0.0002 | 0.0000 | 0.0000 | 0.0000 |
| | 1 | 0.3774 | 0.2702 | 0.1368 | 0.0576 | 0.0211 | 0.0068 | 0.0020 | 0.0005 | 0.0001 | 0.0000 |
| | 2 | 0.1887 | 0.2852 | 0.2293 | 0.1369 | 0.0669 | 0.0278 | 0.0100 | 0.0031 | 0.0008 | 0.0002 |
| | 3 | 0.0596 | 0.1901 | 0.2428 | 0.2054 | 0.1339 | 0.0716 | 0.0323 | 0.0123 | 0.0040 | 0.0011 |
| | 4 | 0.0133 | 0.0898 | 0.1821 | 0.2182 | 0.1897 | 0.1304 | 0.0738 | 0.0350 | 0.0139 | 0.0046 |
| | 5 | 0.0022 | 0.0319 | 0.1028 | 0.1746 | 0.2023 | 0.1789 | 0.1272 | 0.0746 | 0.0365 | 0.0148 |
| | 6 | 0.0003 | 0.0089 | 0.0454 | 0.1091 | 0.1686 | 0.1916 | 0.1712 | 0.1244 | 0.0746 | 0.0370 |
| | 7 | 0.0000 | 0.0020 | 0.0160 | 0.0545 | 0.1124 | 0.1643 | 0.1844 | 0.1659 | 0.1221 | 0.0739 |
| | 8 | 0.0000 | 0.0004 | 0.0046 | 0.0222 | 0.0609 | 0.1144 | 0.1614 | 0.1797 | 0.1623 | 0.1201 |
| | 9 | 0.0000 | 0.0001 | 0.0011 | 0.0074 | 0.0271 | 0.0654 | 0.1158 | 0.1597 | 0.1771 | 0.1602 |
| | 10 | 0.0000 | 0.0000 | 0.0002 | 0.0020 | 0.0099 | 0.0308 | 0.0686 | 0.1171 | 0.1593 | 0.1762 |
| | 11 | 0.0000 | 0.0000 | 0.0000 | 0.0005 | 0.0030 | 0.0120 | 0.0336 | 0.0710 | 0.1185 | 0.1602 |
| | 12 | 0.0000 | 0.0000 | 0.0000 | 0.0001 | 0.0008 | 0.0039 | 0.0136 | 0.0355 | 0.0727 | 0.1201 |
| | 13 | 0.0000 | 0.0000 | 0.0000 | 0.0000 | 0.0002 | 0.0010 | 0.0045 | 0.0146 | 0.0366 | 0.0739 |
| | 14 | 0.0000 | 0.0000 | 0.0000 | 0.0000 | 0.0000 | 0.0002 | 0.0012 | 0.0049 | 0.0150 | 0.0370 |
| | 15 | 0.0000 | 0.0000 | 0.0000 | 0.0000 | 0.0000 | 0.0000 | 0.0003 | 0.0013 | 0.0049 | 0.0148 |
| | 16 | 0.0000 | 0.0000 | 0.0000 | 0.0000 | 0.0000 | 0.0000 | 0.0000 | 0.0003 | 0.0013 | 0.0046 |
| | 17 | 0.0000 | 0.0000 | 0.0000 | 0.0000 | 0.0000 | 0.0000 | 0.0000 | 0.0000 | 0.0002 | 0.0011 |
| | 18 | 0.0000 | 0.0000 | 0.0000 | 0.0000 | 0.0000 | 0.0000 | 0.0000 | 0.0000 | 0.0000 | 0.0002 |
| | 19 | 0.0000 | 0.0000 | 0.0000 | 0.0000 | 0.0000 | 0.0000 | 0.0000 | 0.0000 | 0.0000 | 0.0000 |
| | 20 | 0.0000 | 0.0000 | 0.0000 | 0.0000 | 0.0000 | 0.0000 | 0.0000 | 0.0000 | 0.0000 | 0.0000 |

**Chart 2** A chart of probabilities Prob($Z \leq z$) for the standard normal random variable $Z$ and negative $z$ values

| z | 0.00 | 0.01 | 0.02 | 0.03 | 0.04 | 0.05 | 0.06 | 0.07 | 0.08 | 0.09 |
|---|------|------|------|------|------|------|------|------|------|------|
| −3.4 | 0.0003 | 0.0003 | 0.0003 | 0.0003 | 0.0003 | 0.0003 | 0.0003 | 0.0003 | 0.0003 | 0.0002 |
| −3.3 | 0.0005 | 0.0005 | 0.0005 | 0.0004 | 0.0004 | 0.0004 | 0.0004 | 0.0004 | 0.0004 | 0.0003 |
| −3.2 | 0.0007 | 0.0007 | 0.0006 | 0.0006 | 0.0006 | 0.0006 | 0.0006 | 0.0005 | 0.0005 | 0.0005 |
| −3.1 | 0.0010 | 0.0009 | 0.0009 | 0.0009 | 0.0008 | 0.0008 | 0.0008 | 0.0008 | 0.0007 | 0.0007 |
| −3.0 | 0.0013 | 0.0013 | 0.0013 | 0.0012 | 0.0012 | 0.0011 | 0.0011 | 0.0011 | 0.0010 | 0.0010 |
| −2.9 | 0.0019 | 0.0018 | 0.0018 | 0.0017 | 0.0016 | 0.0016 | 0.0015 | 0.0015 | 0.0014 | 0.0014 |
| −2.8 | 0.0026 | 0.0025 | 0.0024 | 0.0023 | 0.0023 | 0.0022 | 0.0021 | 0.0021 | 0.0020 | 0.0019 |
| −2.7 | 0.0035 | 0.0034 | 0.0033 | 0.0032 | 0.0031 | 0.0030 | 0.0029 | 0.0028 | 0.0027 | 0.0026 |
| −2.6 | 0.0047 | 0.0045 | 0.0044 | 0.0043 | 0.0041 | 0.0040 | 0.0039 | 0.0038 | 0.0037 | 0.0036 |
| −2.5 | 0.0062 | 0.0060 | 0.0059 | 0.0057 | 0.0055 | 0.0054 | 0.0052 | 0.0051 | 0.0049 | 0.0048 |
| −2.4 | 0.0082 | 0.0080 | 0.0078 | 0.0075 | 0.0073 | 0.0071 | 0.0069 | 0.0068 | 0.0066 | 0.0064 |
| −2.3 | 0.0107 | 0.0104 | 0.0102 | 0.0099 | 0.0096 | 0.0094 | 0.0091 | 0.0089 | 0.0087 | 0.0084 |
| −2.2 | 0.0139 | 0.0136 | 0.0132 | 0.0129 | 0.0125 | 0.0122 | 0.0119 | 0.0116 | 0.0113 | 0.0110 |
| −2.1 | 0.0179 | 0.0174 | 0.0170 | 0.0166 | 0.0162 | 0.0158 | 0.0154 | 0.0150 | 0.0146 | 0.0143 |
| −2.0 | 0.0228 | 0.0222 | 0.0217 | 0.0212 | 0.0207 | 0.0202 | 0.0197 | 0.0192 | 0.0188 | 0.0183 |
| −1.9 | 0.0287 | 0.0281 | 0.0274 | 0.0268 | 0.0262 | 0.0256 | 0.0250 | 0.0244 | 0.0239 | 0.0233 |
| −1.8 | 0.0359 | 0.0351 | 0.0344 | 0.0336 | 0.0329 | 0.0322 | 0.0314 | 0.0307 | 0.0301 | 0.0294 |
| −1.7 | 0.0446 | 0.0436 | 0.0427 | 0.0418 | 0.0409 | 0.0401 | 0.0392 | 0.0384 | 0.0375 | 0.0367 |
| −1.6 | 0.0548 | 0.0537 | 0.0526 | 0.0516 | 0.0505 | 0.0495 | 0.0485 | 0.0475 | 0.0465 | 0.0455 |
| −1.5 | 0.0668 | 0.0655 | 0.0643 | 0.0630 | 0.0618 | 0.0606 | 0.0594 | 0.0582 | 0.0571 | 0.0559 |
| −1.4 | 0.0808 | 0.0793 | 0.0778 | 0.0764 | 0.0749 | 0.0735 | 0.0721 | 0.0708 | 0.0694 | 0.0681 |
| −1.3 | 0.0968 | 0.0951 | 0.0934 | 0.0918 | 0.0901 | 0.0885 | 0.0869 | 0.0853 | 0.0838 | 0.0823 |
| −1.2 | 0.1151 | 0.1131 | 0.1112 | 0.1093 | 0.1075 | 0.1056 | 0.1038 | 0.1020 | 0.1003 | 0.0985 |
| −1.1 | 0.1357 | 0.1335 | 0.1314 | 0.1292 | 0.1271 | 0.1251 | 0.1230 | 0.1210 | 0.1190 | 0.1170 |
| −1.0 | 0.1587 | 0.1562 | 0.1539 | 0.1515 | 0.1492 | 0.1469 | 0.1446 | 0.1423 | 0.1401 | 0.1379 |
| −0.9 | 0.1841 | 0.1814 | 0.1788 | 0.1762 | 0.1736 | 0.1711 | 0.1685 | 0.1660 | 0.1635 | 0.1611 |
| −0.8 | 0.2119 | 0.2090 | 0.2061 | 0.2033 | 0.2005 | 0.1977 | 0.1949 | 0.1922 | 0.1894 | 0.1867 |
| −0.7 | 0.2420 | 0.2389 | 0.2358 | 0.2327 | 0.2296 | 0.2266 | 0.2236 | 0.2206 | 0.2177 | 0.2148 |
| −0.6 | 0.2743 | 0.2709 | 0.2676 | 0.2643 | 0.2611 | 0.2578 | 0.2546 | 0.2514 | 0.2483 | 0.2451 |
| −0.5 | 0.3085 | 0.3050 | 0.3015 | 0.2981 | 0.2946 | 0.2912 | 0.2877 | 0.2843 | 0.2810 | 0.2776 |
| −0.4 | 0.3446 | 0.3409 | 0.3372 | 0.3336 | 0.3300 | 0.3264 | 0.3228 | 0.3192 | 0.3156 | 0.3121 |
| −0.3 | 0.3821 | 0.3783 | 0.3745 | 0.3707 | 0.3669 | 0.3632 | 0.3594 | 0.3557 | 0.3520 | 0.3483 |
| −0.2 | 0.4207 | 0.4168 | 0.4129 | 0.4090 | 0.4052 | 0.4013 | 0.3974 | 0.3936 | 0.3897 | 0.3859 |
| −0.1 | 0.4602 | 0.4562 | 0.4522 | 0.4483 | 0.4443 | 0.4404 | 0.4364 | 0.4325 | 0.4286 | 0.4247 |
| 0.0 | 0.5000 | 0.4960 | 0.4920 | 0.4880 | 0.4840 | 0.4801 | 0.4761 | 0.4721 | 0.4681 | 0.4641 |

**Chart 3** A chart of probabilities Prob($Z \leq z$) for the standard normal random variable $Z$ and positive $z$ values

| z | 0.00 | 0.01 | 0.02 | 0.03 | 0.04 | 0.05 | 0.06 | 0.07 | 0.08 | 0.09 |
|---|------|------|------|------|------|------|------|------|------|------|
| 0.0 | 0.5000 | 0.5040 | 0.5080 | 0.5120 | 0.5160 | 0.5199 | 0.5239 | 0.5279 | 0.5319 | 0.5359 |
| 0.1 | 0.5398 | 0.5438 | 0.5478 | 0.5517 | 0.5557 | 0.5596 | 0.5636 | 0.5675 | 0.5714 | 0.5753 |
| 0.2 | 0.5793 | 0.5832 | 0.5871 | 0.5910 | 0.5948 | 0.5987 | 0.6026 | 0.6064 | 0.6103 | 0.6141 |
| 0.3 | 0.6179 | 0.6217 | 0.6255 | 0.6293 | 0.6331 | 0.6368 | 0.6406 | 0.6443 | 0.6480 | 0.6517 |
| 0.4 | 0.6554 | 0.6591 | 0.6628 | 0.6664 | 0.6700 | 0.6736 | 0.6772 | 0.6808 | 0.6844 | 0.6879 |
| 0.5 | 0.6915 | 0.6950 | 0.6985 | 0.7019 | 0.7054 | 0.7088 | 0.7123 | 0.7157 | 0.7190 | 0.7224 |
| 0.6 | 0.7257 | 0.7291 | 0.7324 | 0.7357 | 0.7389 | 0.7422 | 0.7454 | 0.7486 | 0.7517 | 0.7549 |
| 0.7 | 0.7580 | 0.7611 | 0.7642 | 0.7673 | 0.7704 | 0.7734 | 0.7764 | 0.7794 | 0.7823 | 0.7852 |
| 0.8 | 0.7881 | 0.7910 | 0.7939 | 0.7967 | 0.7995 | 0.8023 | 0.8051 | 0.8078 | 0.8106 | 0.8133 |
| 0.9 | 0.8159 | 0.8186 | 0.8212 | 0.8238 | 0.8264 | 0.8289 | 0.8315 | 0.8340 | 0.8365 | 0.8389 |
| 1.0 | 0.8413 | 0.8438 | 0.8461 | 0.8485 | 0.8508 | 0.8531 | 0.8554 | 0.8577 | 0.8599 | 0.8621 |
| 1.1 | 0.8643 | 0.8665 | 0.8686 | 0.8708 | 0.8729 | 0.8749 | 0.8770 | 0.8790 | 0.8810 | 0.8830 |
| 1.2 | 0.8849 | 0.8869 | 0.8888 | 0.8907 | 0.8925 | 0.8944 | 0.8962 | 0.8980 | 0.8997 | 0.9015 |
| 1.3 | 0.9032 | 0.9049 | 0.9066 | 0.9082 | 0.9099 | 0.9115 | 0.9131 | 0.9147 | 0.9162 | 0.9177 |
| 1.4 | 0.9192 | 0.9207 | 0.9222 | 0.9236 | 0.9251 | 0.9265 | 0.9279 | 0.9292 | 0.9306 | 0.9319 |
| 1.5 | 0.9332 | 0.9345 | 0.9357 | 0.9370 | 0.9382 | 0.9394 | 0.9406 | 0.9418 | 0.9429 | 0.9441 |
| 1.6 | 0.9452 | 0.9463 | 0.9474 | 0.9484 | 0.9495 | 0.9505 | 0.9515 | 0.9525 | 0.9535 | 0.9545 |
| 1.7 | 0.9554 | 0.9564 | 0.9573 | 0.9582 | 0.9591 | 0.9599 | 0.9608 | 0.9616 | 0.9625 | 0.9633 |
| 1.8 | 0.9641 | 0.9649 | 0.9656 | 0.9664 | 0.9671 | 0.9678 | 0.9686 | 0.9693 | 0.9699 | 0.9706 |
| 1.9 | 0.9713 | 0.9719 | 0.9726 | 0.9732 | 0.9738 | 0.9744 | 0.9750 | 0.9756 | 0.9761 | 0.9767 |
| 2.0 | 0.9772 | 0.9778 | 0.9783 | 0.9788 | 0.9793 | 0.9798 | 0.9803 | 0.9808 | 0.9812 | 0.9817 |
| 2.1 | 0.9821 | 0.9826 | 0.9830 | 0.9834 | 0.9838 | 0.9842 | 0.9846 | 0.9850 | 0.9854 | 0.9857 |
| 2.2 | 0.9861 | 0.9864 | 0.9868 | 0.9871 | 0.9875 | 0.9878 | 0.9881 | 0.9884 | 0.9887 | 0.9890 |
| 2.3 | 0.9893 | 0.9896 | 0.9898 | 0.9901 | 0.9904 | 0.9906 | 0.9909 | 0.9911 | 0.9913 | 0.9916 |
| 2.4 | 0.9918 | 0.9920 | 0.9922 | 0.9925 | 0.9927 | 0.9929 | 0.9931 | 0.9932 | 0.9934 | 0.9936 |
| 2.5 | 0.9938 | 0.9940 | 0.9941 | 0.9943 | 0.9945 | 0.9946 | 0.9948 | 0.9949 | 0.9951 | 0.9952 |
| 2.6 | 0.9953 | 0.9955 | 0.9956 | 0.9957 | 0.9959 | 0.9960 | 0.9961 | 0.9962 | 0.9963 | 0.9964 |
| 2.7 | 0.9965 | 0.9966 | 0.9967 | 0.9968 | 0.9969 | 0.9970 | 0.9971 | 0.9972 | 0.9973 | 0.9974 |
| 2.8 | 0.9974 | 0.9975 | 0.9976 | 0.9977 | 0.9977 | 0.9978 | 0.9979 | 0.9979 | 0.9980 | 0.9981 |
| 2.9 | 0.9981 | 0.9982 | 0.9982 | 0.9983 | 0.9984 | 0.9984 | 0.9985 | 0.9985 | 0.9986 | 0.9986 |
| 3.0 | 0.9987 | 0.9987 | 0.9987 | 0.9988 | 0.9988 | 0.9989 | 0.9989 | 0.9989 | 0.9990 | 0.9990 |
| 3.1 | 0.9990 | 0.9991 | 0.9991 | 0.9991 | 0.9992 | 0.9992 | 0.9992 | 0.9992 | 0.9993 | 0.9993 |
| 3.2 | 0.9993 | 0.9993 | 0.9994 | 0.9994 | 0.9994 | 0.9994 | 0.9994 | 0.9995 | 0.9995 | 0.9995 |
| 3.3 | 0.9995 | 0.9995 | 0.9995 | 0.9996 | 0.9996 | 0.9996 | 0.9996 | 0.9996 | 0.9996 | 0.9997 |
| 3.4 | 0.9997 | 0.9997 | 0.9997 | 0.9997 | 0.9997 | 0.9997 | 0.9997 | 0.9997 | 0.9997 | 0.9998 |

**Chart 4** A chart of critical points for a one-sided up $t$ test for a given number of degrees of freedom (df) and chosen $\alpha$ level

| df | $\alpha = 0.10$ | $\alpha = 0.05$ | $\alpha = 0.025$ | $\alpha = 0.01$ | $\alpha = 0.005$ | $\alpha = 0.001$ | $\alpha = 0.0005$ |
|---|---|---|---|---|---|---|---|
| 1 | 3.078 | 6.314 | 12.706 | 31.821 | 63.657 | 318.309 | 636.619 |
| 2 | 1.886 | 2.920 | 4.303 | 6.965 | 9.925 | 22.327 | 31.599 |
| 3 | 1.638 | 2.353 | 3.182 | 4.541 | 5.841 | 10.215 | 12.924 |
| 4 | 1.533 | 2.132 | 2.776 | 3.747 | 4.604 | 7.173 | 8.610 |
| 5 | 1.476 | 2.015 | 2.571 | 3.365 | 4.032 | 5.893 | 6.869 |
| 6 | 1.440 | 1.943 | 2.447 | 3.143 | 3.707 | 5.208 | 5.959 |
| 7 | 1.415 | 1.895 | 2.365 | 2.998 | 3.499 | 4.785 | 5.408 |
| 8 | 1.397 | 1.860 | 2.306 | 2.896 | 3.355 | 4.501 | 5.041 |
| 9 | 1.383 | 1.833 | 2.262 | 2.821 | 3.250 | 4.297 | 4.781 |
| 10 | 1.372 | 1.812 | 2.228 | 2.764 | 3.169 | 4.144 | 4.587 |
| 11 | 1.363 | 1.796 | 2.201 | 2.718 | 3.106 | 4.025 | 4.437 |
| 12 | 1.356 | 1.782 | 2.179 | 2.681 | 3.055 | 3.930 | 4.318 |
| 13 | 1.350 | 1.771 | 2.160 | 2.650 | 3.012 | 3.852 | 4.221 |
| 14 | 1.345 | 1.761 | 2.145 | 2.624 | 2.977 | 3.787 | 4.140 |
| 15 | 1.341 | 1.753 | 2.131 | 2.602 | 2.947 | 3.733 | 4.073 |
| 16 | 1.337 | 1.746 | 2.120 | 2.583 | 2.921 | 3.686 | 4.015 |
| 17 | 1.333 | 1.740 | 2.110 | 2.567 | 2.898 | 3.646 | 3.965 |
| 18 | 1.330 | 1.734 | 2.101 | 2.552 | 2.878 | 3.610 | 3.922 |
| 19 | 1.328 | 1.729 | 2.093 | 2.539 | 2.861 | 3.579 | 3.883 |
| 20 | 1.325 | 1.725 | 2.086 | 2.528 | 2.845 | 3.552 | 3.850 |
| 21 | 1.323 | 1.721 | 2.080 | 2.518 | 2.831 | 3.527 | 3.819 |
| 22 | 1.321 | 1.717 | 2.074 | 2.508 | 2.819 | 3.505 | 3.792 |
| 23 | 1.319 | 1.714 | 2.069 | 2.500 | 2.807 | 3.485 | 3.768 |
| 24 | 1.318 | 1.711 | 2.064 | 2.492 | 2.797 | 3.467 | 3.745 |
| 25 | 1.316 | 1.708 | 2.060 | 2.485 | 2.787 | 3.450 | 3.725 |
| 26 | 1.315 | 1.706 | 2.056 | 2.479 | 2.779 | 3.435 | 3.707 |
| 27 | 1.314 | 1.703 | 2.052 | 2.473 | 2.771 | 3.421 | 3.690 |
| 28 | 1.313 | 1.701 | 2.048 | 2.467 | 2.763 | 3.408 | 3.674 |
| 29 | 1.311 | 1.699 | 2.045 | 2.462 | 2.756 | 3.396 | 3.659 |
| 30 | 1.310 | 1.697 | 2.042 | 2.457 | 2.750 | 3.385 | 3.646 |
| 40 | 1.303 | 1.684 | 2.021 | 2.423 | 2.704 | 3.307 | 3.551 |
| 60 | 1.296 | 1.671 | 2.000 | 2.390 | 2.660 | 3.232 | 3.460 |
| 120 | 1.289 | 1.658 | 1.980 | 2.358 | 2.617 | 3.160 | 3.373 |
| Inf | 1.282 | 1.645 | 1.960 | 2.326 | 2.576 | 3.090 | 3.291 |

**Chart 5** A chart of critical points for a chi-square test for a given number of degrees of freedom (df) and chosen $\alpha$ level

| df | $\alpha = 0.10$ | $\alpha = 0.05$ | $\alpha = 0.025$ | $\alpha = 0.01$ | $\alpha = 0.005$ | $\alpha = 0.001$ | $\alpha = 0.0005$ | $\alpha = 0.0001$ |
|---|---|---|---|---|---|---|---|---|
| 1 | 2.7055 | 3.8415 | 5.0239 | 6.6349 | 7.8794 | 10.8276 | 12.1157 | 15.1367 |
| 2 | 4.6052 | 5.9915 | 7.3778 | 9.2103 | 10.5966 | 13.8155 | 15.2018 | 18.4207 |
| 3 | 6.2514 | 7.8147 | 9.3484 | 11.3449 | 12.8382 | 16.2662 | 17.7300 | 21.1075 |

(continued)

**Chart 5** (continued)

| df | $\alpha = 0.10$ | $\alpha = 0.05$ | $\alpha = 0.025$ | $\alpha = 0.01$ | $\alpha = 0.005$ | $\alpha = 0.001$ | $\alpha = 0.0005$ | $\alpha = 0.0001$ |
|-----|-----|-----|-----|-----|-----|-----|-----|-----|
| 4 | 7.7794 | 9.4877 | 11.1433 | 13.2767 | 14.8603 | 18.4668 | 19.9974 | 23.5127 |
| 5 | 9.2364 | 11.0705 | 12.8325 | 15.0863 | 16.7496 | 20.5150 | 22.1053 | 25.7448 |
| 6 | 10.6446 | 12.5916 | 14.4494 | 16.8119 | 18.5476 | 22.4577 | 24.1028 | 27.8563 |
| 7 | 12.0170 | 14.0671 | 16.0128 | 18.4753 | 20.2777 | 24.3219 | 26.0178 | 29.8775 |
| 8 | 13.3616 | 15.5073 | 17.5345 | 20.0902 | 21.9550 | 26.1245 | 27.8680 | 31.8276 |
| 9 | 14.6837 | 16.9190 | 19.0228 | 21.6660 | 23.5894 | 27.8772 | 29.6658 | 33.7199 |
| 10 | 15.9872 | 18.3070 | 20.4832 | 23.2093 | 25.1882 | 29.5883 | 31.4198 | 35.5640 |
| 11 | 17.2750 | 19.6751 | 21.9200 | 24.7250 | 26.7568 | 31.2641 | 33.1366 | 37.3670 |
| 12 | 18.5493 | 21.0261 | 23.3367 | 26.2170 | 28.2995 | 32.9095 | 34.8213 | 39.1344 |
| 13 | 19.8119 | 22.3620 | 24.7356 | 27.6882 | 29.8195 | 34.5282 | 36.4778 | 40.8707 |
| 14 | 21.0641 | 23.6848 | 26.1189 | 29.1412 | 31.3193 | 36.1233 | 38.1094 | 42.5793 |
| 15 | 22.3071 | 24.9958 | 27.4884 | 30.5779 | 32.8013 | 37.6973 | 39.7188 | 44.2632 |
| 16 | 23.5418 | 26.2962 | 28.8454 | 31.9999 | 34.2672 | 39.2524 | 41.3081 | 45.9249 |
| 17 | 24.7690 | 27.5871 | 30.1910 | 33.4087 | 35.7185 | 40.7902 | 42.8792 | 47.5664 |
| 18 | 25.9894 | 28.8693 | 31.5264 | 34.8053 | 37.1565 | 42.3124 | 44.4338 | 49.1894 |
| 19 | 27.2036 | 30.1435 | 32.8523 | 36.1909 | 38.5823 | 43.8202 | 45.9731 | 50.7955 |
| 20 | 28.4120 | 31.4104 | 34.1696 | 37.5662 | 39.9968 | 45.3147 | 47.4985 | 52.3860 |
| 21 | 29.6151 | 32.6706 | 35.4789 | 38.9322 | 41.4011 | 46.7970 | 49.0108 | 53.9620 |
| 22 | 30.8133 | 33.9244 | 36.7807 | 40.2894 | 42.7957 | 48.2679 | 50.5111 | 55.5246 |
| 23 | 32.0069 | 35.1725 | 38.0756 | 41.6384 | 44.1813 | 49.7282 | 52.0002 | 57.0746 |
| 24 | 33.1962 | 36.4150 | 39.3641 | 42.9798 | 45.5585 | 51.1786 | 53.4788 | 58.6130 |
| 25 | 34.3816 | 37.6525 | 40.6465 | 44.3141 | 46.9279 | 52.6197 | 54.9475 | 60.1403 |
| 26 | 35.5632 | 38.8851 | 41.9232 | 45.6417 | 48.2899 | 54.0520 | 56.4069 | 61.6573 |
| 27 | 36.7412 | 40.1133 | 43.1945 | 46.9629 | 49.6449 | 55.4760 | 57.8576 | 63.1645 |
| 28 | 37.9159 | 41.3371 | 44.4608 | 48.2782 | 50.9934 | 56.8923 | 59.3000 | 64.6624 |
| 29 | 39.0875 | 42.5570 | 45.7223 | 49.5879 | 52.3356 | 58.3012 | 60.7346 | 66.1517 |
| 30 | 40.2560 | 43.7730 | 46.9792 | 50.8922 | 53.6720 | 59.7031 | 62.1619 | 67.6326 |
| 31 | 41.4217 | 44.9853 | 48.2319 | 52.1914 | 55.0027 | 61.0983 | 63.5820 | 69.1057 |
| 32 | 42.5847 | 46.1943 | 49.4804 | 53.4858 | 56.3281 | 62.4872 | 64.9955 | 70.5712 |
| 33 | 43.7452 | 47.3999 | 50.7251 | 54.7755 | 57.6484 | 63.8701 | 66.4025 | 72.0296 |
| 34 | 44.9032 | 48.6024 | 51.9660 | 56.0609 | 58.9639 | 65.2472 | 67.8035 | 73.4812 |
| 35 | 46.0588 | 49.8018 | 53.2033 | 57.3421 | 60.2748 | 66.6188 | 69.1986 | 74.9262 |
| 36 | 47.2122 | 50.9985 | 54.4373 | 58.6192 | 61.5812 | 67.9852 | 70.5881 | 76.3650 |
| 37 | 48.3634 | 52.1923 | 55.6680 | 59.8925 | 62.8833 | 69.3465 | 71.9722 | 77.7977 |
| 38 | 49.5126 | 53.3835 | 56.8955 | 61.1621 | 64.1814 | 70.7029 | 73.3512 | 79.2247 |
| 39 | 50.6598 | 54.5722 | 58.1201 | 62.4281 | 65.4756 | 72.0547 | 74.7253 | 80.6462 |
| 40 | 51.8051 | 55.7585 | 59.3417 | 63.6907 | 66.7660 | 73.4020 | 76.0946 | 82.0623 |
| 50 | 63.1671 | 67.5048 | 71.4202 | 76.1539 | 79.4900 | 86.6608 | 89.5605 | 95.9687 |
| 60 | 74.3970 | 79.0819 | 83.2977 | 88.3794 | 91.9517 | 99.6072 | 102.6948 | 109.5029 |
| 70 | 85.5270 | 90.5312 | 95.0232 | 100.4252 | 104.2149 | 112.3169 | 115.5776 | 122.7547 |
| 80 | 96.5782 | 101.8795 | 106.6286 | 112.3288 | 116.3211 | 124.8392 | 128.2613 | 135.7825 |
| 90 | 107.5650 | 113.1453 | 118.1359 | 124.1163 | 128.2989 | 137.2084 | 140.7823 | 148.6273 |
| 100 | 118.4980 | 124.3421 | 129.5612 | 135.8067 | 140.1695 | 149.4493 | 153.1670 | 161.3187 |

# Solutions to Problems

## Chapter 1

**1.1** The answer needed is something like: "The above probability statement shows that if the probability of landing "point up" is 3/4, it is unlikely that it will land "point up" 3082 or more times. Since it did land "point up" 3082 times, we have strong evidence that the probability that it will land "point up" is not 3/4."

**1.2** If that view is correct, it is extremely unlikely to obtain the data value 5202 or a larger one. Therefore we have strong evidence that the view that a newborn is equally likely to be a boy as a girl is incorrect.

**1.3** (a) the weather forecast did not predict rain. (b) he does not have the ace of spades. (c) she has a passport.

## Chapter 2

**2.1** (a) $A^c$ is the event "1, 2, 4 or 5 turns up". (b) $B^c$ is the event "1, 2 or 6 turns up". (c) $A \cup B$ is the event "3, 4, 5 or 6 turns up". (d) $A \cap B$ is the event "3 turns up". $A$ and $B$ are not mutually exclusive: they both occur if 3 turns up.

**2.2** (a) $L \cup O$ is the event that a bird has a long tail, orange beak, or both. (b) $L \cap O$ is the event that a bird has a long tail and an orange beak. (c) $L^C \cap O$ is the event that a bird has a short tail and an orange beak. (d) $L^C \cup O^C$ is the event that a bird has a short tail, a yellow beak, or both.

**2.3** Both $(A \cup B)^c$ and $A^c \cap B^c$ are the event "neither $A$ nor $B$ occurs".

© The Author(s), under exclusive license to Springer Nature Switzerland AG 2023
W. J. Ewens, K. Brumberg, *Introductory Statistics for Data Analysis*,
https://doi.org/10.1007/978-3-031-28189-1

## Chapter 3

**3.1** (a) (i) Prob($A$) = 1/2. (ii) Prob($B$) = 1/3. (iii) Prob($A \cup B$) = 2/3. (iv) Prob($A \cap B$) = 1/6.

(b) Prob($A$) × Prob($B$) = $\frac{1}{2} \times \frac{1}{3} = \frac{1}{6}$. Since this is equal to Prob($A \cap B$), the events $A$ and $B$ are independent.

**3.2** (a) (i) Prob($A$) = $\frac{9}{21}$, (ii) Prob($B$) = $\frac{5}{21}$, (iii) Prob($A \cap B$) = $\frac{3}{21} = \frac{1}{7}$. (iv) Prob($A \cup B$) can be found in two ways. The first of these is to note that the union of $A$ and $B$ is the event that 1, 2, 3 or 5 turns up. Adding the probabilities of these cases we get Prob($A \cup B$) = $\frac{1+2+3+5}{21} = \frac{11}{21}$. The second way is to use Eq. (3.2) to get Prob($A \cup B$) = Prob($A$) + Prob($B$) - Prob($A \cap B$) = $\frac{9+5-3}{21} = \frac{11}{21}$.

(b) Prob($A$) × Prob($B$) = $\frac{9}{21} \times \frac{5}{21} = \frac{45}{441} = \frac{5}{49}$. Since this is not equal to Prob($A \cap B$) calculated in part (a)(iii), the events $A$ and $B$ are not independent.

**3.3** (a) Prob($D$) = $\frac{1}{2}$. (b) Prob($D \cap E$) = $\frac{1}{6}$. (c) Prob($D \cup E$) = $\frac{5}{6}$.

**3.4** (a) The event $A \cup B \cup C$ is the event that a 1, 2, 3, 5 or 6 turns up, and thus has probability $\frac{5}{6}$.

(b) The right-hand side in Eq. (3.10) is $\frac{3+2+2-1-1-1+1}{6} = \frac{5}{6}$. The two calculations agree.

**3.5** (a) The sum will be 2 if and only if a 1 turns up on both rolls. The probability of this is $\frac{1}{6} \times \frac{1}{6} = \frac{1}{36}$.

(b) The sum will be 3 if and only if a 1 turns up on the first roll and a 2 on the second, or if a 2 turns up on the first roll and a 1 on the second. The probability of this is $\frac{1}{6} \times \frac{1}{6} + \frac{1}{6} \times \frac{1}{6} = \frac{2}{36} = \frac{1}{18}$.

(c) The sum will be 4 if and only if a 1 turns up on the first roll and a 3 on the second, or if a 2 turns up both rolls, or if a 3 turns up on the first roll and a 1 on the second. The probability of this is $\frac{1}{6} \times \frac{1}{6} + \frac{1}{6} \times \frac{1}{6} + \frac{1}{6} \times \frac{1}{6} = \frac{3}{36} = \frac{1}{12}$.

**3.6** (a) Prob($C \cap L$) = 0.63 × 0.1 = 0.063. (b) From Eq. (3.2), Prob($C \cup L$) = Prob($C$) + Prob($L$) - Prob($C \cap L$) = 0.63 + 0.1 − 0.063 = 0.667.

**3.7** (a) (i) 0.3 × 0.6 = 0.18. (ii) 0.3 + 0.6 − 0.6 × 0.3 = 0.72, (iii) 0.7 × 0.6 = 0.42, (iv) 0.7 + 0.4 − 0.7 × 0.4 = 0.82.

(b) From Eq. (3.2), Prob($L \cup O$) = Prob($L$) + Prob($O$) − Prob($L \cap O$). Plugging in known values, 0.64 = 0.6 + 0.3 − Prob($L \cap O$), and from this Prob($L \cap O$) = 0.26. This is not equal to Prob($L$) × Prob($O$), which is 0.6 × 0.3 = 0.18, so the two events are not independent.

(c) Prob($L|O$) = $\frac{\text{Prob}(L \cap O)}{\text{Prob}(O)} = \frac{0.26}{0.3} = \frac{13}{15}$. Prob($O|L$) = $\frac{\text{Prob}(L \cap O)}{\text{Prob}(L)} = \frac{0.26}{0.6} = \frac{13}{30}$.

Since Prob($L|O$) $\neq$ Prob($L$) (and similarly Prob($O|L$) $\neq$ Prob($O$)), the two events are not independent.

**3.8** From the hint, Prob($A^c \cap B^c$) = 1 − Prob($A \cup B$). Using Eq. (3.2) on the right hand side for Prob($A \cup B$), we have 1 − Prob($A$) − Prob($B$) + Prob($A \cap B$). From the independence of $A$ and $B$, this is 1 − Prob($A$) − Prob($B$) + Prob($A$) × Prob($B$).

Using algebra and the definition of the complement, this is $\{1 - \mathrm{Prob}(A)\} \times \{1 - \mathrm{Prob}(B)\} = \mathrm{Prob}(A^c) \times \mathrm{Prob}(B^c)$. We have shown $\mathrm{Prob}(A^c \cap B^c) = \mathrm{Prob}(A^c) \times \mathrm{Prob}(B^c)$, which implies that $A^c$ and $B^c$ are independent.

**3.9** (a) Her mammogram is negative. (b) She does not have breast cancer. (c) $\mathrm{Prob}(B|A)$ is the probability that she has breast cancer given that her mammogram is positive. $\mathrm{Prob}(B|A^c)$ is the probability that she has breast cancer given that her mammogram is negative. (d) If these two probabilities are equal the mammogram test is useless.

# Chapter 4

**4.1** Let $X_1$ be the number to turn up on roll 1 and $X_2$ be the number to turn up on roll 2.

As one example, the sum is 9 if and only if (i) $X_1 = 3, X_2 = 6$, or (ii) $X_1 = 4, X_2 = 5$, or (iii) $X_1 = 5, X_2 = 4$, or (iv) $X_1 = 6, X_2 = 3$. The probability of each of these mutually exclusive events is $\frac{1}{6} \times \frac{1}{6} = \frac{1}{36}$, so that $\mathrm{Prob}(X_1 + X_2 = 9)$ is $\frac{4}{36}$.

Continuing in this way, we have:

| Possible values for $T_2$ | 2 | 3 | 4 | 5 | 6 | 7 | 8 | 9 | 10 | 11 | 12 |
|---|---|---|---|---|---|---|---|---|---|---|---|
| Probability | $\frac{1}{36}$ | $\frac{2}{36}$ | $\frac{3}{36}$ | $\frac{4}{36}$ | $\frac{5}{36}$ | $\frac{6}{36}$ | $\frac{5}{36}$ | $\frac{4}{36}$ | $\frac{3}{36}$ | $\frac{2}{36}$ | $\frac{1}{36}$ |

**4.2** From the hint,

| Possible values for $\bar{X}$ | 1 | 1.5 | 2 | 2.5 | 3 | 3.5 | 4 | 4.5 | 5 | 5.5 | 6 |
|---|---|---|---|---|---|---|---|---|---|---|---|
| Probability | $\frac{1}{36}$ | $\frac{2}{36}$ | $\frac{3}{36}$ | $\frac{4}{36}$ | $\frac{5}{36}$ | $\frac{6}{36}$ | $\frac{5}{36}$ | $\frac{4}{36}$ | $\frac{3}{36}$ | $\frac{2}{36}$ | $\frac{1}{36}$ |

**4.3** The probability distribution is

| Possible values | 0 | 1 | 2 |
|---|---|---|---|
| Probabilities | 0.36 | 0.48 | 0.16 |

There are four methods to get this answer (at least). These are:

Method 1: Using direct calculation: To get 0 heads, we need to get a tail and a tail (only one possible ordering). Since the two coin flips are independent, the probability of this is $(1 - 0.4) \times (1 - 0.4) = 0.6^2 = 0.36$. To get exactly 1 head, we need to either get a tail and then a head, or a head and then a tail. The probability of this is $2 \times 0.6 \times 0.4 = 0.48$. To get 2 heads, we need to get a head and then a head. The probability of this is $0.4^2 = 0.16$.

Method 2: Using the binomial formula: $\mathrm{Prob}(0 \text{ heads}) = \binom{2}{0}(0.6)^2(0.4)^0 = 0.36$. $\mathrm{Prob}(1 \text{ head}) = \binom{2}{1}(0.6)^1(0.4)^1 = 0.48$. $\mathrm{Prob}(2 \text{ heads}) = \binom{2}{2}(0.6)^0(0.4)^02 = 0.16$.

Method 3: The binomial chart (Chart 1) with $n = 2$ and $\theta = 0.40$ displays the required probabilities.

Method 4: Using R:

```
dbinom(x = 0, size = 2, prob = 0.4)    # 0 heads
dbinom(x = 1, size = 2, prob = 0.4)    # 1 head
dbinom(x = 2, size = 2, prob = 0.4)    # 2 heads
```

or, we can give dbinom a vector in the x argument and it will return a vector of the corresponding probabilities: dbinom(x = 0:2, size = 2, prob = 0.4).

**4.4** The possible orders are: HHHTT, HHTHT, HHTTH, HTHHT, HTHTH, HTTHH, THHHT, THHTH, THHHT, TTHHH (10 orders). $5! = 5 \times 4 \times 3 \times 2 \times 1 = 120$, $3! = 3 \times 2 \times 1 = 6$, $2! = 2 \times 1 = 2$, so that the required answer is $\binom{5}{3} = \frac{120}{6 \times 2} = 10$. This agrees with the number found by enumeration.

**4.5** The required number is $\binom{7}{3} = \frac{7!}{3! \times 4!} = \frac{5040}{6 \times 24} = 35$.
  In R: choose(n = 7, k = 3).

**4.6** The probability of getting any one specific sequence of heads or tails for a fair coin flipped seven times is $0.5^7 = 0.0078125$. From Problem 4.5 we know there are 35 unique sequences of heads and tails that yield exactly three heads in seven flips. Each has the same probability and the various sequences are all mutually exclusive. Thus the required probability is $35 \times 0.5^7 = 35 \times 0.0078125 = 0.2734375$.

**4.7** The probability of exactly two successes is $\theta^2$ and the probability of exactly one success is $2\theta(1 - \theta)$. Thus $\theta^2 = 2\theta(1 - \theta)$. Since $\theta \neq 0$ we can divide through by $\theta$ to get $\theta = 2(1 - \theta)$. Solving this we get $\theta = \frac{2}{3}$.

**4.8** The six committees are AB, AC, AD, BC, BD, CD.

**4.9** There are 35 committees (from Problem 4.5). These can be found systematically by starting with ABC, then changing the third member in turn to D, E, F, G, then changing the second member to C, D, E, F and G and so on.

**4.10** Choosing the $x$ people on the committee is the same as choosing the $n - x$ people who are not on the committee. Therefore the number of ways of choosing $n - x$ people, namely $\binom{n}{n-x}$, is the same as the number of ways of choosing $x$ people, namely $\binom{n}{x}$.

**4.11** We must reorganize the problem since the binomial chart only lists values of $\theta$ less than or equal to 0.5. Having 7 successes out of 12 trials with probability of success equal to 0.7 can be reframed as having 5 failures out of 12 trials with probability of failure equal to 0.3. The binomial chart shows that the required probability is 0.1585.
  From the binomial distribution formula the required probability is $\binom{12}{7}(0.7)^7$ $(0.3)^5 = 0.15849579....$ Given that the chart is accurate to four decimal places only, the answers agree.

**4.12** (a) From the chart, the required probability is 0.2007 (to four decimal place accuracy).

Using the binomial probability formula, $\text{Prob}(X = 5) = \binom{10}{5}(0.4)^5(0.6)^5 = 252 \times 0.01024 \times 0.07776 \approx 0.2007$.

In R: `dbinom(x = 5, size = 10, prob = 0.4)`.

(b) From the chart, the required probability is $0.2150 + 0.2508 + 0.2007 + 0.1115 = 0.7780$. Using the binomial probability formula, the required probability is $\binom{10}{3}(0.4)^3(0.6)^7 + \binom{10}{4}(0.4)^4(0.6)^6 + \binom{10}{5}(0.4)^5(0.6)^5 + \binom{10}{6}(0.4)^6(0.6)^4 \approx 0.7780$.

In R:

```
dbinom(x = 3, size = 10, prob = 0.4) + dbinom(x = 4, size
   = 10, prob = 0.4) + dbinom(x = 5, size = 10, prob = 0.4)
 +   dbinom(x = 6, size = 10, prob = 0.4)
```

or, more concisely, `sum( dbinom(x = 3:6, size = 10, prob = 0.4) )`. We can also use the function `pbinom()`, which will add up the probabilities that X is equal to q or fewer. We can calculate the probability that X is equal to 3, 4, 5, or 6 by calculating the probability that X is equal to 6 or fewer and then subtracting the probability that X is equal to 2 or fewer: `pbinom(q = 6, size = 10, prob = 0.4, lower.tail = TRUE) - pbinom(q = 2, size = 10, prob = 0.4, lower.tail = TRUE)`.

(c) From the chart: $0.0060 + \ldots + 0.2007 = 0.8337$.

From the binomial probability formula: $\binom{10}{0}(0.4)^0(0.6)^{10} + \ldots + \binom{10}{5}(0.4)^5(0.6)^5 \approx 0.8337$.

In R: either `dbinom(x = 0, size = 10, prob = 0.4) + ... + dbinom(x = 5, size = 10, prob = 0.4)` or `sum( dbinom(x = 0:5, size = 10, prob = 0.4) )` or `pbinom(q = 5, size = 10, prob = 0.4, lower.tail = TRUE)`.

**4.13** Using Method 1, there are three possible ways of getting exactly four heads: (i) one head in the morning, three in the afternoon, (ii) two heads in the morning, two heads in the afternoon, and (iii) three heads in the morning, one head in the afternoon. The probabilities of these three possible ways are:

(i) $\binom{3}{1}(0.4)^1(0.6)^2 \times \binom{3}{3}(0.4)^3(0.6)^0 = 0.432 \times 0.064 = 0.027648$,

(ii) $\binom{3}{2}(0.4)^2(0.6)^1 \times \binom{3}{2}(0.4)^2(0.6)^1 = 0.288 \times 0.288 = 0.082944$,

(iii) $\binom{3}{3}(0.4)^3(0.6)^0 \times \binom{3}{1}(0.4)^1(0.6)^2 = 0.064 \times 0.432 = 0.027648$.

Adding these three probabilities we get $0.13824$.

Using Method 2, The probability of four heads from six flips is $\binom{6}{4}(0.4)^4(0.6)^2 = 15 \times 0.0256 \times 0.36 = 0.13824$. The two calculations agree. The calculation is much easier using Method 2.

**4.14** The calculation can be done by Method 1, since the morning calculation (with $\theta_1 = 0.4$) can be done separately from the afternoon calculation (with $\theta_2 = 0.6$) and then the two calculations combined to give the requires probability. The calculation cannot be done by Method 2 since the probability of head is not the same on all six flips, so that the answer cannot be found by one single binomial calculation, since the binomial distribution calculation requires the same probability of head on all flips.

**4.15** From Eq. (4.19), $\mu = 1 \times 0.1 + 2 \times 0.3 + 3 \times 0.1 + 4 \times 0.4 + 5 \times 0.05 + 6 \times 0.05 = 3.15$.

In R: `1 * 0.1 + 2 * 0.3 + 3 * 0.1 + 4 * 0.4 + 5 * 0.05 + 6 * 0.05`.

Note: An easier way to not make mistakes when using R, but involving more coding, would be the following:

```
X <- 1:6    # "<-" assigns a value
probs <- c(0.1, 0.3, 0.1, 0.4, 0.05, 0.05)    # "c(...)" creates a vector
sum(probs)    # Check that probabilities sum to 1 to make sure we didn't
  make any typos
sum(X * probs)    # When R multiplies two vectors using "*", it does it
  element by element
```

**4.16** From Eq. (4.35), the variance is $1^2 \times 0.1 + 2^2 \times 0.3 + 3^2 \times 0.1 + 4^2 \times 0.4 + 5^2 \times 0.05 + 6^2 \times 0.05 - 3.15^2 = 1.73$.

In    R:    `1^2 * 0.1 + 2^2 * 0.3 + 3^2 * 0.1 + 4^2 * 0.4 + 5^2 * 0.05 + 6^2 * 0.05 - 3.15^2`.

Instead using `X` and `probs` from the previous solution, we can also do `sum(X^2 * probs) - 3.15^2` since R squares vectors element by element.

**4.17** (a) Using the long formula (4.19) for a mean and the probabilities as given in the binomial chart, the mean is $0 \times 0.1250 + 1 \times 0.3750 + 2 \times 0.3750 + 3 \times 0.1250 = 1.5$.

In    R:    `0 * dbinom(x = 0, size = 3, prob = 0.5) + ...` `3 * dbinom(x = 3, size = 3, prob = 0.5)`    or,    more    concisely, `sum( (0:3) * dbinom(x = 0:3, size = 3, prob = 0.5) )`.

(b) Using the short formula for a mean of a binomial random variable ($n\theta$) the mean is $3 \times 0.5 = 1.5$.

(c) The answers agree.

**4.18** (a) Using the alternative long formula for a variance (4.35) and the probabilities as given in the binomial chart, the variance is $0^2 \times 0.1250 + ... + 3^2 \times 0.1250 - (1.5)^2 = 0.375 + 1.5 + 1.125 - 2.25 = 0.75$. In R: `0^2 * dbinom(x = 0, size = 3, prob = 0.5) + ... + 3^2 * dbinom(x = 3, size = 3, prob = 0.5) - 1.5^2` or `sum( (0:3)^2 * dbinom(x = 0:3, size = 3, prob = 0.5) ) - 1.5^2`.

(b) Using the short formula for a variance of a binomial random variable, the variance is $3 \times 0.5 \times (1 - 0.5) = 0.75$. The answers agree.

**4.19** Mean $= 0 \times (1 - \theta)^2 + 1 \times 2 \times \theta(1 - \theta) + 2 \times \theta^2 = 2\theta - 2\theta^2 + 2\theta^2 = 2\theta$.

**4.20** The mean of $X$ is $5000 \times 0.9 = 4500$. The variance of $X$ is $5000 \times 0.9 \times 0.1 = 450$.

**4.21** (a) The support of $X$ is $\{0, 1, 2, 3, 4\}$.

(b) The probabilities are Prob(0) = $\frac{\binom{5}{0}\binom{6}{4}}{\binom{11}{4}}$ = $\frac{3}{66}$, Prob(1) = $\frac{\binom{5}{1}\binom{6}{3}}{\binom{11}{4}}$ = $\frac{20}{66}$, Prob(2) =

$\frac{\binom{5}{2}\binom{6}{2}}{\binom{11}{4}}$ = $\frac{30}{66}$, Prob(3) = $\frac{\binom{5}{3}\binom{6}{1}}{\binom{11}{4}}$ = $\frac{12}{66}$, Prob(4) = $\frac{\binom{5}{4}\binom{6}{0}}{\binom{11}{4}}$ = $\frac{1}{66}$. These probabilities

add to 1. In R: dhyper(x = 0:4, m = 5, n = 6, k = 4).

(c) From Eq. (4.19), the mean of $X$ is $\frac{1\times20+2\times30+3\times12+4\times1}{66}$ = $\frac{120}{66}$ = $\frac{20}{11}$.

This agrees with the value $\frac{4\times5}{11}$ = $\frac{20}{11}$ found from Eq. (4.29). In R:

sum( 0:4 * dhyper(x = 0:4, m = 5, n = 6, k = 4) ).

From Eq. (4.35), the variance of $X$ is $\frac{1\times20+4\times30+9\times12+16\times1}{66}$ − $\frac{400}{121}$ = $4 - \frac{400}{121}$ =

$\frac{84}{121}$. This agrees with the value $\frac{4\times5\times6\times7}{11^2\times10}$ = $\frac{84}{121}$ found from Eq. (4.34). In R:

sum( (0:4)^2 * dhyper(x = 0:4, m = 5, n = 6, k = 4))
- (20/11)^2.

**4.22** (a) The support of $X$ is $\{1, 2, 3, 4\}$.

(b) The probabilities are Prob(1) = $\frac{\binom{5}{1}\binom{3}{3}}{\binom{8}{4}}$ = $\frac{5}{70}$, Prob(2) = $\frac{\binom{5}{2}\binom{3}{2}}{\binom{8}{4}}$ = $\frac{30}{70}$, Prob(3)

= $\frac{\binom{5}{3}\binom{3}{1}}{\binom{8}{4}}$ = $\frac{30}{70}$, Prob(4) = $\frac{\binom{5}{4}\binom{3}{0}}{\binom{8}{4}}$ = $\frac{5}{70}$. These probabilities add to 1. In R:

dhyper(x = 1:4, m = 5, n = 3, k = 4).

(c) From Eq. (4.19), the mean of $X$ is $\frac{1\times5+2\times30+3\times30+4\times5}{70}$ − $\frac{175}{70}$ = $\frac{5}{2}$.

This agrees with the value $\frac{4\times5}{8}$ = $\frac{5}{2}$ found from Eq. (4.29). In R:

sum( 1:4 * dhyper(x = 1:4, m = 5, n = 3, k = 4) ).

From Eq. (4.35), the variance of $X$ is $\frac{1\times20+4\times30+9\times30+16\times5}{70}$ − $\frac{25}{4}$ = $\frac{190}{28} - \frac{175}{28}$ =

$\frac{15}{28}$. This agrees with the value $\frac{4\times5\times3\times4}{8^2\times7}$ = $\frac{15}{28}$ found from Eq. (4.34). In R:

sum( (1:4)^2 * dhyper(x = 1:4, m = 5, n = 3, k = 4) ) - 2.5^2.

**4.23** Define the number of red marbles initially in the urn as $r$ and the number of blue marbles initially in the urn as $b$, with $r + b = n$. The number of marbles drawn ($d$ in Eq. (4.9)) is $n - 1$.

There are only two possibilities for $X$. One is that all the red marbles were drawn (along with all but 1 of the blue marbles), such that $X = r$ with probability $\frac{\binom{r}{r}\binom{b}{b-1}}{\binom{n}{n-1}}$ = $\frac{b}{n}$, and the other is that all but 1 of the red marbles were drawn (along

with all the blue marbles), such that $X = r - 1$ with probability $\frac{\binom{r}{r-1}\binom{b}{b}}{\binom{n}{n-1}}$ = $\frac{r}{n}$.

From Eq. (4.19) the mean of $X$ is $r\frac{b}{n} + (r - 1)\frac{r}{n} = r\frac{n-1}{n} = \frac{dr}{n}$. This agrees with the value found from Eq. (4.29).

From Eq. (4.35) the variance of $X$ is $r^2\frac{b}{n} + (r - 1)^2\frac{r}{n} - (\frac{(n-1)r}{n})^2 = \frac{rb}{n^2}$. This agrees with the value found from Eq. (4.34).

**4.24** (a) The probability is $\frac{\binom{6}{6}\binom{34}{0}}{\binom{40}{6}}$ = $\frac{1}{\binom{40}{6}}$ $\approx 0.00000026$. In R, dhyper(x = 6,

m = 6, n = 34, k = 6).

(b) The probability is $\frac{\binom{6}{6}\binom{34}{0}}{\binom{40}{6}} + \frac{\binom{6}{5}\binom{34}{1}}{\binom{40}{6}} \approx 0.00000026 + 0.0000531 \approx 0.0000534.$

In R,

```
sum(dhyper(x = 5:6, m = 6, n = 34, k = 6)) or
phyper(q = 4, m = 6, n = 34, k = 6, lower.tail = FALSE).
```

## Chapter 5

**5.1** (a) (i) From Eq. (4.19), the mean of $T_2$ is $2 \times \frac{1}{36} + 3 \times \frac{2}{36} + \cdots + 12 \times \frac{1}{36} = 7.$

(a) (ii) From Eq. (4.35), the variance of $T_2$ is $2^2 \times \frac{1}{36} + 3^2 \times \frac{2}{36} + \cdots + 12^2 \times \frac{1}{36} - 7^2 = \frac{35}{6}.$

(b) The mean of $T_2$ is twice the mean of $X_1$. The variance of $T_2$ is twice the variance of $X_1$.

**5.2** (a) (i) The mean of $\bar{X}$ is $1 \times \frac{1}{36} + 1.5 \times \frac{2}{36} + 2 \times \frac{3}{36} + \cdots + 6 \times \frac{1}{36} = 3.5.$

(a) (ii) The variance of $\bar{X}$ is $1^2 \times \frac{1}{36} + 1.5^2 \times \frac{2}{36} + 2^2 \times \frac{3}{36} + \cdots + 6^2 \times \frac{1}{36} - 3.5^2 = \frac{35}{24}.$

(b) The mean of $\bar{X}$ is equal the mean of $X_1$. The variance of $\bar{X}$ is half the variance of $X_1$.

**5.3** (a) The mean of $T_2$ is $2 \times 3.5 = 7$. The variance $= 2 \times \frac{35}{12} = \frac{35}{6}$. They agree with the values found from the long formulas. The calculations are much easier with the short formulas.

(b) The mean of $\bar{X}$ is 3.5. The variance of $\bar{X}$ is $\frac{35/12}{2} = \frac{35}{24}$. They agree with the values found from the long formulas. The calculations are much easier with the short formulas.

**5.4** The mean of $T_4$ is $4(1/1296) + 5(4/1296) + \cdots + 24(1/1296) = 14$. The variance of $T_4$ is $4^2(1/1296) + 5^2(4/1298) + \ldots + (24)^2(1/1296) - (14)^2 = 35/3.$

**5.5** The mean of $T_4$ is $4 \times 3.5 = 14$. The variance of $T_4$ is $4 \times 35/12 = 35/3$. These agree with the answers to Problem 5.4, and are much easier to calculate.

**5.6** (a) The probability distribution of $\bar{X}$ is:

| Possible values of $\bar{X}$ | 1 | 5/4 | 3/2 | 7/4 | 2 | 9/4 | 5/2 | 11/4 | 3 | 13/4 | 7/2 |
|---|---|---|---|---|---|---|---|---|---|---|---|
| Probabilities | $\frac{1}{1296}$ | $\frac{4}{1296}$ | $\frac{10}{1296}$ | $\frac{20}{1296}$ | $\frac{35}{1296}$ | $\frac{56}{1296}$ | $\frac{80}{1296}$ | $\frac{104}{1296}$ | $\frac{125}{1296}$ | $\frac{140}{1296}$ | $\frac{146}{1296}$ |

| Possible values of $\bar{X}$ | 15/4 | 4 | 17/4 | 9/2 | 19/4 | 5 | 21/4 | 11/2 | 23/4 | 6 |
|---|---|---|---|---|---|---|---|---|---|---|
| Probabilities | $\frac{140}{1296}$ | $\frac{125}{1296}$ | $\frac{104}{1296}$ | $\frac{80}{1296}$ | $\frac{56}{1296}$ | $\frac{35}{1296}$ | $\frac{20}{1296}$ | $\frac{10}{1296}$ | $\frac{4}{1296}$ | $\frac{1}{1296}$ |

(b) The mean of $\bar{X}$ is $1(1/1296) + (5/4)(4/1296) + \cdots + 6(1/1296) = 3.5$. The variance of $\bar{X}$ is $1^2(1/1296) + (5/4)^2(4/1296) + \cdots + 6^2(1/1296) - (3.5)^2 = 35/48$. (Or by the other formula).

(c) The mean of $\bar{X}$ is 3.5. The variance of $\bar{X}$ is 35/48. These agree with the values found from the long formulas and are much easier to calculate.

**5.7** (a) The mean of $T_{2000}$ is $2000 \times 3.5 = 7000$. The variance of $T_{2000}$ is $2000 \times \frac{35}{12} = \frac{70,000}{12}$.

(b) The mean of $\bar{X}_{2000} = 3.5$. The variance of $\bar{X}_{2000}$ is $\frac{35/12}{2000} = \frac{35}{24,000}$.

**5.8** (a) The mean of $T_{4000}$ is $4000 \times 3.5 = 14,000$. The variance of $T_{4000}$ is $4000 \times \frac{35}{12} = \frac{140,000}{12}$.

(b) The mean of $\bar{X}_{4000} = 3.5$. The variance of $\bar{X}_{4000}$ is $\frac{35/12}{4000} = \frac{35}{48,000}$.

**5.9** (a) The mean of $T_{6000}$ is $6000 \times 3.5 = 21,000$. The variance of $T_{6000}$ is $6000 \times \frac{35}{12} = \frac{210,000}{12}$.

(b) The mean of $\bar{X}_{6000}$ is 3.5. The variance of $\bar{X}_{6000}$ is $\frac{35/12}{6000} = \frac{35}{72,000}$.

**5.10** The means are all the same and that makes sense. Each average is "aiming at the same target" 3.5. The variances of the $\bar{X}$'s decrease as the number of rolls increases. This implies that the sample averages (once the die has been rolled) tend closer to 3.5 as the number of rolls increases.

**5.11** (a) The probability distribution $D$ is:

| Possible values of $D$ | −5 | −4 | −3 | −2 | −1 | 0 | 1 | 2 | 3 | 4 | 5 |
|---|---|---|---|---|---|---|---|---|---|---|---|
| Probabilities | $\frac{1}{36}$ | $\frac{2}{36}$ | $\frac{3}{36}$ | $\frac{4}{36}$ | $\frac{5}{36}$ | $\frac{6}{36}$ | $\frac{5}{36}$ | $\frac{4}{36}$ | $\frac{3}{36}$ | $\frac{2}{36}$ | $\frac{1}{36}$ |

(b) The mean is $(-5)\frac{1}{36} + (-4)\frac{2}{36} + \cdots + 5\frac{1}{36} = 0$. The variance is $(-5)^2\frac{1}{36} + (-4)^2\frac{2}{36} + \cdots + 5^2\frac{1}{36} - 0^2 = 35/6$.

(c) The mean is 0. The variance is $2 \times \frac{35}{12} = \frac{35}{6}$. The calculations agree and are easier with the short formulas.

**5.12** From the formulas in Eq. (5.6), the mean of $D$ is $7 - 10 = -3$ and the variance of $D$ is $16 + 9 = 25$.

**5.13** From the first equation in (5.7), the mean of $D$ is $125 - 118 = 7$. From the second equation in (5.7), the variance of $D$ is $\frac{25}{100} + \frac{36}{144} = \frac{1}{4} + \frac{1}{4} = \frac{1}{2}$.

**5.14** Mean of $D = 0$, variance of $D = \frac{\theta(1-\theta)}{300} + \frac{\theta(1-\theta)}{200} = \frac{\theta(1-\theta)}{120}$.

**5.15** From the equations in (5.10), the mean is $0.4 - 0.3 = 0.1$ and the variance is $\frac{0.4 \times 0.6}{300} + \frac{0.3 \times 0.7}{200} = 0.00185$.

**5.16** (a) The probability distribution of $U$ is:

| Possible values | 0 | $\frac{1}{2}$ | 1 |
|---|---|---|---|
| Probabilities | $\frac{1}{4}$ | $\frac{1}{2}$ | $\frac{1}{4}$ |

The probability distribution of $V$ is:

| Possible values | 0 | $\frac{1}{4}$ | $\frac{1}{2}$ | $\frac{3}{4}$ | 1 |
|---|---|---|---|---|---|
| Probabilities | $\frac{1}{16}$ | $\frac{4}{16}$ | $\frac{6}{16}$ | $\frac{4}{16}$ | $\frac{1}{16}$ |

(b) By the short formulas, the mean of both U and V is $\frac{1}{2}$, the variance of U is $\frac{1}{2} \times \frac{1}{2}/2 = \frac{1}{8}$, and the variance of V is $\frac{1}{2} \times \frac{1}{2}/4 = \frac{1}{16}$.

(c) The possible value of $D$ are $-1, -\frac{3}{4}, -\frac{1}{2}, -\frac{1}{4}, 0, \frac{1}{4}, \frac{1}{2}, \frac{3}{4}$ and 1. There are 15 $U, V$ value combinations and we have to consider all of them to find the probability distribution of $D$. As one example, there are three $(U, V)$ combinations that lead to the value $D = 0$: $U = V = 0$ (probability $\frac{1}{4} \times \frac{1}{16} = \frac{1}{64}$), $U = V = 1/2$ (probability $\frac{1}{2} \times \frac{6}{16} = \frac{12}{64}$), $U = V = 1$ (probability $\frac{1}{4} \times \frac{1}{16} = \frac{1}{64}$). Thus the total probability that $D = 0$ is $\frac{1}{64} + \frac{12}{64} + \frac{1}{64} = \frac{14}{64}$. Similarly for other cases. The eventual probability distribution for $D$ is:

| Possible value of D: | $-1$ | $-\frac{3}{4}$ | $-\frac{1}{2}$ | $-\frac{1}{4}$ | 0 | $\frac{1}{4}$ | $\frac{1}{2}$ | $\frac{3}{4}$ | 1 |
|---|---|---|---|---|---|---|---|---|---|
| Probability: | $\frac{1}{64}$ | $\frac{4}{64}$ | $\frac{8}{64}$ | $\frac{12}{64}$ | $\frac{14}{64}$ | $\frac{12}{64}$ | $\frac{8}{64}$ | $\frac{4}{64}$ | $\frac{1}{64}$ |

(d) The mean of $D$ is $-1 \times \frac{1}{64} + ... + 1 \times \frac{1}{64} = 0$ and the variance of $D$ is $(-1)^2 \times \frac{1}{64} + ... + 1^2 \times \frac{1}{64} - 0^2 = \frac{3}{16}$.

(e) Using any set of short formulas, we find that the mean of $D = \frac{1}{2} - \frac{1}{2} = 0$ and the variance of $D$ is $\frac{1}{8} + \frac{1}{16} = \frac{3}{16}$.

**5.17** From Eq. (5.10), the mean of $D = 0.5 - 0.3 = 0.2$, The variance of $D = \frac{0.5^2}{10} + \frac{0.3 \times 0.7}{15} = 0.039$.

# Chapter 6

**6.1** From the Z chart, the answers are

(a) 0.9066. In R: pnorm(q = 1.32).
(b) $0.9066 - 0.5000 = 0.4066$. In R: pnorm(q = 1.32) - pnorm(q = 0).
(c) $0.5000 - 0.3300 = 0.1700$. In R: pnorm(q = 0) - pnorm(q = -0.44).
(d) $0.9147 - 0.7324 = 0.1823$. In R: pnorm(q = 1.37) - pnorm(0.62).
(e) $1 - 0.8790 = 0.1210$. In R: pnorm(q = 1.17, lower.tail = FALSE).
(f) $1 - 0.1038 = 0.8962$. In R: pnorm(q = -1.26, lower.tail = FALSE).

**6.2** In all parts of this question, we have to create a Z by subtracting the mean of 3 and dividing by the standard deviation 2. In detail:

(a) Prob$(-\infty < X \leq 4.14) = $ Prob$(\frac{X-3}{2} \leq \frac{4.14-3}{2}) = $ Prob$(Z \leq 0.57) = 0.7157$.
In R: pnorm(q = (4.14 - 3)/2 or pnorm(q = 4.14, mean = 3, sd = 2)).

(b) $\text{Prob}(-\infty < X \le 2.24) = \text{Prob}(\frac{X-3}{2} \le \frac{2.24-3}{2}) = \text{Prob}(Z \le -0.38) = 0.3520$.
In R: pnorm(q = (2.24 - 3)/2 or pnorm(q = 2.24, mean = 3,
sd = 2)).

(c) $\text{Prob}(X \ge 3.68) = \text{Prob}(\frac{X-3}{2} \ge \frac{3.68-3}{2}) = \text{Prob}(Z \ge 0.34) = 1 - 0.6331 = 0.3669$.
In R: pnorm(q = (3.68 - 3)/2, lower.tail = FALSE) or
pnorm(q = 3.68, mean = 3, sd = 2, lower.tail = FALSE).

(d) $\text{Prob}(X \ge 2.56) = \text{Prob}(\frac{X-3}{2} \ge \frac{2.56-3}{2}) = \text{Prob}(Z \ge -0.22) = 1 - 0.4129 = 0.5871$.
In R: pnorm(q = (2.56 - 3)/2, lower.tail = FALSE) or
pnorm(q = 2.56, mean = 3, sd = 2, lower.tail = FALSE).

(e) $\text{Prob}(1.76 \le X \le 2.48) = \text{Prob}(\frac{1.76-3}{2} \le \frac{X-3}{2} \le \frac{2.48-3}{2}) = \text{Prob}(-0.62 \le Z \le -0.26) = 0.3974 - 0.2676 = 0.1298$.
In R: pnorm(q = (2.48 - 3)/2) - pnorm(q = (1.76 - 3)/2) or
pnorm(q = 2.48, mean = 3, sd = 2) - pnorm(q = 1.76,
mean = 3, sd = 2).

(f) $\text{Prob}(3.66 \le X \le 4.42) = \text{Prob}(\frac{3.66-3}{2} \le \frac{X-3}{2} \le \frac{4.42-3}{2}) = \text{Prob}(0.33 \le Z \le 0.71) = 0.7611 - 0.6293 = 0.1318$.
In R: pnorm(q = (4.42 - 3)/2) - pnorm(q = (3.66 - 3)/2) or
pnorm(q = 4.42, mean = 3, sd = 2) - pnorm(q = 3.66,
mean = 3, sd = 2).

**6.3** (a) From the Z chart, $a = 0.55$. In R: qnorm(p = 0.7088).

(b) From the Z chart, $b = -0.43$. In R: qnorm(p = 0.3336).

(c) $\text{Prob}(-\infty < Z \le c) = 1 - 0.3372 = 0.6628$. From the Z chart, $c = 0.42$. In R: qnorm(p = 0.3372, lower.tail = FALSE).

(d) $\text{Prob}(-\infty < Z \le d) = 1 - 0.8485 = 0.1515$. From the Z chart, $d = -1.03$. In R: qnorm(p = 0.8485, lower.tail = FALSE).

(e) From the symmetry of the Z chart, $\text{Prob}(0 \le Z \le e) = \frac{1}{2} \times 0.3830 = 0.1915$. From this, $\text{Prob}(-\infty \le Z \le e) = 0.5000 + 0.1915 = 0.6915$. From the Z chart, $e = 0.5$. In R: qnorm(p = 0.5 + 0.3830/2).

(f) From the symmetry of the z chart, $\text{Prob}(0 \le Z \le f) = \frac{1}{2} \times 0.3472 = 0.1736$. From this, $\text{Prob}(-\infty \le Z \le f) = 0.5000 + 0.1736 = 0.6736$. From the Z chart, $f = 0.45$. In R: qnorm(p = 0.5 + 0.3472/2).

**6.4** In all parts of this question we have to create a $Z$ by subtracting the mean of 3 and dividing by the standard deviation 2. This standardization procedure is carried out in all the answers below.

(a) Given that $\text{Prob}(-\infty < X \le a) = 0.7088$, $\text{Prob}(-\infty < \frac{X-3}{2} \le \frac{a-3}{2}) = 0.7088$. This implies that $\text{Prob}(-\infty < Z \le \frac{a-3}{2}) = 0.7088$. From the Z chart, $\frac{a-3}{2} = 0.55$. From this, $a = 4.1$. In R: qnorm(p = 0.7088) * 2 + 3 or qnorm(p = 0.7088, mean = 3, sd = 2).

(b) Given that $\text{Prob}(-\infty < X \le b) = 0.3336$ we get $\text{Prob}(-\infty < \frac{X-3}{2} \le \frac{b-3}{2}) = 0.3336$. This implies that $\text{Prob}(-\infty < Z \le \frac{b-3}{2}) = 0.3336$. From the Z chart,

$\frac{b-3}{2} = -0.43$. From this, $b = 2.14$. In R: qnorm(p = 0.3336) * 2 + 3 or qnorm(p = 0.3336, mean = 3, sd = 2).

(c) Prob( $-\infty \leq X \leq c$ ) $= 1 - 0.3372 = 0.6628$. This implies that Prob($-\infty < \frac{X-3}{2} < \frac{c-3}{2}$) $= 0.6628$. From this, $\frac{c-3}{2} = 0.42$, so that $c = 3.84$. In R: qnorm(p = 0.3372, lower.tail = FALSE) * 2 + 3 or qnorm(p = 0.3372, mean = 3, sd = 2, lower.tail = FALSE).

(d) Prob( $-\infty \leq X \leq d$ ) $=1 - 0.8485 = 0.1515$. This implies that Prob($-\infty < \frac{X-3}{2} < \frac{d-3}{2}$) $= 0.1515$. From the $Z$ chart, $\frac{d-3}{2} = -1.03$. From this, $d = 0.94$. In R: qnorm(p = 0.8485, lower.tail = FALSE) * 2 + 3 or qnorm(p = 0.8485, mean = 3, sd = 2, lower.tail = FALSE).

**6.5** (a) Prob($X > 5$) $= $ Prob($\frac{X-2}{5} > \frac{5-2}{5}$) $=$ Prob($Z > 0.6$) $= 1-0.7257 = 0.2743$.

(b) Prob($X < 1$) $=$ Prob($\frac{X-2}{5} < \frac{1-2}{5}$) $=$ Prob($Z < -0.2$) $= 0.4207$.

(c) From part (a), Prob($X < 5$)$=1 - 0.2753 = 0.7257$. From part (b), Prob($X < 1$)$=0.4207$. Therefore Prob($1 < X < 5$)$=$Prob($X < 5$)$-$Prob($X < 1$)$= 0.7257 - 0.4207 = 0.3050$.

(d) Since Prob($X \leq b$)$=0.5987$, Prob($\frac{X-2}{5} \leq \frac{b-2}{5}$)$=0.5987$. Therefore Prob($Z \leq \frac{b-2}{5}$)$=0.5987$.

From the $Z$ chart, Prob($Z \leq 0.25$) $= 0.5987$. Therefore $\frac{b-2}{5} = 0.25$, so that $b = 3.25$.

**6.6** The standardization procedure shows that Prob($\frac{\mu-k\sigma-\mu}{\sigma} \leq \frac{X-\mu}{\sigma} \leq \frac{\mu+k\sigma-\mu}{\sigma}$) $= 0.5160$. Simplifying the extreme ends of these inequalities, we obtain Prob($-k \leq Z \leq k$) $= 0.5160$. From the symmetry of the $Z$ distribution around 0, Prob($0 \leq Z \leq k$) $= \frac{1}{2} \times 0.5160 = 0.2580$. Since Prob($-\infty \leq Z \leq 0$) $= 0.5000$, Prob($-\infty \leq Z \leq k$)$= 0.5000 + 0.2580 = 0.7580$. From the $Z$ chart, $k = 0.7$.

**6.7** Prob($X > Y$) $=$ Prob($X - Y > 0$) $=$ Prob($D > 0$), where $D = X - Y$.

The mean of $D$ is $5-2 = 3$ and the variance of $D$ is $3+6 = 9$, so that the standard deviation of $D$ is 3 Therefore Prob($X-Y > 0$) $=$ Prob($D > 0$) $= 1-$Prob($D < 0$) $= 1 -$ Prob($\frac{D-3}{3} < \frac{-3}{3}$) $= 1 -$ Prob($Z < -1$) $= 1 - 0.1587 = 0.8413$.

**6.8** (a) Prob($X_1 \geq 3.0$) $=$ Prob($\frac{X_1-2.5}{0.6} \geq \frac{3.0-2.5}{0.6}$) $\approx$ Prob($Z \geq 0.83$) $= 0.2033$.

(b) The mean of $\bar{X}$ is 2.5 and that the variance of $\bar{X}$ is $0.36/4 = 0.09$, so that the standard deviation of $\bar{X}$ is 0.3. Therefore Prob($\bar{X} \geq 3$) $=$ Prob($\frac{\bar{X}-2.5}{0.3} \geq \frac{3-2.5}{0.3}$) $\approx$ Prob($Z \geq 1.67$ ) $= 0.0475$.

(c) The answers make sense. As the sample size increases, the variance of the average decreases, so that it becomes less likely that the data average will deviate from the mean.

**6.9** (a) Prob($X < 2$) $=$ Prob($\frac{X-2.75}{0.79} < \frac{2-2.75}{0.79}$) $\approx$ Prob($Z < -0.95$) $= 0.1711$.

(b) The variance of the average $\bar{X}$ is $0.625/4 = 0.15625$. The standard deviation of $\bar{X}$ is thus approximately 0.395. Therefore Prob($\bar{X} < 2$) $=$ Prob($\frac{\bar{X}-2.75}{0.395} < \frac{2-2.75}{0.395}$) $\approx$ Prob($Z < -1.90$) $= 0.0287$.

(c) The answers make sense. As the sample size increases, the variance of the average decreases, so that it becomes less likely that the data average will deviate from the mean.

**6.10** (a) If $X_p$ is the weight of a platypus taken at random and $X_m$ is the weight of a muskrat taken at random, then $\text{Prob}(X_m > X_p) = \text{Prob}(X_m - X_p > 0) = \text{Prob}(D > 0)$, where $D$ $(= X_m - X_p)$ is a random variable having a normal distribution with mean 0.25 and variance $0.36 + 0.625 = 0.985$. Thus upon standardizing, $\text{Prob}(D > 0) = \text{Prob}(\frac{D-0.25}{\sqrt{0.985}} > \frac{0-0.25}{\sqrt{0.985}}) \approx \text{Prob}(Z > -0.25) = 0.5987$.

(b) If $\bar{X}_m$ is the average weight of four muskrats taken at random and $\bar{X}_p$ is the average weight of four platypuses taken at random, then $\text{Prob}(\bar{X}_m > \bar{X}_p) = \text{Prob}(\bar{X}_m - \bar{X}_p > 0) = \text{Prob}(D > 0)$ where $D$ $(= \bar{X}_m - \bar{X}_p)$ is a random variable having a normal distribution with mean 0.25 and variance $0.985/4 = 0.24625$. Thus upon standardizing, $\text{Prob}(D > 0) = \text{Prob}(\frac{D-0.25}{\sqrt{0.24625}} > \frac{0-0.25}{\sqrt{0.24625}}) \approx \text{Prob}(Z > -0.50) = 0.6915$.

(c) The answers make sense. As the sample size increases, the variance of $D$ decreases, so that it becomes more likely that the $D$, whose mean is 0.25, exceeds zero.

**6.11** (a) The mean of $\bar{X}$ is 5 and the variance of $\bar{X}$ is $16/5 = 3.2$. Therefore
$$\text{Prob}(\bar{X} > 6) = \text{Prob}(\frac{\bar{X}-5}{\sqrt{3.2}} > \frac{6-5}{\sqrt{3.2}}) \approx \text{Prob}(Z > 0.56) = 0.2877.$$

(b) The mean of $T_5$ is $5 \times 5 = 25$, and the variance of $T_5$ is $5 \times 16 = 80$. Therefore
$$\text{Prob}(T_5 > 30) = \text{Prob}(\frac{T-25}{\sqrt{80}} > \frac{30-25}{\sqrt{80}}) \approx \text{Prob}(Z > 0.56) = 1 - \text{Prob}(Z < 0.56) = 1 - 0.7123 = 0.2877.$$

(c) The answer are identical since the events $\bar{X} > 6$ and $T_5 > 30$ are equivalent events.

**6.12** (a) The mean of $\bar{X}_{200}$ is 3.5 and the variance of $\bar{X}_{200}$ is $\frac{35}{12 \times 200} \approx 0.0145833$, so that the standard deviation of $\bar{X}_{200}$ is approximately 0.1208. From Eq. (6.37), $a$ is $3.5 - 1.96 \times 0.1208 = 3.2632$ and $b$ is $3.5 + 1.96 \times 0.1208 = 3.7368$.

(b) The mean of $\bar{X}_{500}$ is 3.5 and the variance of $\bar{X}_{500}$ is $\frac{35}{12 \times 500} \approx 0.005833$, so that the standard deviation of $\bar{X}_{500}$ is approximately 0.0764. From Eq. (6.37), $c$ is $3.5 - 1.96 \times 0.0764 = 3.3502$ and $d$ is $3.5 + 1.96 \times 0.0764 = 3.6497$.

(c) The mean of $\bar{X}_{1000}$ is 3.5 and the variance of $\bar{X}_{1000}$ is $\frac{35}{12 \times 1000} \approx 0.00291666$, so that the standard deviation of $\bar{X}_{1000}$ is approximately 0.0540. From Eq. (6.37), $e$ is 3.39242 and $f$ is 3.6058.

(d) The respective values make sense. As the number of rolls increases, the variance of the average of the numbers turning up decreases and it becomes more and more likely that the average will be close to the mean (of 3.5).

**6.13** (a) The mean of $P$ is 0.5 and the variance of $P$ is $0.5 \times 0.5/500 = 0.0005$. Therefore, the standard deviation of $P$ is $\sqrt{0.0005} \approx 0.02236$. Thus $a = 0.5 - 1.96 \times 0.02236 = 0.4562$, $b = 0.5 + 1.96 \times 0.02258 = 0.5438$.

(b) The mean of $P$ is 0.5 and the variance of $P$ is $0.5 \times 0.5/5000 = 0.00005$. Therefore the standard deviation of $P$ is $\sqrt{0.0005} \approx 0.00707$. Thus $c = 0.5 - 1.96 \times 0.00707 = 0.4861, d = 0.5 + 1.96 \times 0.00707 = 0.51539$.

(c) The interval from $c$ to $d$ is shorter than the interval from $a$ to $b$. This occurs because the variance of $P$ is smaller for 5000 flips than it is for 500 flips, leading to a distribution of $P$ more tightly concentrated around 0.5.

**6.14** (a) The mean of $\bar{X}$ is 160 and the variance of $\bar{X}$ is $64/4 = 16$. The standard deviation of $\bar{X}$ is then 4. Therefore, $\text{Prob}(160 - 1.96 \times 4 < \bar{X} < 160 + 1.96 \times 4) = 0.95$, which gives $a = 152.16$ and $b = 167.84$.

(b) The mean of $\bar{X}$ is 160 and the variance of $\bar{X}$ is $64/16 = 4$. The standard deviation of $\bar{X}$ is then 2. Therefore, $\text{Prob}(160 - 1.96 \times 2 < \bar{X} < 160 + 1.96 \times 2) = 0.95$, which gives $c = 156.08$ and $d = 163.92$.

(c) The mean of $\bar{X}$ is 160 and the variance of $\bar{X}$ is $64/64 = 1$. The standard deviation of $\bar{X}$ is then 1. Therefore, $\text{Prob}(160 - 1.96 < \bar{X} < 160 + 1.96) = 0.95$, which gives $e = 158.04$ and $f = 161.96$.

**6.15** Let $X$ be the random number of heads we will see in 2000 flips of the coin. If the coin is fair, the mean of $X$ is $2000 \times \frac{1}{2} = 1000$ and the variance of $X$ is $2000 \times \frac{1}{4} = 500$. From this, $\text{Prob}(X \geq 1072) = \text{Prob}(\frac{X-1000}{\sqrt{500}} \geq \frac{1072-1000}{\sqrt{500}}) \approx \text{Prob}(Z \geq 3.22) = 0.0006$.

**6.16** Let $P$ be the random proportion of heads in 500 flips of the coin. If the coin is fair, the mean of $P$ is 0.5 and the variance of $X$ is $\frac{0.5 \times 0.5}{500} = 0.0005$ From this, $\text{Prob}(P \geq 0.52) = \text{Prob}(\frac{P-0.5}{\sqrt{0.0005}} \geq \frac{0.52-0.5}{\sqrt{0.0005}}) \approx \text{Prob}(Z \geq 0.89) = 0.1867$.

**6.17** (a) The probability as given by the binomial chart is $0.1650 + 0.1797 + 0.1597 + 0.1171 + 0.0710 + 0.0355 = 0.7280$.

(b) $X$ has mean 8 and variance 4.8. Upon standardizing, $\text{Prob}(7 \leq X \leq 12)$ is $\text{Prob}\left(\frac{7-8}{\sqrt{4.8}} \leq \frac{X-8}{\sqrt{4.8}} \leq \frac{12-8}{\sqrt{4.8}}\right) \approx \text{Prob}(-0.46 \leq Z \leq 1.86) = 0.6640$.

(c) With a continuity correction the approximating is $\text{Prob}(6.5 \leq X \leq 12.5)$. Upon standardizing, this is $\text{Prob}\left(\frac{6.5-8}{\sqrt{4.8}} \leq \frac{X-8}{\sqrt{4.8}} \leq \frac{12.5-8}{\sqrt{4.8}}\right) \approx \text{Prob}(-0.68 \leq Z \leq 2.05) \approx 0.7315$.

(d) The approximation using the continuity correction is more accurate than the approximation when the continuity correction is not used.

**6.18** (a) Upon standardizing, the required probability as approximated by the normal distribution is $\text{Prob}\left(\frac{13-14}{\sqrt{35/3}} \leq \frac{T_4-14}{\sqrt{35/3}} \leq \frac{15-14}{\sqrt{35/3}}\right) \approx \text{Prob}(-0.29 \leq Z \leq +0.29) = 0.2282$.

(b) Upon standardizing, the required probability is $\text{Prob}\left(\frac{12.5-14}{\sqrt{35/3}} \leq \frac{T_4-14}{\sqrt{35/3}} \leq \frac{15.5-14}{\sqrt{35/3}}\right) \approx \text{Prob}(-0.44 \leq Z \leq +0.44) = 0.3400$.

(c) The approximation using the continuity correction is more accurate than the approximation not using the continuity correction.

# Chapter 8

**8.1** The estimate of $\theta$ is $5265/10{,}000 = 0.5265$. The approximate 95% confidence interval is $0.5265 - 1/\sqrt{10{,}000}$ to $0.5265 + 1/\sqrt{10{,}000}$, which is 0.5165 to 0.5365.

**8.2** (a) The margin of error $= 0.05 = 1/\sqrt{n}$, giving $n = 400$.
(b) They would need $0.02 = 1/\sqrt{n}$, giving $n = 2500$.
(c) They would need $0.01 = 2/\sqrt{n}$, giving $n = 40{,}000$.

**8.3** The estimate of $\theta$ is $1300/2500 = 0.52$. From interval (8.4), the bounds are $0.52 - 1.96\sqrt{(0.52)(0.48)/2500}$ to $0.52 + 1.96\sqrt{(0.52)(0.48)/2500}$. These are 0.5004 and 0.5396.

From interval (8.6), the bounds of the confidence interval are $0.52 - \sqrt{1/2500}$ to $0.52 + \sqrt{1/2500}$. These are 0.50 and 0.54, and are thus slightly wider than the bounds as given by interval (8.4).

**8.4** (a) From Eq. (8.9), the estimate of $\mu$ is $\bar{x} = 22.25$.
(b) From Eq. (8.14), the approximate confidence interval is $22.25 - 1.96(9.6019)/\sqrt{20}$ to $22.25 + 1.96(9.6019)/\sqrt{20}$, that is, from 18.04 to 26.46.
Note: See Problem (13.15) for a more precise answer.

**8.5** From Eq. (8.9), the estimate of $\mu$ is $\bar{x} = (127 + \ldots + 138)/6 = 133.8333$.
From Eq. (8.13), the estimate of $\sigma^2$ is $s^2 = [(127)^2 + \ldots + (138)^2 - 6(133.8333)^2]/5 = 92.16667$, so that $s = \sqrt{92.16667} = 9.600347$. Thus from Eq. (8.14), the approximate 95% confidence interval is $133.83333 - 1.96(9.600347)\sqrt{1/6}$ to $133.8333 + 1.96(9.600347)\sqrt{1/6}$, or approximately 126.15 to 141.52.
Note: See Problem (13.16) for a more precise answer.
In R:

```
x <- c(127, 144, 140, 136, 118, 138)   # Load in the data values
xbar <- mean(x);   xbar # Data average
n <- length(x)
s2 <- (sum(x^2) - n * xbar^2) / (n-1)
s <- sqrt(s2) # Estimate of sigma using formulas
s <- sd(x) # Alternatively, R has a shortcut
xbar - 1.96 * s / sqrt(n) # Lower bound
xbar + 1.96 * s / sqrt(n) # Upper bound
```

**8.6** From Eq. (8.9), the estimate of $\mu$ is $\bar{x} = 6.615$. From Eq. (8.14), the approximate 95% confidence interval is $6.615 - 1.96(0.0593)$ to $6.615 + 1.96(0.0593)$, or approximately from 6.50 to 6.73.
Note: See Problem (13.17) for a more precise answer.

**8.7** (a) From Eq. (8.19), the estimate is of $\theta_1 - \theta_2$ is $p_1 - p_2 = 375/1000 - 345/1000 = 0.030$. From Eq. (8.23), the approximate confidence 95% confidence interval is from $0.030 - \sqrt{1/1000 + 1/1000} = 0.030 - 0.045 = -0.015$ to $0.030 + \sqrt{1/1000 + 1/1000} = 0.030 + 0.045 = 0.075$.

(b) From Eq. (8.19), the estimate is of $\theta_1 - \theta_2$ is $3700/10{,}000 - 3350/10{,}000 = 0.035$.

From Eq. (8.23), the approximate conservative confidence interval is from $0.035 - \sqrt{1/10{,}000 + 1/10{,}000} = 0.035 - 0.014 = 0.021$ to $0.035 + \sqrt{1/10{,}000 + 1/10{,}000} = 0.035 + 0.014 = 0.049$.

(c) The estimates of $\theta_1 - \theta_2$ are close to each other, and this makes sense because they are both unbiased estimates of $\theta_1 - \theta_2$. The width of the confidence interval in part (a) is $0.045 + 0.045 = 0.090$. The width of the confidence interval in part (b) is $0.014 + 0.014 = 0.028$. Therefore the confidence interval in part (b) is much shorter than that in part (a), and this arises because of the larger sample size in part (b).

**8.8** From the data, $p_1 = 640/1000 = 0.640$ and $p_2 = 670/1200 = 0.558$. Since $0.3 < p_1, p_2 < 0.7$, we are justified in using the approximate confidence interval (8.23). This leads to the approximate confidence interval $0.640 - 0.558 - \sqrt{1/1200 + 1/1000}$ to $0.640 - 0.558 + \sqrt{1/1200 + 1/1000}$. This yields an approximate confidence interval from $0.04$ to $0.13$.

**8.9** (a) Such a comparison does not make sense, since the numbers of men and women in the sample are not equal, so it is not a fair comparison.

(b) We estimate $\theta_1 - \theta_2$ by $p_1 - p_2 = 348/2000 - 294/1500 = 0.174 - 0.196 = -0.022$.

(c) Since both $p_1$ and $p_2$ lie outside the interval $0.3$ to $0.7$ we do not use the conservative formula (8.23), and instead we use use the confidence interval (8.22). This gives a confidence interval from
$$-0.022 - 1.96\sqrt{(0.174)(0.826)/2000 + (0.196)(0.804)/1500} = -0.022 - 0.027 = -0.049 \text{ to } -0.022 + 0.027 = 0.005.$$

**8.10** (a) From Eq. (8.26), we estimate $\mu_1 - \mu_2$ by $\bar{x}_1 - \bar{x}_2$, which is $133.200 - 126.125 = 7.075$.

(b) The 95% confidence interval is $7.075 - 1.96\sqrt{79.7333/10 + 83.5536/8}$ to $7.075 + 1.96\sqrt{79.7333/10 + 83.5536/8}$, that is from $-1.34$ to $15.49$.

Note: See Problem (13.18) for a more precise answer.

**8.11** (a) We estimate $\mu_1 - \mu_2$ by $\bar{x}_1 - \bar{x}_2 = 7.075$, as in Problem 8.10.

(b) There are two (equivalent) ways to answer this. The first way is to compute $7.075 - 1.96\sqrt{79.7333/160 + 83.5536/128}$ to $7.075 + 1.96\sqrt{79.7333/160 + 83.5536/128}$, which gives a confidence interval from $4.97$ to $9.18$.

The second way is to note that for both samples the sample size has increased by a factor of 16. This implies that the width of the confidence interval decreases by a factor of 4. This leads to the confidence interval $7.075 - 1.96\dfrac{\sqrt{79.7333/10 + 83.5536/8}}{4}$ to $7.075 + 1.96\dfrac{\sqrt{79.7333/10 + 83.5536/8}}{4}$, which also gives a confidence interval from $4.97$ to $9.18$.

(c) The estimate of $\mu_1 - \mu_2$ does not change. However, the width of the confidence interval is much smaller (in fact by a factor of four) in this question than the width in Problem 8.10 and this occurs because of the increased sample size in Problem 8.11.

Note: See Problem (13.19) for a more precise answer.

**8.12** (a) Using Eqs. (8.48) and (8.49), $b = 93.53/464.9 = 0.2011831 \approx 0.20$, $a = 11.57 - (0.2011831)(22.1) = 7.123854 \approx 7.12$. The regression line is therefore approximately $y = 7.124 + 0.201x$.

In R:

```
age <- c(33,32,14,20,15,16,30,17,21,23)
weight <- c(12.9,13.8,8.2,12.2,8.5,12.9,13.7,11.2,11.9,10.4)
model <- lm(weight ~ age)
model$coefficients
```

(b) The line approximately "skewers" through the data points.

In R:

```
plot(age, weight, main = "Age of Infant Girls and Their
        Weights", xlab = "Age (months)", ylab = "Weight (kg)",
        xlim = c(10, 40), ylim = c(7, 15), pch = 16)
abline(model)
```

(c) From Eq. (8.50), $s_r^2 = 35.841 - (0.2011831)^2 \times 464.9/8 = 2.12804$. Thus $s_r = 1.45878$. From Eq. (8.51) the confidence interval is $0.201 - \frac{1.96(1.45878)}{\sqrt{464.9}}$ to $0.201 + \frac{1.96(1.45878)}{\sqrt{464.9}}$, or approximately from 0.07 to 0.33.

In R, either confint.default(model, parm = "age") or

```
modelsummary <- summary(model)
model$coefficients["age"] - 1.96 * modelsummary$
  coefficients["age", "Std. Error"]
model$coefficients["age"] + 1.96 * modelsummary$
  coefficients["age", "Std. Error"]
```

Note: See Problem (13.20) for a more precise answer.

**8.13** (a) The line "skewers through" the data points.

In R:

```
x <- c(16, 16, 16, 18, 18, 20, 22, 24, 24, 26, 26, 26)
y <- c(76.2, 77.1, 75.7, 78.1, 77.8, 79.2, 80.2, 82.5,
     80.7, 83.1, 82.2, 83.6)
plot(x, y, main = "Amount of Water and Plant Growth Height",
    xlab = "Amount of Water", ylab = "Growth Height",
    pch = 16)
abline(lm(y ~ x))
```

(b) From Eq. (8.52), the confidence interval is from $0.65 - 2.576 \times 0.045252$   to $0.65 + 2.576 \times 0.045252$, that is, approximately from 0.53 to 0.77.

In R:

```
model <- lm(y ~ x)
confint.default(model, parm = "x", level = 0.99)
```

Note: See Problem (13.21) for a more precise answer.

**8.14** (a) From Eq. (8.48), the estimate of $\beta$ is $b = s_{xy}/s_{xx} = 610/210 \approx 2.905$. From Eq. (8.49), the estimate of $\alpha$ is $a = \bar{y} - b\bar{x} = 43.75 - 2.905 \times 10 \approx 14.700$. Thus the estimated mean growth height is approximately $14.700 + 2.905x$.

In R:

```
x <- c(5, 10, 20, 8, 4, 6, 12, 15)
y <- c(27, 47, 73, 40, 30, 28, 46, 59)
lm(y ~ x)$coef
```

(b) To calculate the 95% confidence interval for $\beta$ we first need to calculate $s_r$. Equation (8.50) shows that $s_r^2 = (1835.5 - (2.905)^2 \times 210)/6 = 10.551$, so that $s_r \approx 3.248$. Therefore, the approximate 95% confidence interval for $\beta$ is $2.905 - 1.96 \times 3.248/\sqrt{210}$   to   $2.905 + 1.96 \times 3.248/\sqrt{210}$, or from 2.47 to 3.34. In R: `confint.default(lm(y ~ x), parm = "x")`.

Note: See Problem (13.22) for a more precise answer.

# Chapter 9

**9.1** (a) In all three cases the proportion is 0.55.

(b) (i) The mean of $X$ is 20, the variance of $X$ is 10, so upon using a normal approximation to the binomial and standardizing, the required probability is approximately $\text{Prob}(Z \geq (22 - 20)/\sqrt{10}) \approx \text{Prob}(Z \geq 0.63) = 0.2643$.

(b) (ii) The mean of $X$ is 50, the variance of $X$ is 25, so upon using a normal approximation to the binomial and standardizing, the required probability is approximately $\text{Prob}(Z \geq (55 - 50)/\sqrt{25}) \approx \text{Prob}(Z \geq 1) = 0.1587$.

(b) (iii) The mean of $X$ is 100, the variance of $X$ is 50, so upon using a normal approximation to the binomial and standardizing, the required probability is approximately $\text{Prob}(Z \geq (110 - 100)/\sqrt{50}) \approx \text{Prob}(Z \geq 1.41) = 0.0793$.

(c) Giving the proportion on its own without giving the number of flips is useless.

**9.2** (a) We give the $c_2$ calculation throughout this problem, and then give the $c_1$ result by symmetry.

If $X$ is the number of times that a head turns up and if the coin is fair, the mean of $X$ is $50,000 \times 0.5 = 25,000$ and the variance of $X$ is $50,000 \times 0.5 \times 0.5 = 12,500$. Therefore, we require that $\text{Prob}(X \geq c_2|\theta = 0.5)$ is equal to 0.025. From this, $\text{Prob}\left(\frac{X-25,000}{\sqrt{12,500}} \geq \frac{c_2-25,000}{\sqrt{12,500}}\right) = 0.025$, so that upon using a normal approximation to the binomial and standardizing, $\text{Prob}\left(Z \geq \frac{c_2 - 25,000}{\sqrt{12,500}}\right) = 0.025$. Equation (6.17) shows $\text{Prob}(Z \geq 1.96) = 0.025$. This gives $(c_2 - 25,000)/\sqrt{12,500} = 1.96$, and from this $c_2 = 25,219.13$. Rounding up, $c_2 = 25,220$.

By symmetry, since $c_2$ is 220 greater than the null hypothesis mean of 25,000, $c_1$ will be 220 less than this mean. Thus $c_1 = 25,000 - 220 = 24,780$.

In R, we can find $c_2$ by standardizing manually with

`qnorm(0.025, lower.tail = FALSE) * sqrt(12500) + 25000`

or by specifying the mean and standard deviation with

`qnorm(0.025, mean = 25000, sd = sqrt(12500), lower.tail`
`= FALSE)`.

(b) As in part (a), but with 1.96 replaced by 2.576, found from Eqs. (6.21) and (6.22). This gives $c_2 = 25,288.05$, or, rounding up, 25,289. By symmetry, $c_1 = 24,711$.

**9.3** (a) Let $a$ be the critical point. Upon standardizing, we get $\text{Prob}((X - 200)/10 > (a - 200)/10) = 0.05$ which gives $\text{Prob}(Z > (a - 200)/10) = 0.05$. From Eq. (6.12), $(a - 200)/10 = 1.645$, giving $a = 216.45$. Rounding up, $a = 217$.

(b) Let $b$ be the critical point. Upon standardizing, we get $\text{Prob}((X - 200)/10 > (b - 200)/10) = 0.01$, which gives $\text{Prob}(Z > (b - 200)/10) = 0.01$. From Eq. (6.19), $(b - 200)/10 = 2.326$, giving $b = 223.26$. Rounding up, $b = 224$.

**9.4** (a) Let $x$ be the number of cures observed in the clinical trial. Then we will reject the null hypothesis if $x \geq a$, where $a$ is chosen so that if the null hypothesis is true, $\text{Prob}(X \geq a) = 0.01$, where $X$ is the random number of cures before the clinical trial is conducted.

If the null hypothesis is true, the mean of $X$ is $2000 \times 0.8 = 1600$ and the variance of $X$ is $2000 \times 0.8 \times 0.2 = 320$. Thus the standard deviation of $X$ is $\sqrt{320} \approx 17.89$.

We want $\text{Prob}(X \geq a|\theta = 0.8) = 0.01$. This gives $\text{Prob}\left(\frac{X - 1600}{17.89} \geq \frac{a - 1600}{17.89}\right) = 0.01$, so that upon using a normal approximation to the binomial and standardizing, $\text{Prob}\left(Z \geq \frac{a - 1600}{17.89}\right) = 0.01$. From Eq. (6.19), $(a - 1600)/17.89$, giving $a = 1641.12$. Rounding up, the critical point is 1642.

In R: `qnorm(0.01, mean = 1600, sd = 17.89, lower.tail`
`= FALSE)`.

(b) Since the observed number of cures (1634) is less than the critical point, we do not have enough evidence to reject the null hypothesis.

(c) The $P$-value is $\text{Prob}(X \geq 1634)$ given that the null hypothesis is true. Standardizing, the $P$-value is $\text{Prob}\left(\frac{X - 1600}{17.88854} \geq \frac{1634 - 1600}{17.88854}\right) \approx \text{Prob}(Z \geq 1.90) = 0.0287$. Since the $P$-value exceeds the chosen Type I error 0.01, we do not have enough evidence to reject the null hypothesis. This agrees with the conclusion reached in part (b).

In R: pnorm(1634, mean = 1600, sd = 17.89, lower.tail
= FALSE) or prop.test(x = 1634, n = 2000, p = 0.8,
alternative = "greater", conf.level = 0.99, correct = FALSE).

(d) Since the observed number of cures (1648) is greater than the critical point, we can reject the null hypothesis and claim that we have significant evidence that the new medicine is superior to the current one.

(e) The $P$-value is Prob($X \geq 1648$) given that the null hypothesis is true. Upon standardizing, this is Prob$\left(\frac{X-1600}{17.88854} \geq \frac{1648-1600}{17.88854}\right) \approx$ Prob($Z \geq 2.68$) = 0.0037. Since the $P$-value is less than the chosen Type I error 0.01, we have enough evidence to reject the null hypothesis. This agrees with the conclusion reached in part (d).

In   R,   pnorm(1648, mean = 1600, sd = 17.89, lower.tail   =
FALSE) or prop.test(x = 1648, n = 2000, p = 0.8,
alternative = "greater", conf.level = 0.99, correct = FALSE).

**9.5** (a) Let $p$ be the proportion of cures observed in the clinical trial. We will reject the null hypothesis if $p \geq b$, where $b$ is chosen so that if the null hypothesis is true, Prob($P \geq b$) = 0.01, where $P$ is the random proportion of cures before the clinical trial is conducted.

If the null hypothesis is true, the mean of $P$ is 0.8 and the variance of $P$ is $0.8 \times 0.2/2000 = 0.00008$, so that the standard deviation of $P$ is approximately 0.0089443.

If the null hypothesis is true, then upon using the normal approximation to the binomial and standardizing, we get Prob$\left(Z \geq \frac{b-0.8}{0.0089443}\right) = 0.01$. From Eq. (6.19), $(b - 0.8)/0.0089443 = 2.326$. From this, $b = 0.820844$.

In   R:   qnorm(0.01, mean = 0.8, sd = 0.0089443, lower.tail
= FALSE).

(b) Since the counts are 2000 times larger than the proportions, the "numbers" critical point should be 2000 times larger than the "proportions" critical point. Since $2000 \times 0.820844 = 1641.6$, this requirement is satisfied.

**9.6** (a) Let $p$ be the proportion of heads observed. Then we will reject the null hypothesis if $p \leq a$ or if $p \geq b$, where $a$ and $b$ are chosen so that if the coin is fair, Prob($P \leq a$) = 0.025, Prob($P \geq b$) = 0.025. If the null hypothesis is true, $P$ has mean 0.5 and variance $0.5 \times 0.5/1600 = 0.00015625$, and thus standard deviation 0.0125.

We thus have Prob($P \geq b|\theta = 0.5$) = 0.025. From this, Prob$\left(\frac{P-0.5}{0.0125} \geq \frac{b-0.5}{0.0125}\right) = 0.025$.

Therefore Prob$\left(Z \geq \frac{b-0.5}{0.0125}\right) = 0.025$. From Eq. (6.17), $(b - 0.5)/0.0125 = 1.96$, giving $b = 0.5245$. By symmetry, $a = 0.5 - 0.0245 = 0.4755$.

In   R:   qnorm(0.025, mean = 0.5, sd = 0.0125, lower.tail
= FALSE).

(b) Since the observed proportion of heads, $p = 844/1600 = 0.5275$, exceeds the upper critical point 0.5245, we have enough evidence to reject the null hypothesis and claim that we have significant evidence that the coin is unfair.

(c) Since this is a two-sided test, the $P$-value is $\text{Prob}(P \geq 0.5275) + \text{Prob}(P \leq 0.4725)$ assuming that the coin is fair. Upon standardizing, the $P$-value is $\text{Prob}(Z \geq (0.5275 - 0.5)/0.0125) + \text{Prob}(Z \leq (0.4725 - 0.5)/0.0125) = \text{Prob}(Z \geq 2.2) + \text{Prob}(Z \leq -2.2) = 0.0278$. Since this is less than the chosen numerical value 0.05 of the Type 1 error, we have enough evidence to reject the null hypothesis. This agrees with the decision reached in part (b).

In R: `pnorm(0.5275, mean = 0.5, sd = 0.0125, lower.tail = FALSE) +`
`pnorm(0.4725, mean = 0.5, sd = 0.0125, lower.tail = TRUE)` or
`prop.test(x = 844, n = 1600, p = 0.5,`
`alternative = "two.sided", conf.level = 0.95,          correct = FALSE)`.

**9.7** (a) Denote the probability that the number 29 comes up by $\theta$. Under the null hypothesis, $\theta = \frac{1}{38}$ and under the alternative hypothesis, $\theta > \frac{1}{38}$.

The test statistic is $p$, the proportion of times that 29 came up. Under the null hypothesis and using the normal distribution approximation to the distribution of $P$, the "before the experiment" random variable, $P$, has mean $\frac{1}{38}$ and variance $\frac{\frac{1}{38} \times \frac{37}{38}}{420} \approx 0.000061$. If the critical point is denoted by $c$, we require $\text{Prob}((P > c | H_0 \text{ true}) = 0.05$. Standardizing and using the normal distribution approximation, this gives $\text{Prob}\left(Z > \frac{c - \frac{1}{38}}{\sqrt{0.000061}}\right) = 0.05$, so that $\text{Prob}\left(Z < \frac{c - \frac{1}{38}}{\sqrt{0.000061}}\right) = 1 - 0.05 = 0.95$. From Eq. (6.11), $\frac{c - \frac{1}{38}}{\sqrt{0.000061}} = 1.645$. From this, $c = 0.03916$.

In   R:   `qnorm(0.05, mean = 1/38, sd = sqrt(1/38 * 37/38 / 420), lower.tail = FALSE)`

We observe $p = \frac{14}{420} \approx 0.0333$. Since $p$ is less than the critical point $C = 0.03916$ and the test is one-sided up, we do not have enough evidence to reject the null hypothesis.

(b) We denote $X$ as the number of times that the number 29 will come up, and use the observed number $x$ of times that the number 29 did come up as the test statistic. If the null hypothesis is true, $X$ approximately has mean $420 \times \frac{1}{38}$ and variance $420 \times \frac{1}{38} \times \frac{37}{38}$.

We observe $x = 14$. The $P$-value is $\text{Prob}(X > 14 | H_0 \text{ true})$. Standardizing and using the normal distribution approximation, this is approximately $\text{Prob}\left(Z > \frac{14 - 420 \times \frac{1}{38}}{\sqrt{420 \times \frac{1}{38} \times \frac{37}{38}}}\right) = 1 - \text{Prob}\left(Z < \frac{14 - 420 \times \frac{1}{38}}{\sqrt{420 \times \frac{1}{38} \times \frac{37}{38}}}\right) \approx 1 - \text{Prob}(Z < 0.90) = 0.1841$. Since the $P$-value is greater than $\alpha = 0.05$, we do not have enough evidence to reject the null hypothesis.

In R: there are several options. We can manually calculate the P-value, either manually standardizing or providing the mean and standard deviation:
`pnorm((14 - 1/38 * 420) / sqrt(420 * 1/38 * 37/38), lower.tail = FALSE)` or
`pnorm(14, mean = 1/38 * 420, sd = sqrt(420 * 1/38 * 37/38), lower.tail = FALSE)`. We can also run the whole test in R: `prop.test(14, 420, p = 1/38, alternative = "greater", correct = FALSE)`. If we do this, we should at least state the test statistic and P-values before writing a conclusion. Since R will print out the test statistic as a proportion, we will need to convert it back to a count:
`prop.test(14, 420, p = 1/38, alternative = "greater", correct = FALSE)$estimate * 420`. We can then print out the P-value with
`prop.test(14, 420, p = 1/38, alternative = "greater", correct = FALSE)$p.value`.

**9.8** We will reject the null hypothesis if the observed number $x$ of successes is greater than or equal to the critical point $c$, where $c$ is chosen so that $\text{Prob}(X \geq c) = 0.05$ if the null hypothesis is true. Under the null hypothesis, $X$ has mean 1120 and variance 336, so upon using the normal distribution approximation and standardizing, $\text{Prob}\left(\frac{X-1120}{\sqrt{336}} > \frac{c-1120}{\sqrt{336}}\right) = 0.05$. This gives $\frac{c-1120}{\sqrt{336}} = 1.645$, and from this $c = 1150.15$, or rounding up, $c = 1151$.

(a) Suppose first that $\theta = 0.71$. If $X$ is the number of successes, the power of the test is $\text{Prob}(X \geq 1151)$ given that $\theta = 0.71$. If $\theta = 0.71$, the mean of $X$ is 1136 and the variance of $X$ is 329.44. Upon using the normal distribution approximation and standardizing, the power of the test is approximately $\text{Prob}\left(\frac{X-1136}{\sqrt{329.44}} \geq \frac{1151-1136}{\sqrt{329.44}}\right)$. This is $\text{Prob}(Z \geq 0.826) \approx 0.204$.

(b) Suppose next that $\theta = 0.72$. If $X$ is the number of successes, the power of the test is $\text{Prob}(X \geq 1151)$ given that $\theta = 0.72$. If $\theta = 0.72$, the mean of $X$ is 1152 and the variance of $X$ is 322.56. Upon using the normal distribution approximation and standardizing, the power of the test is approximately $\text{Prob}\left(\frac{X-1152}{\sqrt{322.56}} \geq \frac{1151-1152}{\sqrt{322.56}}\right)$. This is $\text{Prob}(Z \geq 0.0557) \approx 0.4261$.

(c) Suppose next that $\theta = 0.73$. If $X$ is the number of successes, the power of the test is $\text{Prob}(X \geq 1151)$ given that $\theta = 0.73$. If $\theta = 0.73$, the mean of $X$ is 1168 and the variance of $X$ is 315.36. Upon using the normal distribution approximation and standardizing, the power of the test is approximately $\text{Prob}\left(\frac{X-1168}{\sqrt{315.36}} \geq \frac{1151-1168}{\sqrt{315.36}}\right)$. This is $\text{Prob}(Z \geq -0.957) \approx 0.827$.

(d) Suppose next that $\theta = 0.74$. If $X$ is the number of successes, the power of the test is $\text{Prob}(X \geq 1151)$ given that $\theta = 0.74$. If $\theta = 0.74$, the mean of $X$ is 1184 and the variance of $X$ is 307.84. Upon using the normal distribution approximation and standardizing, the power of the test is approximately $\text{Prob}\left(\frac{X-1184}{\sqrt{307.84}} \geq \frac{1151-1184}{\sqrt{307.84}}\right)$. This is $\text{Prob}(Z \geq -1.88) \approx 0.9699$.

(e) Suppose finally that $\theta = 0.75$. If $X$ is the number of successes, the power of the test is $\text{Prob}(X \geq 1151)$ given that $\theta = 0.75$. If $\theta = 0.75$, the mean of

$X$ is 1200 and the variance of $X$ is 300. Upon using the normal distribution approximation and standardizing, the power of the test is approximately $\text{Prob}\left(\frac{X-1200}{\sqrt{300}} \geq \frac{1151-1200}{\sqrt{300}}\right)$. This is $\text{Prob}(Z \geq -2.83) \approx 0.9977$.

**9.9** We reject the null hypothesis if the observed number $x$ of successes is greater than or equal to the critical point $c$, where $c$ is chosen so that $\text{Prob}(X \geq c) = 0.05$ if the null hypothesis is true. Under the null hypothesis, $X$ has mean 280 and variance 84, so upon using the normal distribution approximation and standardizing, $\text{Prob}\left(\frac{X-280}{\sqrt{84}} > \frac{c-280}{\sqrt{84}}\right) = 0.05$. This gives $\frac{c-280}{\sqrt{84}} = 1.645$, and from this $c = 295.08$, or rounding up, $c = 296$.

(a) Suppose first that $\theta = 0.71$. If $X$ is the number of successes, the power of the test is $\text{Prob}(X \geq 296)$ given that $\theta = 0.71$. If $\theta = 0.71$, the mean of $X$ is 284 and the variance of $X$ is 82.36. Upon using the normal distribution approximation and standardizing, the power of the test is approximately $\text{Prob}\left(\frac{X-284}{\sqrt{82.36}} \geq \frac{296-284}{\sqrt{82.36}}\right)$. This is $\text{Prob}(Z \geq 1.32) \approx 0.064$.

(b) Suppose next that $\theta = 0.72$. If $X$ is the number of successes, the power of the test is $\text{Prob}(X \geq 296)$ given that $\theta = 0.72$. If $\theta = 0.72$, the mean of $X$ is 288 and the variance of $X$ is 80.64. Upon using the normal distribution approximation and standardizing, the power of the test is approximately $\text{Prob}\left(\frac{X-288}{\sqrt{80.64}} \geq \frac{296-288}{\sqrt{80.64}}\right)$. This is $\text{Prob}(Z \geq 0.89) \approx 0.187$.

(c) Suppose next that $\theta = 0.73$. If $X$ is the number of successes, the power of the test is $\text{Prob}(X \geq 296)$ given that $\theta = 0.73$. If $\theta = 0.73$, the mean of $X$ is 292 and the variance of $X$ is 78.84. Upon using the normal distribution approximation and standardizing, the power of the test is approximately $\text{Prob}\left(\frac{X-292}{\sqrt{78.84}} \geq \frac{296-292}{\sqrt{78.84}}\right)$. This is $\text{Prob}(Z \geq 0.45) \approx 0.326$.

(d) Suppose next that $\theta = 0.74$. If $X$ is the number of successes, the power of the test is $\text{Prob}(X \geq 296)$ given that $\theta = 0.74$. If $\theta = 0.74$, the mean of $X$ is 296 and the variance of $X$ is 76.94. Upon using the normal distribution approximation and standardizing, the power of the test is approximately $\text{Prob}\left(\frac{X-296}{\sqrt{76.94}} \geq \frac{296-296}{\sqrt{76.94}}\right)$. This is $\text{Prob}(Z \geq 0) = 0.5$.

(e) Suppose finally that $\theta = 0.75$. If $X$ is the number of successes, the power of the test is $\text{Prob}(X \geq 296)$ given that $\theta = 0.75$. If $\theta = 0.75$, the mean of $X$ is 300 and the variance of $X$ is 75. Upon using the normal distribution approximation and standardizing, the power of the test is approximately $\text{Prob}\left(\frac{X-300}{\sqrt{75}} \geq \frac{296-300}{\sqrt{75}}\right)$. This is $\text{Prob}(Z \geq -0.46) \approx 0.677$.

**9.10** (a) From the answer to Problem 9.6, we will reject the null hypothesis if $p \leq 0.4755$ or if $p \geq 0.5245$. The power of the test is then $\text{Prob}(P \leq 0.4755) + \text{Prob}(P \geq 0.5245)$, given that the probability of heads is $\theta$.

(i) If $\theta = 0.51$, the mean of $P$ is 0.51 and the variance of $P$ is 0.000156187. Upon standardizing, the power of the test is $\text{Prob}\left(\dfrac{P-0.51}{\sqrt{0.000156187}}\right.$

$\left.\le \dfrac{0.4755-0.51}{\sqrt{0.000156187}}\right) + \text{Prob}\left(\dfrac{P-0.51}{\sqrt{0.000156187}} \ge \dfrac{0.5245-0.51}{\sqrt{0.000156187}}\right)$.

This is approximately $\text{Prob}(Z \le -2.76) + \text{Prob}(Z \ge 1.16) \approx +0.0029 + 0.1230 = 0.1256$.

(ii) If $\theta = 0.52$, the mean of $P$ is 0.52 and the variance of $P$ is 0.000156. Upon standardizing, the power of the test is $\text{Prob}\left(\dfrac{P-0.52}{\sqrt{0.000156}} \le \dfrac{0.4755-0.52}{\sqrt{0.000156}}\right) +$

$\text{Prob}\left(\dfrac{P-0.52}{\sqrt{0.000156}} \ge \dfrac{0.5245-0.52}{\sqrt{0.000156}}\right)$. This is approximately $\text{Prob}(Z \le -3.56) + \text{Prob}(Z \ge 0.36) \approx 0 + 0.359 = 0.359$.

(iii) If $\theta = 0.53$, the mean of $P$ is 0.53 and the variance of $P$ is 0.000155687. Upon standardizing, the power of the test is $\text{Prob}\left(\dfrac{P-0.53}{\sqrt{0.000155687}}\right.$

$\left.\le \dfrac{0.4755-0.53}{\sqrt{0.000155687}}\right) + \text{Prob}\left(\dfrac{P-0.53}{\sqrt{0.000155687}} \ge \dfrac{0.5245-0.53}{\sqrt{0.000155687}}\right)$. This is approximately $\text{Prob}(Z \le -4.4) + \text{Prob}(Z \ge -0.439) \approx 0 + 0.676 = 0.676$.

(iv) If $\theta = 0.54$, the mean of $P$ is 0.54 and the variance of $P$ is 0.00015256. Upon standardizing, the power of the test is $\text{Prob}\left(\dfrac{P-0.54}{\sqrt{0.00015256}}\right.$

$\left.\le \dfrac{0.4755-0.54}{\sqrt{0.00015256}}\right) + \text{Prob}\left(\dfrac{P-0.54}{\sqrt{0.00015256}} \ge \dfrac{0.5245-0.54}{\sqrt{0.00015256}}\right)$. This is approximately $\text{Prob}(Z \le -4.73) + \text{Prob}(Z \ge -1.24) \approx 0 + 0.892 = 0.8925$.

(v) If $\theta = 0.55$, the mean of $P$ is 0.55 and the variance of $P$ is 0.000154687. Upon standardizing, the power of the test is $\text{Prob}\left(\dfrac{P-0.55}{\sqrt{0.000154687}}\right.$

$\left.\le \dfrac{0.4755-0.55}{\sqrt{0.000154687}}\right) + \text{Prob}\left(\dfrac{P-0.55}{\sqrt{0.000154687}} \ge \dfrac{0.5245-0.55}{\sqrt{0.000154687}}\right)$. This is approximately $\text{Prob}(Z \le -5.99) + \text{Prob}(Z \ge -2.05) \approx 0 + 0.980 = 0.980$.

(b) The power curve is symmetric around $\theta = 0.5$.

# Chapter 10

**10.1** (a) Define $\theta_1$ as the probability that a trained mouse will make the correct decision and $\theta_2$ as the probability that an untrained mouse will make the correct decision. The null hypothesis is that trained mice are equally likely to make a correct decision as are untrained mice, that is, that $\theta_1 = \theta_2 = \theta$ (unspecified). The alternative hypothesis is that trained mice are more likely to make a correct decision than are untrained mice, that is, that $\theta_1 > \theta_2$.

(b) It is first necessary to consider the formula for $z$ as given in Eq. (10.4). If the alternative hypothesis is true, we would expect the proportion of trained mice making a correct decision $(o_{11}/r_1)$ to be greater than the proportion of untrained mice making a correct decision $(o_{21}/r_2)$. This implies that, if the alternative hypothesis is true, we would expect $z$ to be positive. Therefore the test is one-sided up.

(c) From the computationally convenient Eq. (10.5), $z = \dfrac{(8 \times 7 - 5 \times 6)\sqrt{26}}{\sqrt{14 \times 12 \times 13 \times 13}} = 0.79$.

In R, we can use `prop.test()` and then take the square root of the "X-squared" statistic it prints out to get the $z$ statistic.

```
tab <- matrix(c(8, 6, 5, 7), nrow = 2, byrow = TRUE,
              dimnames = list(c("Trained", "Untrained"),
              c("Correct", "Incorrect")))
prop.test(tab, correct = FALSE, alternative = "greater")
sqrt(0.61905)
```

(d) Since this is a one-sided up test, the critical point is 1.645 (from Eq. (6.14)). Since the value of $z$ is less than 1.645, we do not have enough evidence to reject the null hypothesis. In R: `qnorm(0.05, lower.tail = FALSE)`.

(e) For a one-sided up test, the $P$-value is $\mathrm{Prob}(Z \geq 0.79) = 0.2148$. This exceeds the chosen value 0.05 of $\alpha$, so we do not have enough evidence to reject the null hypothesis. In R, the `prop.test()` print out includes a $P$-value. Alternatively, it can be calculated manually: `pnorm(0.79, lower.tail = FALSE)`.

(f) They agree. They must agree since doing the test via Approach 1 is equivalent to doing the test via Approach 2.

**10.2** (a) The percentages are the same in both data sets.

(b) From Eq. (10.5), $z = \dfrac{(80 \times 70 - 50 \times 60)\sqrt{260}}{\sqrt{140 \times 120 \times 130 \times 130}} = 2.49$.

In R:

```
tab <- matrix(c(80, 60, 50, 70), nrow = 2, byrow = TRUE,
              dimnames = list(c("Trained", "Untrained"),
              c("Correct", "Incorrect")))
prop.test(tab, correct = FALSE, alternative = "greater")
sqrt(6.1905)
```

(c) The critical point is 1.645 (the same as for data set 1). Since the value of $z$ exceeds this critical point, we have enough evidence to reject the null hypothesis.

(d) The $P$-value is $\mathrm{Prob}(Z \geq 2.49) = 0.0064$. Since this is less than 0.05, we have enough evidence to reject the null hypothesis. In R: `pnorm(2.49, lower.tail = FALSE)`.

(e) They agree. They must agree since doing the test via Approach 1 is equivalent to doing the test via Approach 2.

(f) We do not reach the same conclusion. The reason is that the actual numbers matter, not the percentages, and the numbers differ between the two data sets.

**10.3** (a) Define $\theta_1$ as the probability that a child is cured by the proposed medicine and $\theta_2$ as the probability that an adult is cured by the proposed medicine. The null hypothesis is that $\theta_1 = \theta_2 = \theta$ (unspecified). The alternative hypothesis is that $\theta_1 \neq \theta_2$.

(b) The test is two-sided since we have no prior view as to whether adults or children have the higher cure probability.

(c) From Eq. (10.5), $z = \dfrac{(116 \times 23 - 137 \times 24)\sqrt{300}}{\sqrt{253 \times 47 \times 140 \times 160}} = -0.66$.

In R, we can use $\texttt{prop.test()}$ and then take the negative square root of the "X-squared" statistic it prints out. We need the negative square root because the cure rate among children is less than the cure rate among adults so our statistic should be negative.

```
tab <- matrix(c(116, 24, 137, 23), nrow = 2, byrow = TRUE,
              dimnames = list(c("Children", "Adults"),
              c("Cured", "Not cured")))
prop.test(tab, correct = FALSE, alternative = "two.sided")
-sqrt(0.43295)
```

(d) Since the test is two-sided and the value of $\alpha$ is 0.05, there are two critical points, a "down" critical point $-1.96$ and an "up" critical point $+1.96$ (see Eq. (6.16)). Since the value of $z$ is not less than or equal to $-1.96$ and is not greater than or equal to $+1.96$, we do not have enough evidence to reject the null hypothesis. In R: $\texttt{qnorm(0.025, lower.tail = TRUE)}$ and $\texttt{qnorm(0.025, lower.tail = FALSE)}$.

(e) The $P$-value is Prob$(Z \leq -0.66)$ + Prob$(Z \geq +0.66)$ = 0.2546 + 0.2546 = 0.5092. Since this exceeds 0.05, we do not have enough evidence to reject the null hypothesis. In R: $\texttt{pnorm(-0.66, lower.tail = TRUE)}$ + $\texttt{pnorm(0.66, lower.tail = FALSE)}$.

(f) They agree, since doing the test via Approach 1 is equivalent to doing it via Approach 2.

**10.4** (a) Define $\theta_1$ as the probability that a vaccinated person will contract the disease and $\theta_2$ as the probability that a person given the placebo will contract the disease. The null hypothesis is that a vaccinated person is equally likely to contract the disease as is a person given the placebo, that is, that $\theta_1 = \theta_2 = \theta$ (unspecified). The alternative hypothesis is that a vaccinated person is less likely to contract the disease than a person given the placebo is, that is, that $\theta_1 < \theta_2$.

(b) To answer this question, we first have to consider the formula for $z$ as given in (10.4). If the alternative hypothesis is true, we would expect the proportion of vaccinated people contracting the disease $(o_{11}/r_1)$ to be less than the proportion of people given the placebo contracting the disease $(o_{21}/r_2)$. This implies that if the alternative hypothesis is true, we would expect $z$ to be negative. Therefore the test is one-sided down.

(c) From the computationally convenient Eq. (10.5),

$$z = \frac{(50 \times 9850 - 150 \times 9950)\sqrt{20{,}000}}{\sqrt{10{,}000 \times 10{,}000 \times 2\,00 \times 19{,}800}} \approx -7.1.$$

In R, we can use `prop.test()` and then take the negative square root of the "X-squared" statistic it prints out. We need the negative square root because the statistic should be negative since the illness rate is lower amongst the vaccine group than the placebo group.

```
tab <- matrix(c(50, 9950, 150, 9850), nrow = 2, byrow = TRUE,
              dimnames = list(c("Vaccine", "Placebo"),
              c("Sick", "Not sick")))
prop.test(tab, correct = FALSE, alternative = "less")
-sqrt(50.505)
```

(d) Since this is a one-sided down test, there is only one critical point, namely a "down" critical point. From Eq. (6.19) and the fact that $\alpha = 0.01$, this is $-2.326$. Since the value of $z$ is less than $-2.326$ we have enough evidence to reject the null hypothesis. In R: `qnorm(0.01, lower.tail = TRUE)`.

(e) The $z$ value $-7.1$ is "off the chart", and the $P$-value is therefore less than the smallest value on the chart (0.0002). This is less than 0.01, so we have enough evidence to reject the null hypothesis. In R: `pnorm(-7.1, lower.tail = TRUE)`.

(f) They agree, since doing the test via Approach 1 is equivalent to doing the test via Approach 2.

**10.5** The null hypothesis is $\theta_1 = \theta_2$ and the alternative hypothesis is $\theta_1 > \theta_2$.

The formula for $z$ as given in Eq. (10.4) shows that the test is one-sided up. From the computationally convenient Eq. (10.5),

$$z = \frac{(15995 \times 200 - 15800 \times 5)\sqrt{32000}}{\sqrt{16000 \times 16000 \times 31795 \times 205}} = 13.663.$$

From Eq. (6.19), the critical point for this one-sided up test is 2.326. Since $z > 2.326$ we have enough evidence to reject the null hypothesis.

In R, we can calculate the critical point for Approach 1 with `qnorm(0.01, lower.tail = FALSE)` or the P-value for Approach 2 with `pnorm(13.663, lower.tail = FALSE)`. We can also take the full R approach:

```
tab <- matrix(c(15995, 5, 15800, 200), nrow = 2, byrow = TRUE,
              dimnames = list(c("Vaccine", "Placebo"),
              c("Virus", "No virus")))
prop.test(tab, correct = FALSE, alternative = "greater")
```

The $P$-value is much smaller than $\alpha = 0.01$ so we have enough evidence to reject the null hypothesis by Approach 2 as well.

**10.6** (a) The exact $P$-value is $\dfrac{\binom{10}{8}\binom{10}{5}}{\binom{20}{13}} + \dfrac{\binom{10}{9}\binom{10}{4}}{\binom{20}{13}} + \dfrac{\binom{10}{10}\binom{10}{3}}{\binom{20}{13}} = \dfrac{13350}{77520} \approx 0.172.$

In R:

```
sum(dhyper(x = 8:10, m = 13, n = 7, k = 10))    or    1-phyper
(q = 7, m = 13, n = 7, k = 10) or
phyper(q = 7, m = 13, n = 7, k = 10, lower.tail = FALSE).
```

Finally, we can use the built in `fisher.test()` function: `fisher.test (x = matrix(c(8, 5, 2, 5), nrow = 2), alternative = "greater")`.

(b) The value of $z$ is approximately 1.41, leading to a $P$-value of approximately 0.079. In R:

```
prop.test(c(8, 5), c(10, 10), alternative = "greater",
correct = FALSE).
```

(c) The value of $z$ is approximately 9.94, leading to a $P$-value of approximately 0.174. In R:

```
prop.test(c(8, 5), c(10, 10), alternative = "greater",
correct = TRUE).
```

(d) The approximation using a continuity correction is more accurate than the approximation that does not use a continuity correction.

**10.7** (a) The exact $P$-value is

$$\frac{\binom{14}{10}\binom{14}{6}}{\binom{28}{16}} + \frac{\binom{14}{11}\binom{14}{5}}{\binom{28}{16}} + \frac{\binom{14}{12}\binom{14}{4}}{\binom{28}{16}} + \frac{\binom{14}{13}\binom{14}{3}}{\binom{28}{16}} + \frac{\binom{14}{14}\binom{14}{2}}{\binom{28}{16}} = \frac{3831009}{304217755} \approx 0.126.$$

In R, we can do `sum(dhyper(x = 10:14, m = 16, n = 12, k = 14))` or

```
1 - phyper(q = 9, m = 16, n = 12, k = 14) or
phyper(q = 9, m = 16, n = 12, k = 14, lower.tail = FALSE).
```

Finally, we can also use the built in `fisher.test()` function: `fisher.test (x = matrix(c(10, 6, 4, 8), nrow = 2), alternative = "greater")`.

(b) The value of $z$ is approximately 1.53, leading to a $P$-value of approximately 0.063. In R:

```
prop.test(c(10, 6), c(14, 14), alternative = "greater",
correct = TRUE).
```

(c) The value of $z$ is approximately 1.15, leading to a $P$-value of approximately 0.125. In R:

```
prop.test(c(10, 6), c(14, 14), alternative = "greater",
correct = TRUE).
```

(d) The approximation using a continuity correction is more accurate than the approximation that does not use a continuity correction.

# Chapter 11

**11.1** The value of the first test statistic is $\dfrac{(10 \times 14 - 16 \times 8)^2 \times 48}{26 \times 22 \times 18 \times 30} = 0.022378$.

To calculate the second test statistic, we first calculate

$e_{11} = 26 \times 18/48 = 9.75$, $e_{12} = 26 \times 30/48 = 16.25$, $e_{21} = 22 \times 18/48 = 8.25$,

$e_{22} = 22 \times 30/48 = 13.75$.

The value of the second test statistic is then

$(10-9.75)^2/9.75+(16-16.25)^2/16.25+(8-8.25)^2/8.25+(14-13.75)^2/13.75$,
which is $= 0.0064103 + 0.0038462 + 0.0075758 + 0.0045455 = 0.022378$. The
two values therefore agree.

In R, we can double check that we got the right answer for both formulas:

```
tab <- matrix(c(10, 16, 8, 14), nrow = 2, byrow = TRUE,
              dimnames = list(c("Row 1", "Row 2"), c("Col 1",
              "Col 2")))
prop.test(tab, correct = FALSE, alternative = "two.sided")
```

**11.2** (a) There are $(5 - 1) \times (7 - 1) = 4 \times 6 = 24$ degrees of freedom.
(b) Since $\alpha = 0.05$, the critical point in the chi-square chart for 24 degrees of
freedom is 36.4150, so since 38.33 exceeds this, we have enough evidence to
reject the null hypothesis. In R:
`qchisq(0.05, df = 24, lower.tail = FALSE)`.
(c) It cannot be found exactly from the chi-square chart. It can only be found by
using a computer package. In R: `pchisq(38.33, df = 24, lower.tail`
`= FALSE)`.

**11.3** (a) There are $(4 - 1) \times (6 - 1) = 3 \times 5 = 15$ degrees of freedom.
(b) Since $\alpha = 0.01$, the critical point for 15 degrees of freedom is 30.5779. Since
28.68 is less than this, we do not have enough evidence to reject the null
hypothesis. In R: `qchisq(0.01, df = 15, lower.tail = FALSE)`.
(c) It cannot be found exactly from the chi-square chart. It can only be found by
using a computer package. In R: `pchisq(28.68, df = 15, lower.tail`
`= FALSE)`.

**11.4** The (null hypothesis) expected numbers are:

| severity of disorder | blood type | | | | total |
| --- | --- | --- | --- | --- | --- |
| | O | A | B | AB | |
| absent | 541.20 | 212.96 | 96.8 | 469.04 | 1320 |
| mild | 43.05 | 16.94 | 7.70 | 37.31 | 105 |
| severe | 30.75 | 12.10 | 5.50 | 26.65 | 75 |
| total | 615 | 242 | 110 | 533 | 1500 |

(For example, $e_{23} = r_2 \times c_3/n = 105 \times 110/1500 = 7.70$.) The value of $\chi^2$ is $(529 - 541.20)^2/541.20 + \ldots + (31 - 26.65)^2/26.65 = 12.352$. There are six degrees of freedom, so the $\alpha = 0.05$ critical point is 12.592. Since $12.352 < 12.592$, we do not have enough evidence to reject the null hypothesis.

In R:

```
qchisq(0.05, df = 6, lower.tail = FALSE) # Critical value
pchisq(12.352, df = 6, lower.tail = FALSE) # Manual P-value
tab <- matrix(c(529, 220, 95, 476, 58, 13, 8, 26, 28, 9, 7, 31),
              nrow = 3, byrow = TRUE, dimnames = list(c("Absent",
              "Mild", "Severe"), c("O", "A", "B", "AB")))
chisq.test(tab) # Full R approach
```

**11.5** The null hypothesis is that there is no association between the defective status and the machine used. The alternative hypothesis is that there is some association between the defective status and the machine used.

The (null hypothesis) expected numbers are:

| | machine A | machine B | machine C | total |
|---|---|---|---|---|
| defective | $\frac{26 \times 62}{200} = 8.06$ | $\frac{26 \times 68}{200} = 8.84$ | $\frac{26 \times 70}{200} = 9.1$ | 26 |
| non-defective | $\frac{174 \times 62}{200} = 53.94$ | $\frac{174 \times 68}{200} = 59.16$ | $\frac{174 \times 70}{200} = 60.90$ | 174 |
| total | 62 | 68 | 70 | 200 |

From this, $\chi^2 = 0.0004467 + 0.9124 + 0.9241 + 0.0000667 + 0.1363 + 0.1381 \approx 2.11$. From the chi-square chart for $\alpha = 0.05$ and $(2 - 1) \times (3 - 1) = 2$ degrees of freedom, the critical point is 5.9915. Since the observed $\chi^2$ is less than the critical point, we do not have enough evidence to reject the null hypothesis.

In R:

```
qchisq(0.05, df = 2, lower.tail = FALSE) # Critical point
pchisq(2.11, df = 2, lower.tail = FALSE) # Manual P-value
tab <- matrix(c(8, 6, 12, 54, 62, 58), nrow = 2, byrow = TRUE,
              dimnames = list(c("Defective", "Non-defective"),
              c("Machine A", "Machine B", "Machine C")))
chisq.test(tab)  # Full R approach
```

# Chapter 12

**12.1** Under the null hypothesis, the mean number of times that any number turns up is 1000. The value of $\chi^2$ is $\dfrac{(9)^2 + (16)^2 + (38)^2 + (12)^2 + (2)^2 + (21)^2}{1000} = 2.37$. Since $\alpha = 0.05$, the critical point of $\chi^2$ with five degrees of freedom is 11.0705, so we do not have enough evidence to reject the null hypothesis.

In R: `chisq.test(c(1009, 984, 1038, 988, 1002, 979), p = rep(1/6, 6))`.

**12.2** Under the null hypothesis, the respective expected numbers are $250, 500$ and $250$, so the value of $\chi^2$ is

$$\frac{(-40)^2}{250} + \frac{(-16)^2}{500} + \frac{(56)^2}{250} = 19.456.$$

Since $\alpha = 0.05$, the critical point of $\chi^2$ with two degrees of freedom is $5.9915$, so we have enough evidence to reject the null hypothesis.

In R: `chisq.test(c(210, 484, 306), p = c(1/4, 1/2, 1/4))`.

**12.3** We estimate $\theta$ by $\dfrac{484 + 612}{2000} = 0.548$. Under the null hypothesis, the expected numbers are then, respectively, $1000(0.452)^2$, $2000(0.548)(0.452)$ and $1000(0.548)^2$, that is, $204.3040$, $495.3920$ and $300.3040$. The value of $\chi^2$ is then $\dfrac{(210 - 204.3040)^2}{204.3040} + \dfrac{(484 - 495.3920)^2}{495.3920} + \dfrac{(306 - 300.3040)^2}{300.3040} = 0.5288$. Since $\alpha = 0.05$, the critical point of $\chi^2$ with one degree of freedom is $3.8415$, so we do not have enough evidence to reject the null hypothesis.

In R, we can calculate the value of $\chi^2$ with the `chisq.test()` function, but this function does not know that we estimated a parameter and so will have an incorrect amount of degrees of freedom when calculating the $P$-value. We thus need to calculate the $P$-value manually with the `pchisq()` function:

```
thetahat <- (484+2*306)/2000
chisq.test(c(210, 484, 306), p = c((1-thetahat)^2, 2*thetahat*
    (1-thetahat), thetahat^2))
pchisq(0.52881, df = 1, lower.tail = FALSE)
```

**12.4** Under the null hypothesis, the respective expected numbers are $250, 750, 750$ and $250$, so the value of $\chi^2$ is $\dfrac{(-6)^2}{250} + \dfrac{(32)^2}{750} + \dfrac{(-8)^2}{750} + \dfrac{(-18)^2}{250} = 2.8907$. Since $\alpha = 0.01$, the critical point of $\chi^2$ with three degrees of freedom is $11.3449$, so we do not have enough evidence to reject the null hypothesis.

In R: `chisq.test(c(244, 782, 742, 232), p = c(1/8, 3/8, 3/8, 1/8))`.

# Chapter 13

**13.1** (a) From the values of $\bar{x}$ and $s$ given, and using Eq. (13.3), $t = (6.63125 - 6.5)/[0.21437/\sqrt{8}] = 1.7317$. This is a one-sided up test, so the critical point is $1.895$ (7 degrees of freedom, $\alpha = 0.05$). Since the observed value of $t$ does not exceed this value, we do not have enough evidence to reject the null hypothesis.
In R: `qt(0.95, df = 7)`.

Alternatively, using R and Approach 2, we would find a P-value of 0.06347, which exceeds the $\alpha = 0.05$ level and thus we do not reject the null hypothesis: pt(1.7317, df = 7, lower.tail = FALSE).

We can also do the full R approach with

t.test(x = c(6.39, 6.75, 6.60, 6.43, 6.65, 7.05, 6.47, 6.71), alternative = "greater", mu = 6.5).

(b) From the information given and Eq. (13.3), $t = (6.65 - 6.5)/[0.2/\sqrt{25}] = 3.75$. This is a one-sided up test, and since $\alpha = 0.05$, the critical point is 2.492 (24 degrees of freedom). Since the observed value of $t$ exceeds this value, we have enough evidence to reject the null hypothesis. In R: qt(0.01, df = 24, lower.tail = FALSE).

In R, we could calculate a $P$-value instead of a critical point: pt(3.75, df = 24, lower.tail = FALSE). Since the $P$-value is 0.00049, which is less than $\alpha = 0.01$, we have significant evidence to reject the null hypothesis.

**13.2** (a) From the value of $s^2$ given, $s = 0.05$. From Eq. (13.3), $t = (14.985 - 15.000)/[0.05/\sqrt{25}] = -1.5$. With $\alpha = 0.05$, the critical points are $-2.064$ and $+2.064$ (24 degrees of freedom). Since the value of $t$ is not less than $-2.064$ and is not greater than $+2.064$, we do not have enough evidence to reject the null hypothesis. In R, qt(0.025, df = 24, lower.tail = TRUE) and qt(0.025, df = 24, lower.tail = FALSE).

In R, we could calculate a two-sided $P$-value instead of two critical points: pt(-1.5, df = 24) + pt(1.5, df = 24, lower.tail = FALSE). Since the $P$-value is 0.147, which is greater than $\alpha = 0.05$, we do not have significant evidence to reject the null hypothesis.

(b) We still have $s = 0.05$. From Eq. (13.3), $t = (14.975 - 15.000)/[0.05/\sqrt{25}] = -2.5$. The critical points have not changed. Since the value of $t$ is less than $-2.064$, we have enough evidence to reject the null hypothesis.

In R, we could calculate a two-sided $P$-value instead of two critical points: pt(-2.5, df = 24) + pt(2.5, df = 24, lower.tail = FALSE). Since the $P$-value is 0.0197, which is less than $\alpha = 0.05$, we have significant evidence to reject the null hypothesis.

(c) From the values given, $s = 0.03$. From Eq. (13.3), $t = (14.985 - 15.000)/[0.03/\sqrt{25}] = -2.5$. The critical points have not changed. Since the value of $t$ is less than $-2.064$, we have enough evidence to reject the null hypothesis. In R, the $P$-value would also remain the same.

**13.3** (a) From the values given, $s = 0.05$. From Eq. (13.3), $t = (4.98 - 5.00)/[0.05/\sqrt{16}] = -1.6$. This is a one-sided down test, so that since $\alpha = 0.05$, the critical point is $-1.753$ (15 degrees of freedom). Since the observed value of $t$ is not less than this value, we do not have enough evidence to reject the null hypothesis.

(b) From the values given and using From Eq. (13.3), $t = (4.98-5.00)/[0.04/\sqrt{16}]$ $= -2$. This is a one-sided down test, so that with $\alpha = 0.05$, the critical point is $-1.753$ (15 degrees of freedom). Since the observed value of $t$ is less than this value, we have enough evidence to reject the null hypothesis.

(c) The difference between the two conclusions is caused by the different values of $s$ in the two cases. The "noise" is larger in part (a) than it is in part (b), so that the signal-to-noise ratio is smaller in part (a) than it is in part (b), resulting in a smaller (and not significant) value of $t$ in part (a) and a significant value in part (b).

**13.4** (a) (i) From Eq. (13.3), the value of $t$ is $(8.42 - 8.5)/[0.16/\sqrt{9}] = -1.5$.

(a) (ii) There are 8 degrees of freedom, so the (two-sided) critical points are $+2.306$ and $-2.306$. Since the value of $t$ lies within these critical points, we do not have enough evidence to reject the null hypothesis. In R: `qt(0.025, df = 8, lower.tail = TRUE)` and `qt(0.025, df = 8, lower.tail = FALSE)`.

In R, we could calculate a two-sided $P$-value instead of two critical points: `pt(-1.5, df = 8) + pt(1.5, df = 8, lower.tail = FALSE)`. Since the $P$-value is 0.172, which is greater than $\alpha = 0.05$, we do not have significant evidence to reject the null hypothesis.

(b) From Eq. (13.3), the value of $t$ is $(8.42 - 8.5)/[0.16/\sqrt{25}] = -2.5$. There are 24 degrees of freedom, so the (two-sided) critical points are $+2.064$ and $-2.064$. Since the value of $t$ is below the "down" critical point, we have enough evidence to reject the null hypothesis. In R: `qt(0.025, df = 24, lower.tail = TRUE)` and `qt(0.025, df = 24, lower.tail = FALSE)`.

In R, we could calculate a two-sided $P$-value instead of two critical points: `pt(-2.5, df = 24) + pt(2.5, df = 24, lower.tail = FALSE)`. Since the $P$-value is 0.0197, which is less than $\alpha\ (= 0.05)$, we have enough evidence to reject the null hypothesis.

(c) There are two reasons for the differing conclusions. The main one is the sample size. The larger sample size leads to a larger value of $t$ in part (b) compared to part (a). (This ultimately derives from the formula for the variance of an average.) Another reason is that the critical points are different for the two different sample sizes, due to differing degrees of freedom.

**13.5** Computing $t$, we have $\bar{x} = \dfrac{27.9 + 27.5 + 30.5 + 23.8 + 26.4 + 28.9}{6} = 27.5$, and

$$s^2 = \frac{27.9^2 + 27.5^2 + 30.5^2 + 23.8^2 + 26.4^2 + 28.9^2 - 6 \times 27.5^2}{5} = 5.204,\ \text{so}$$

that $s = 2.28$. From Eq. (13.3), $t = \dfrac{27.5 - 26.9}{2.28/\sqrt{6}} = 0.6446$. There are $n - 1 = 6 - 1 = 5$ degrees of freedom. The critical point (five degrees of freedom, $\alpha = 0.05$) is 2.015 from the $t$ chart (in R: `qt(0.05, df = 5, lower.tail = FALSE)`).

Since the observed value of $t$ is less than the critical point and the test is one-sided up, we do not have enough evidence to reject the null hypothesis.

In R:

```
x <- c(27.9, 27.5, 30.5, 23.8, 26.4, 28.9)
(mean(x) - 26.9) / (sd(x) / sqrt(6)) # Manually calculate t
# Can also pull the t statistic and P-value from the t.test()
t.test(x, mu = 26.9, alternative = "greater")
t.test(x, mu = 26.9, alternative = "greater")$statistic
t.test(x, mu = 26.9, alternative = "greater")$p.value
```

**13.6** (a) From the data given, $t_2 = (474 - 428)/[32\sqrt{(1/9 + 1/11)}] = 3.20$. This is a one-sided up test, so that with $\alpha = 0.01$, the critical point is 2.552 (18 degrees of freedom). Since the observed value of $t_2$ exceeds this value, we reject the null hypothesis.

(b) Since the value of $t_1$ is the negative of the value of $t_2$, the answer to part (a) shows that $t_1 = -3.20$. With $t_1$ as the test statistic, the test is one-sided down and the critical point is $-2.552$ (18 degrees of freedom). Since the observed value of $t_1$ is less than this value, we reject the null hypothesis. This is the same conclusion as that reached with $t_2$ as the test statistic.

**13.7** (a) From the data given, $\bar{x}_2 - \bar{x}_1 = 0.992857$. Since $s_1^2 = 0.339$ and $s_2^2 = 0.669527$, the value of $s^2$ is 0.5192875 (from Eq. (13.13)). From this, s = 0.720616. Therefore the denominator in Eq. (13.13) is $0.720616\sqrt{(1/6 + 1/7)} = 0.400914$.

The value of $t_2$ as calculated from Eq. (13.15) is $0.992857/0.400914 \approx 2.48$. There are $n + m - 2 = 6 + 7 - 2 = 11$ degrees of freedom, and since this is a one-sided up test with $\alpha = 0.05$, we will reject the null hypothesis if $t_2$ is equal to or exceeds 1.796. Since $t_2$ does exceed 1.796, we have enough evidence to reject the null hypothesis.

In R:

```
# Since the question does not have the full data set, we
have to use the manual formulas
n1 <- 6;  n2 <- 7;  x1bar <- 8.75;  x2bar <- 9.742857;
s1sq <- 0.339;  s2sq <- 0.669527
num <- x2bar - x1bar
ssq <- ((n1-1) * s1sq + (n2-1) * s2sq) / (n1 + n2 - 2)
s <- sqrt(ssq)
den <- s * sqrt(1/n1 + 1/n2)
t2 <- num / den; t2
qt(0.05, df = n1 + n2 - 2, lower.tail = FALSE)
# Critical point for Approach 1
pt(t2, df = n1 + n2 - 2, lower.tail = FALSE)
# P-value for Approach 2
```

If we use R and Approach 2, we find the $P$-value of 0.015 to be less than $\alpha = 0.05$, so we have significant evidence to reject the null hypothesis.

(b) When $\alpha = 0.01$, we will reject the null hypothesis if $t_2$ exceeds 2.718. Since the value of $t_2$ is less than 2.718, we do not have enough evidence to reject the null hypothesis. In R, for the critical point: qt(0.01, df = n1 + n2 - 2, lower.tail = FALSE). The $P$-value from R is greater than 0.01, so we do not have enough evidence by Approach 2.

**13.8** With the above data, $s^2 = \dfrac{5 \times 5.204 + 6 \times 3.1329}{11} = 4.0743$, so that $s = 2.01849$. From this, $t_1 = \dfrac{27.5 - 29.94}{2.01849 \times \sqrt{\frac{1}{6} + \frac{1}{7}}} = -2.17$. There are 11 degrees of freedom so the two critical points are $-2.201$ and $+2.201$. Since $t_1$ is not less than $-2.201$ or greater than 2.201, we do not have enough evidence to reject the null hypothesis.

In R:

```
qt(0.025, df = 11);   qt(0.025, df = 11, lower.tail = FALSE)
# Critical points
# Manually calculate t value
x1 <- c(27.9, 27.5, 30.5, 23.8, 26.4, 28.9)
x2 <- c(30.9, 28.3, 30.7, 26.7, 30.7, 30.6, 31.7)
s_sq <- (5 * var(x1) + 6 * var(x2)) / 11
s <- sqrt(s_sq)
t <- (mean(x1)-mean(x2)) / (s * sqrt(1/6 + 1/7)); t
pt(t, df = 11) + pt(-t, df = 11, lower.tail = FALSE) # P-value
# OR: run the test fully in R and look at the t-statistic or P-value
t.test(x1, x2, alternative = "two.sided", var.equal = TRUE)
t.test(x1, x2, alternative = "two.sided", var.equal = TRUE)$statistic
t.test(x1, x2, alternative = "two.sided", var.equal = TRUE)$p.value
```

**13.9** (a) We first calculate the difference values as the "after the operation" temperature values minus the "before the operation" temperature values. These are $d_1 = 0.1, d_2 = 0.2, d_3 = 0.2, d_4 = 0.1, d_5 = 0.2, d_6 = 0.1, d_7 = 0.2, d_8 = 0.2, d_9 = 0.2, d_{10} = 0.2$. From this, $\bar{d} = 0.17$ and $s_d^2 = (0.1)^2 + \ldots + (0.2)^2 - 10 \times (0.17)^2)/9 = 0.002333$, computed using Eq. (13.20). Therefore $s_d = \sqrt{0.002333} = 0.04830$. From Eq. (13.27), $t = 0.17/[0.04830/\sqrt{10}] = 0.17/0.01522753 = 11.1291$.

This is a one-sided up test. Since the value of $t$ exceeds the one-sided up $\alpha = 0.01$ critical point for 9 degrees of freedom, namely 2.821, we have enough evidence to reject the null hypothesis and claim that we have significant evidence that temperatures tend to go up after the operation.

This is a different conclusion from that reached in Sect. 13.1, even though the "before the operation" average 98.6 is the same that in Sect. 13.1.

In R:

```
before <- c(98.8, 98.4, 99.1, 98.6, 98.5, 98.3, 98.8, 98.3, 98.6,
    98.6)
after <- c(98.9, 98.6, 99.3, 98.7, 98.7, 98.4, 99.0, 98.5, 98.8,
    98.8)
n <- length(before)
d <- after - before;   dbar <- mean(d);   s2 <- var(d);   s <- sd(d)
# Manual formulae
t <- dbar / (s / sqrt(n));   t
qt(0.01, df = n - 1, lower.tail = FALSE) # Critical point
pt(t, df = n - 1, lower.tail = FALSE) # P-value for Approach 2
# Since we have the whole data set, we can use t.test()
t.test(after, before, alternative = "greater", paired = TRUE,
    conf.level = 0.99)
```

Under Approach 2, the $P$-value of $7.295 \times 10^{-7}$ is much less than $\alpha = 0.01$ and thus we have very significant evidence to reject the null hypothesis.

(b) The value of $t_2$ as calculated from (13.15) is $(98.77 - 98.6)/[0.25397$ $\sqrt{1/10 + 1/10}] = 1.496767$. This is a one-sided up test and the critical point of $t$ for a one-sided up test with 18 degrees of freedom and $\alpha = 0.01$ is 2.552. The observed value of $t_2$ is less than this critical point, so we do not have enough evidence to reject the null hypothesis.

In R:

```
x1bar <- 98.6;   x2bar <- 98.77;   s2 <- 0.0645;   s <- 0.25397
    # Manually
t <- (x2bar - x1bar) / (s * sqrt(1/n + 1/n));   t
qt(0.01, df = 10 + 10 - 2, lower.tail = FALSE)
    # Critical point for Approach 1
pt(t, df = 10 + 10 - 2, lower.tail = FALSE)
    # P-value for Approach 2
# Using built in function instead
t.test(after, before, alternative = "greater", var.equal
    = TRUE, paired = FALSE, conf.level = 0.99)
```

Under Approach 2, the $P$-value (0.07589) is not less than $\alpha = 0.01$ and thus we do not have enough evidence to reject the null hypothesis.

(c) The value of the $t$ statistic found in part (a) is far larger than that calculated in part (b). The reason for this is that the natural person-to-person variation in temperature, which adds to the denominator of the $t_2$ statistic calculated in part (b), is eliminated when the paired $t$ test of part (a) is used, thus giving a sharper result than that for the unpaired two-sample $t$ test.

**13.10** We arbitrarily think of the sisters as group 1 and the brothers as group 2. The differences between the brother and sister readings are $128 - 124 = 4, \ldots, 125 - 121 = 4$, so that $\bar{d} = 4.0$. Next, $s_d^2 = [(4)^2 + (6)^2 + \ldots + (4)^2 - 10(4.00)^2]/9 = 24.0000$. From this, $s_d = 4.898979$. From Eq. (13.21), the value of $t_d$ is $4.00/[4.89897/\sqrt{10}] = 2.582$. There are nine degrees of freedom, and because of the nature of the alternative hypothesis, the test is one-sided up. Since the value of $t_d$ exceeds the $\alpha = 0.05$ critical point 1.833, we have enough evidence to reject the null hypothesis.

In R:

```
sister <- c(124, 131, 109, 133, 104, 137, 122, 106, 153, 121)
brother <- c(128, 137, 114, 126, 116, 138, 125, 110, 161, 125)
n <- length(sister)
d <- brother - sister;   dbar <- mean(d);  s2 <- var(d);
s <- sd(d) t <- dbar / (s / sqrt(n));   t  # Manually
qt(0.05, df = n - 1, lower.tail = FALSE) # Critical point
pt(t, df = n - 1, lower.tail = FALSE) # P-value for Approach 2
# Using built-in function instead
t.test(brother, sister, alternative = "greater", paired
    = TRUE, conf.level = 0.95)
```

Using Approach 2, we see the P-value of 0.07589 is not less than $\alpha = 0.01$ and thus we do not have significant evidence to reject the null.

**13.11** (a) From the more convenient Eq. (13.26) instead of the equivalent Eq. (13.24), $t = \frac{b\sqrt{s_{xx}}}{s_r} = \frac{0.2011831\sqrt{464.9}}{1.45878} = 2.97$. There are $n - 2 = 8$ degrees of freedom, and since $\alpha = 0.05$ and the test is one-sided up, the critical point is 1.860. Since the observed value of $t$ exceeds this critical point, we have enough evidence to reject the null hypothesis.

In R:

```
age <- c(33,32,14,20,15,16,30,17,21,23)
weight <- c(12.9,13.8,8.2,12.2,8.5,12.9,13.7,11.2,11.9,10.4)
model <- lm(weight ~ age);  summary(model)
```

We find the $t$ value of 2.974 in the coefficients table for "age". The model summary also shows us a two- sided $P$-value. To get the one-sided $P$-value from this, we divide by 2. This yields $0.01777/2 = 0.0089$. Since this $P$-value is less than $\alpha = 0.05$, we also reject using Approach 2. We can also find this same $P$-value using the pt() function: `pt(2.974, df = 8, lower.tail = FALSE)`.

(b) From Eq. (13.27), $t = \frac{(b-\beta_0)\sqrt{s_{xx}}}{s_r} = \frac{(0.2011831-0.25)\sqrt{464.9}}{1.45878} = -0.72$. Since this test is now one-sided down, the critical point is $-1.860$. Since the observed value of $t$ is not less than or equal to this critical point, we do not have enough evidence to reject the null hypothesis.

R will not calculate this $t$ value or a $P$-value by default, but we can acquire these with a bit of effort.

```
t <- (model$coefficients["age"] - 0.25) / summary(model)
    $coefficients["age", "Std. Error"]
t
pt(t, df = 8)
```

**13.12** (a) From the data, $\bar{x} = 2.5$, $\bar{y} = 8$, $s_{xx} = 5$, $s_{xy} = 10$ and $s_{yy} = 22.56$. This gives $b = s_{xy}/s_{xx} = 2$ and $a = \bar{y} - b\bar{x} = 8 - 2 \times 2.5 = 3$. The regression line is therefore $y = 3 + 2x$. It does "skewer through" the data points.

In R, we find the linear model coefficients in the model summary:

```
x <- 1:4;   y <- c(5.8, 6.2, 8.2, 11.8)
model <- lm(y ~ x);   model
summary(model)
plot(x, y, xlab = "Amount of water", ylab = "Growth height",
      main = "Part a", pch = 16, xlim = c(0.5, 4.5),
      ylim = c(5, 13))
abline(model)
```

(b) $s_r^2 = \dfrac{s_{yy} - b^2 s_{xx}}{n-2} = \dfrac{22.56 - 20}{2} = 1.28$, so that $t = \dfrac{b\sqrt{s_{xx}}}{s_r} = \dfrac{2\sqrt{5}}{\sqrt{1.28}} \approx$

3.95. The critical point for the one-sided up test with $\alpha = 0.05$ and $n - 2 = 4 - 2 = 2$ degrees of freedom is 2.920, so we have enough evidence to reject the null hypothesis.

In R, we can find the corresponding $t$ value in the model summary. We can divide the two-sided $P$-value by 2 to get the one-sided $P$-value of 0.029. Since this is less than $\alpha = 0.05$, we also reject the null hypothesis under Approach 2:

```
summary(model)
summary(model)$coefficients["x", "Pr(>|t|)"]/2
```

(c) From the data, $\bar{x} = 2.5$ and $\bar{y} = 8$, $s_{xx} = 5$, $s_{xy} = 10$ and $s_{yy} = 25.76$. This gives $b = 2$ and $a = 3$, so that the regression line is $y = 3 + 2x$, the same as in part (a) of the problem. It does "skewer through" the data points.

In R:

```
x_new <- 1:4;   y_new <- c(6.2, 5.8, 7.8, 12.2)
model_new <- lm(y_new ~ x_new);   model_new
summary(model_new)
plot(x_new, y_new, xlab = "Amount of water", ylab
= "Growth height", main = "Part b", pch = 16, col = "Red",
      xlim = c(0.5, 4.5), ylim = c(5, 13))
abline(model)
```

(d) $s_r^2 = (25.76 - 20)/2 = 2.88$ and from Eq. (13.26), $t = 2\sqrt{5}/\sqrt{2.88} = 2.64$. The critical point is 2.920 (as in part (b) of the problem), so we do not have enough evidence to reject the null hypothesis.

In R, we find the $t$ value in the model summary. We divide the two-sided $P$-value by 2 to get the one-sided $P$-value of 0.059. Since this is greater than $\alpha = 0.05$, we do not have enough evidence to reject the null hypothesis using Approach 2:

```
summary(model_new)
summary(model_new)$coefficients["x_new", "Pr(>|t|)"]/2
```

(e) The scatter of the data points around the regression line is larger in part (c) than it is in part (a), and this has resulted in a larger value of $s_r^2$ and ultimately in a smaller value of $t$. This led to a rejection of the null hypothesis in part (b) but not a rejection of the null hypothesis in part (d). (This is despite the fact that the regression line is the same in both examples.)

```
plot(x, y, xlab = "Amount of water", ylab = "Growth height",
     main = "Comparison of two data sets", pch = 16,
     xlim = c(0.5, 4.5), ylim = c(5, 13))
abline(model)
points(x_new, y_new, col = "Red", pch = 16)
```

**13.13** (a) From the data, $\bar{x} = 2$, $\bar{y} = 5$, $s_{xx} = 2$, $s_{xy} = 6$, $s_{yy} = 18$, so that $b = 3$ and $a = -1$. The regression line is thus $y = 3x - 1$. When $x = 1$, the regression line gives $y = 2$, which is the data value of $y$. When $x = 3$, the regression line gives $y = 8$, which is the data value of $y$. Thus the regression line goes through the two data points.

(b) $s_r^2 = (18 - 32 \times 2)/(2 - 2) = (18 - 18)/0 = 0/0$, which is meaningless.

**13.14** From the data, $b = 610/210 = 2.905$, $s_r^2 = \dfrac{1829.875 - 2.905^2 \times 210}{6} = $

$9.660$, so that $s_r = 3.108$. From this, $t = \dfrac{2.905}{3.108/\sqrt{210}} \approx 13.545$. The observed value of $t$ exceeds the critical point 2.447, so we have enough evidence to reject the null hypothesis.

In R:

```
# Critical points for Approach 1
qt(0.025, df = 6);   qt(0.025, df = 6, lower.tail = FALSE)
# Full R approach
income <- c(5, 10, 20, 8, 4, 6, 12, 15);   pizza <- c(27, 46,
73, 40, 30, 28, 46, 59)
summary(lm(pizza ~ income))
```

The $P$-value is much smaller than $\alpha = 0.05$ and we thus have significant evidence to reject the null hypothesis by Approach 2, in agreement with the conclusion using Approach 1.

**13.15** (a) From Eq. (8.9), the estimate of $\mu$ remains at $\bar{x} = 22.25$.

(b) From Eq. (13.31), the exact confidence interval is $22.25 - 2.093(9.6019)/\sqrt{20}$ to $22.25 + 2.093(9.6019)/\sqrt{20}$, or approximately 17.76 to 26.74. To find $t_{0.025, \nu}$ in R instead of the $t$ chart:
```
qt(0.025, df = 19, lower.tail = FALSE).
```

**13.16** The estimate of $\mu$ remains at 133.8333 and the value of $s$ remains at 9.600347. Thus from Eq. (13.31), the exact 95% confidence interval is $133.83333 - 2.571(9.600347)/\sqrt{6}$ to $133.8333 + 2.571(9.600347)/\sqrt{6}$, or approximately 123.76 to 143.91. To find $t_{0.025, \nu}$ in R instead of the $t$ chart:
```
qt(0.025, df = 5, lower.tail = FALSE).
```

**13.17** The estimate of $\mu$ remains at 6.615 and the value of $s/\sqrt{10}$ remains at 0.0593. From Eq. (13.31), the exact 95% confidence interval is $6.615 - 2.262(0.0593)$ to $6.615 + 2.262(0.0593)$, or approximately from 6.48 to 6.75. To find $t_{0.025,\nu}$ in R instead of the $t$ chart:
`qt(0.025, df = 9, lower.tail = FALSE)`.

**13.18** (a) The estimate $\mu_1 - \mu_2$ remains at 7.075.

(b) Since $s_1^2$ and $s_2^2$ are close to each other, we first assume that $\sigma_1^2 = \sigma_2^2$. From Eq. (13.13), we compute $s^2$ to be 81.4047, so that $s = 9.0225$. There are 16 degrees of freedom and $t_{0.025,16} = 2.120$, so that the exact 95% confidence interval is $7.075 - 2.120s\sqrt{\frac{1}{10} + \frac{1}{8}}$ to $7.075 + 2.120s\sqrt{\frac{1}{10} + \frac{1}{8}}$ that is, approximately from $-2.00$ to 16.15. To find $t_{0.025,\nu}$ in R instead of the $t$ chart:
`qt(0.025, df = 16, lower.tail = FALSE)`.

If we had not been willing to assume that $\sigma_1^2 = \sigma_2^2$, we would use Eq. (13.35). This requires an approximate degrees of freedom calculation from Eq. (13.19). With $s_1^2 = 79.7333$ and $s_2^2 = 83.5536$, Eq. (13.19) gives $\nu \approx 14.98$, so rounding down we use $\nu = 14$. Next, $t_{0.025,14} = 2.145$. Finally, $\sqrt{s_1^2/n + s_2^2/m} = 4.2916$. Equation (13.35) then gives then approximate 95% confidence interval as $7.075 - 2.145 \times 4.2916$ to $7.075 + 2.145 \times 4.2916$, that is, approximately from $-2.13$ to 16.28. The two confidence intervals are fairly close to each other.

**13.19** (b) With $m = 160$ and $n = 128$, there are effectively infinitely many degrees of freedom. If we assume that $\sigma_1^2 = \sigma_2^2$, the confidence interval is $7.075 - 1.96s\sqrt{\frac{1}{160} + \frac{1}{128}}$ to $7.075 + 1.96s\sqrt{\frac{1}{160} + \frac{1}{128}}$. From Eq. (13.13), we calculate the pooled $s^2 = \frac{159 \times 79.7333 + 127 \times 83.5536}{160 + 128 - 2} = 81.4297$, yielding $s = 9.0238$. The confidence interval is then approximately from 4.98 to 9.17. If we do not assume that $\sigma_1^2 = \sigma_2^2$, there are again effectively infinitely many degrees of freedom and $\sqrt{s_1^2/n + s_2^2/m} = 1.0729$. The approximate 95% confidence interval becomes $7.075 - 1.96 \times 1.0729$ to $7.075 + 1.96 \times 1.0729$, that is, approximately from 4.97 to 9.18. The two confidence intervals are very close to each other.

**13.20** (c) From Eq. (13.34) and its solution, the exact confidence interval is $0.201 - \frac{2.306(1.45878)}{\sqrt{464.9}}$ to $0.201 + \frac{2.306(1.45878)}{\sqrt{464.9}}$, that is, approximately from 0.04 to 0.36. To find $t_{0.025,\nu}$ in R instead of the $t$ chart:
`qt(0.025, df = 8, lower.tail = FALSE)`

**13.21** (b) Since an exact 99% confidence interval is wanted, we use a number from the $\alpha = 0.005$ column of the $t$ chart. With $n = 12$, so that $\nu = 10$, the exact 99% confidence interval is $0.65 - 3.169 \times 0.045252$ to $0.65 + 3.169 \times 0.045252$, that is, approximately from 0.51 to 0.79. To find $t_{0.005,\nu}$ in R instead of the $t$ chart:
`qt(0.005, df = 10, lower.tail = FALSE)`

**13.22** (b) From the answer to Problem 8.14, $b = 2.905, s_r = 3.248$ and $s_{xx} = 210$. Also, $n = 8$. From Eq. (13.34) the exact 95% confidence interval is $2.905 -$

$\frac{2.447(3.3248)}{\sqrt{210}}$ to $2.905 + \frac{2.447(3.3248)}{\sqrt{210}}$, that is, approximately from 2.34 to 3.47. To find $t_{0.025,\nu}$ in R instead of the $t$ chart:

`qt(0.025, df = 6, lower.tail = FALSE)`

## Chapter 14

**14.1** $T^+$ will equal 0 if and only if all data values are less than $\mu$ (probability $\frac{1}{2^n}$). Similarly $T^+$ will equal $\frac{n(n-1)}{2}$ if and if only if all data values exceed $\mu$ (probability $\frac{1}{2^n}$). $T^+$ will equal 1 if and only if all data values except one are less than $\mu$, and the single data value exceeding $\mu$ is the closest of all data values to $\mu$ (and thus corresponds to rank 1). This has probability $\binom{n}{n-1}2^n \times \frac{1}{n} = \frac{1}{2^n}$. $T^+$ will equal $\frac{n(n-1)}{2} - 1$ if and only if all data values except one exceed $\mu$, and the single data value less than $\mu$ is the closest of all data values to $\mu$ (and thus corresponds to rank 1). This has probability $\binom{n}{n-1}2^n \times \frac{1}{n} = \frac{1}{2^n}$.

**14.2** The possible values of $T^+$ are 0, 1, 2 and 3, and from the answer to problem 14.1, each has null hypothesis probability $\frac{1}{4}$. From this, the null hypothesis mean of $T^+$ is 1.5 and the null hypothesis variance of $T^+$ is 1.25. These agree with the values given in Sect. 14.2 for the case $n = 2$.

**14.3** (a) There are $\binom{6}{3} = 20$ possible orderings of $x$ and $y$ values, each having null hypothesis probability $\frac{1}{20}$. Consideration of all these orderings shows that the possible values of $W$ are 6, 7, 8, 9, 10, 11, 12, 13, 14 and 15 with respective null hypothesis probabilities $\frac{1}{20}, \frac{1}{20}, \frac{2}{20}, \frac{3}{20}, \frac{3}{20}, \frac{3}{20}, \frac{3}{20}, \frac{2}{20}, \frac{1}{20}$ and $\frac{1}{20}$. These add to 1.

(b) Calculations using Eqs. (4.20) and (4.36) show that the mean of $W$ is 10.5 and the variance of $W$ is 5.25, and these agree with the values found from Eq. (14.8) upon putting $n = m = 3$.

**14.4** Under the null hypothesis, the mean of $W$ is $\frac{3 \times 8}{2} = 12$ and the variance of $W$ is $\frac{3 \times 4 \times 8}{12} = 8$ (both from Eqs. (14.8)). The approximating probability without a continuity correction is then $\text{Prob}(Z \geq \frac{17-12}{\sqrt{8}}) \approx 0.039$. The approximating probability using a continuity correction is $\text{Prob}(Z \geq \frac{16.5-12}{\sqrt{8}}) \approx 0.056$. The approximation using a continuity correction is far more accurate than the approximation which does not use a continuity correction.

**14.5** Under the null hypothesis, the mean of $W$ is 39 and the variance of $W$ is also 39 (both from Eqs. (14.8)). The approximating probability without a continuity correction is $\text{Prob}(Z \geq \frac{50-39}{\sqrt{39}}) \approx 0.039$. The approximating probability using a continuity correction is $\text{Prob}(Z \geq \frac{49.5-39}{\sqrt{39}}) \approx 0.047$. The approximating probability using a continuity correction is very accurate, and is more accurate than the approximation found when a continuity correction is not used.

**14.6** Under the null hypothesis, the mean of $W$ is 26 and the variance of $W$ is $\frac{104}{3}$ (both from Eqs. (14.8)). The approximating probability without a continuity correction is then $\text{Prob}(Z \geq \frac{36-26}{\sqrt{\frac{104}{3}}}) \approx 0.045$. The approximating probability using a continuity correction is $\text{Prob}(Z \geq \frac{35.5-26}{\sqrt{\frac{104}{3}}}) \approx 0.054$. The approximating probability using a continuity correction is very accurate, and is more accurate than the approximation found when a continuity correction is not used.

**14.7** Under the null hypothesis, the mean of $W$ is 105 and the variance of $W$ is 175 (both from Eqs. (14.8)). The approximating probability without a continuity correction is then $\text{Prob}(Z \geq \frac{127-105}{\sqrt{175}}) \approx 0.045$. The approximating probability using a continuity correction is $\text{Prob}(Z \geq \frac{126.5-105}{\sqrt{175}}) \approx 0.052$. The approximating probability using a continuity correction is very accurate, and is more accurate than the approximation found when a continuity correction is not used.

# Index

© The Author(s), under exclusive license to Springer Nature Switzerland AG 2023
W. J. Ewens, K. Brumberg, *Introductory Statistics for Data Analysis*,
https://doi.org/10.1007/978-3-031-28189-1

Printed in the United States
by Baker & Taylor Publisher Services